Genetic Disorders Sourcebook, 1st Edition

Genetic Disorders Sourcebook, 2nd Edition

Head Trauma Sourcebook

Headache Sourcebook

Health Insurance Sourcebook

Health Reference Series Cumulative Index 1999

Healthy Aging Sourcebook

Healthy Children Sourcebook

Healthy Heart Sourcebook for Women

Heart Diseases & Disorders Sourcebook, 2nd Edition

Household Safety Sourcebook

Immune System Disorders Sourcebook

Infant & Toddler Health Sourcebook

Injury & Trauma Sourcebook

Kidney & Urinary Tract Diseases & Disorders Sourcebook

Learning Disabilities Sourcebook, 1st Edition

Learning Disabilities Sourcebook, 2nd Edition

Liver Disorders Sourcebook

Lung Disorders Sourcebook

Medical Tests Sourcebook

Men's Health Concerns Sourcebook

Mental Health Disorders Sourcebook, 1st Edition

Mental Health Disorders Sourcebook, 2nd Edition

Mental Retardation Sourcebook

Movement Disorders Sourcebook

Obesity Sourcebook

Ophthalmic Disorders Sourcebook

Oral Health Sourcebook

Osteoporosis Sourcebook

Pain Sourcebook, 1st Edition

Pain Sourcebook, 2nd Edition

Pediatric Cancer Sourcebook

Physical & Mental Issues in Aging Sourcebook

Podiatry Sourcebook

Pregnancy & Birth Sourcebook

Prostate Cancer

Public Health Sourcebook

Reconstructive & Cosmetic Surgery Sourcebook

Rehabilitation Sourcebook

Respiratory Diseases & Disorders Sourcebook

Sexually Transmitted Diseases Sourcebook, 1st Edition

Sexually Transmitted Diseases Sourcebook, 2nd Edition

Skin Disorders Sourcebook

Sleep Disorders Sourcebook

Sports Injuries Sourcebook, 1st Edition

Sports Injuries Sourcebook, 2nd Edition

Stress-Related Disorders Sourcebook

Substance Abuse Sourcebook

Surgery Sourcebook

Transplantation Sourcebook

Traveler's Health Sourcebook

Vegetarian Sourcebook

Women's Health Concerns Sourcebook

Workplace Health & Safety Sourcebook

Worldwide Health Sourcebook

Teen Health Series

Diet Information for Teens

Drug Information for Teens

Mental Health Information for Teens

Sexual Health Information for Teens

Health Reference Series

Second Edition

Alternative Medicine
SOURCEBOOK

*Basic Consumer Health Information about
Alternative and Complementary Medical Practices,
Including Acupuncture, Chiropractic, Herbal
Medicine, Homeopathy, Naturopathic Medicine,
Mind-Body Interventions, Ayurveda, and Other
Non-Western Medical Traditions*

*Along with Facts about such Specific Therapies as
Massage Therapy, Aromatherapy, Qigong, Hypnosis,
Prayer, Dance, and Art Therapies, a Glossary, and
Resources for Further Information*

Edited by
Dawn D. Matthews

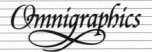

Omnigraphics

615 Griswold Street • Detroit, MI 48226

Because this page cannot legibly accommodate all the copyright notices, the Bibliographic Note portion of the Preface constitutes an extension of the copyright notice.

Edited by Dawn D. Matthews

Health Reference Series

Karen Bellenir, *Managing Editor*
David A. Cooke, MD, *Medical Consultant*
Elizabeth Barbour, *Permissions Associate*
Dawn Matthews, *Verification Assistant*
Carol Munson, *Permissions Assistant*
Laura Pleva Nielsen, *Index Editor*
Ed Index, Services for Publishers, *Indexers*

* * *

Omnigraphics, Inc.

Matthew P. Barbour, *Senior Vice President*
Kay Gill, *Vice President Directories*
Kevin Hayes, *Operations Manager*
David P. Bianco, *Marketing Consultant*

* * *

Peter E. Ruffner, *President and Publisher*

Frederick G. Ruffner, Jr., *Chairman*

Copyright © 2002 Omnigraphics, Inc.

ISBN 0-7808-0605-0

Library of Congress Cataloging-in-Publication Data

Alternative medicine sourcebook : basic consumer health information about alternative and complementary medical practices, including acupuncture, chiropractic, herbal medicine, homeopathy, naturopathic medicine, mind-body interventions, ayurveda, and other non-Western medical traditions; along with facts about such specific therapies as massage therapy, aromatherapy, qigong, hypnosis, prayer, dance, and art therapies, a glossary, and resources for further information / edited by Dawn D. Matthews.-- 2nd ed.
  p. cm.-- (Health reference series)
  Includes bibliographical references and index.
  ISBN 0-7808-0605-0 (lib. bdg. : alk. paper)
  1. Alternative medicine. I. Matthews, Dawn D. II. Health reference series (Unnumbered)

R733 .A475 2002
615.5--dc21
                                                                        2002070376

This book is printed on acid-free paper meeting the ANSI Z39.48 Standard. The infinity symbol that appears above indicates that the paper in this book meets that standard.

Printed in the United States

Table of Contents

Part III: Mind-Body Interventions

Part IV: Dietary Interventions

Part V: Other Alternative Therapies

Part VI: Alternative Treatments for Specific Diseases and Conditions

Part VII: Controversial Cancer Treatments

Part VIII: Skeptical Points of View

Part IX: Additional Help and Information

Preface

About This Book

Complementary and alternative medicine (CAM) refers to the use of treatments and health care practices that are not widely taught in traditional medical schools. "Alternative therapies" are those that are used instead of conventional treatments; "complementary therapies" are those that are used in conjunction with conventional treatments. For some people, the choice to pursue CAM is a philosophical decision based on what they consider to be a more "natural" way to treat illness or disease; to others, it is a last resort. Whatever the individual reasons, however, research indicates that the use of CAM is increasing. In 1990, statistics suggested that 34 percent of the general population used CAM services; by 1997 the figure had risen to 42 percent.

This book contains important information for those considering the use of CAM. It describes practices such as acupuncture, chiropractic, homeopathy, naturopathy, ayurveda, and many others. It provides discussions about the effectiveness of CAM in treating such diseases and disorders as cancer, diabetes, hepatitis C, headaches, menopause, and pain. It also offers suggestions for people to use when considering the safety and effectiveness of a therapy or treatment, the expertise and qualifications of the healthcare practitioner, and the quality of service delivery. A glossary of related terms and chapters describing additional resources round out this volume's coverage.

How to Use This Book

This book is divided into parts and chapters. Parts focus on broad areas of interest. Chapters are devoted to single topics within a part.

Part I: Introduction contains an overview of complementary and alternative medicine (CAM) practices, and it presents facts about selecting among various CAM programs.

Part II: Alternative Medical Systems contains information on various systems of alternative medicine, including acupuncture, herbal medicine, homeopathy, yoga, and others. A chapter discussing the major domains of complementary and alternative medicine defines how the different forms of CAM are grouped.

Part III: Mind-Body Interventions discusses the use of the mind to control the body. Meditation and relaxation, biofeedback, guided imagery, hypnosis, and prayer are examples of the interventions included in this section.

Part IV: Dietary Interventions contains information about the use of special dietary therapies, including fasting, detoxification diets, and dietary supplements. It discusses the effectiveness of various vitamin, mineral, and herbal supplements such as folate, St. John's wort, Vitamin B_{12} and others.

Part V: Other Alternative Therapies includes information on various popular alternative therapies. It contains chapters on aromatherapy, art therapy, massage therapy, qigong and t'ai chi, reflexology, and many others.

Part VI: Alternative Treatments for Specific Diseases and Conditions contains information on alternative therapies currently being used for the treatment of some specific diseases, including cancer, diabetes, and hepatitis C. It also offers information on the use of alternative therapies in the treatment of chronic ailments, including headaches, pain, and some of the symptoms of menopause.

Part VII: Controversial Cancer Treatments discusses the use of controversial drug therapies. It contains chapters with information about such substances as 714X, shark cartilage, coenzyme Q10, and laetrile.

Part VIII: Skeptical Points of View presents examples of how proponents of conventional medical practices sometimes critique CAM practices. A chapter defining "quackery"—the promotion of dubious medical practices—provides information that can help readers recognize and avoid questionable treatments.

Part IX: Additional Help and Information contains a glossary of related terms and descriptions of additional resources for obtaining more information. A chapter with information about health insurance for alternative medicine is also included.

Bibliographic Note

This volume contains documents and excerpts from publications issued by the following U.S. government agencies: Centers for Disease Control and Prevention (CDC); Food and Drug Administration (FDA); National Center for Complementary and Alternative Medicine (NCCAM); National Institute of Diabetes and Digestive Diseases (NIDDK); National Institute of Environmental Health Sciences (NIEHS); National Institutes of Health (NIH); National Institute of Mental Health (NIMH); and National Library of Medicine (NLM).

In addition, this volume contains copyrighted documents from the following organizations and individuals: Alberta Rolfing; Alternative Health Benefit Services; American Art Therapy Association; American Association of Acupuncture and Bio-Energetic Medicine; American Chiropractic Association; American Massage Therapy Association; American Society of Clinical Hypnosis; Association of Reflexologists; Atlantic Institute of Aromatherapy; Ayurvedic Institute; Being Alive; Celestial Arts/Ten Speed Press; Leon Chaitow, N.D., D.O.; Crossing Press; Larry Dossey, M.D.; Elsevier Science; Donna Farhi; Marian Goldberg; Elson Haas, M.D.; Healthology, Inc.; Herbs for Health Magazine; Homeopathy Home; Roger Jahnke, O.M.D.; George T. Lewith; H.J. Kraner/New World Library; International Center for Reiki; Mary and Michael Morton; National Coalition of Arts Therapies Associations; Quackwatch; and Daniel Redwood, D.C.

Acknowledgements

Special thanks go to Liz Barbour for her outstanding work on this book. And many thanks also go to Bruce and Karen Bellenir for their ongoing help and support.

Note from the Editor

This book is part of Omnigraphics' *Health Reference Series*. The series provides basic information about a broad range of medical concerns. It is not intended to serve as a tool for diagnosing illness, in prescribing treatments, or as a substitute for the physician/patient relationship. All persons concerned about medical symptoms or the possibility of disease are encouraged to seek professional care from an appropriate health care provider.

Our Advisory Board

The *Health Reference Series* is reviewed by an Advisory Board comprised of librarians from public, academic, and medical libraries. We would like to thank the following board members for providing guidance to the development of this series:

Dr. Lynda Baker, Associate Professor of Library and Information Science, Wayne State University, Detroit, MI

Nancy Bulgarelli, William Beaumont Hospital Library, Royal Oak, MI

Karen Imarasio, Bloomfield Township Public Library, Bloomfield Township, MI

Karen Morgan, Mardigian Library, University of Michigan-Dearborn, Dearborn, MI

Rosemary Orlando, St. Clair Shores Public Library, St. Clair Shores, MI

Medical Consultant

Medical consultation services are provided to the *Health Reference Series* editors by David A. Cooke, M.D. Dr. Cooke is a graduate of Brandeis University, and he received his M.D. degree from the University of Michigan. He completed residency training at the University of Wisconsin Hospital and Clinics. He is board-certified in Internal Medicine. Dr. Cooke currently works as part of the University of Michigan Health System and practices in Brighton, MI. In his free time, he enjoys writing, science fiction, and spending time with his family.

Health Reference Series *Update Policy*

The inaugural book in the *Health Reference Series* was the first edition of *Cancer Sourcebook* published in 1992. Since then, the *Series* has been enthusiastically received by librarians and in the medical community. In order to maintain the standard of providing high-quality health information for the layperson the editorial staff at Omnigraphics felt it was necessary to implement a policy of updating volumes when warranted.

Medical researchers have been making tremendous strides, and it is the purpose of the *Health Reference Series* to stay current with the most recent advances. Each decision to update a volume will be made on an individual basis. Some of the considerations will include how much new information is available and the feedback we receive from people who use the books. If there is a topic you would like to see added to the update list, or an area of medical concern you feel has not been adequately addressed, please write to:

Editor
Health Reference Series
Omnigraphics, Inc.
615 Griswold Street
Detroit, MI 48226

The commitment to providing on-going coverage of important medical developments has also led to some format changes in the *Health Reference Series*. Each new volume on a topic is individually titled and called a "First Edition." Subsequent updates will carry sequential edition numbers. To help avoid confusion and to provide maximum flexibility in our ability to respond to informational needs, the practice of consecutively numbering each volume has been discontinued.

Part One

Introduction

Chapter 1

Are You Considering Complementary and Alternative Medicine?

What Is Complementary and Alternative Medicine?

Complementary and alternative medicine (CAM) covers a broad range of healing philosophies, approaches, and therapies. Generally, it is defined as those treatments and health care practices not taught widely in medical schools, not generally used in hospitals, and not usually reimbursed by medical insurance companies.

Many therapies are termed "holistic," which generally means that the health care practitioner considers the whole person, including physical, mental, emotional, and spiritual aspects. Many therapies are also known as "preventive," which means that the practitioner educates and treats the person to prevent health problems from arising, rather than treating symptoms after problems have occurred.

People use these treatments and therapies in a variety of ways. Therapies are used alone (often referred to as alternative), in combination with other alternative therapies, or in addition to conventional therapies (sometimes referred to as complementary).

Some approaches are consistent with physiological principles of Western medicine, while others constitute healing systems with a different origin. While some therapies are far outside the realm of

Text in this chapter is excerpted from the following undated fact sheets "What Is Complementary and Alternative Medicine?" and "Considering CAM?" from National Center for Complementary and Alternative Medicine (NCCAM), cited January 2002.

accepted Western medical theory and practice, others are becoming established in mainstream medicine.

How Can I Find More Information about Complementary and Alternative Medical Practices?

Ask your health care provider about complementary and alternative medical treatments and practices in general, and about those particular practices used for your specific health problems. Increasingly, health care providers are becoming familiar with alternative treatments or are able to refer you to someone who is. For scientific information about the safety and effectiveness of a particular treatment, ask your health care provider to obtain valid information for you.

If your health care provider cannot provide information, medical libraries, public libraries, and popular bookstores are good places to find information about particular complementary and alternative medical practices.

Other resources for information are the 25 Institutes and Centers (ICs) at the National Institutes of Health (NIH). For information on a wide range of specific diseases or medical conditions, call 301-496-4000 and ask the operator to direct you to the appropriate NIH office. Also, you may want to ask practitioners of complementary and alternative health care about their practices. Many practitioners belong to a growing number of professional associations, educational organizations, and research institutions that provide information about complementary and alternative medical practices. Many organizations are developing Internet Web sites. Most internet browser programs will have a mechanism for searching the World Wide Web by keyword or concept.

Remember that these organizations may advocate a specific therapy or treatment and may be unable to provide complete and objective health information.

CAM on PubMed

If you have access to a computer with an Internet connection, you may be able to search medical libraries and databases for specific conditions and alternative treatments. CAM on PubMed, developed jointly by the National Library of Medicine and the National Center for Complementary and Alternative Medicine, contains bibliographic citations (1966-present) related to complementary and alternative medicine. These citations are a subset of the National Library of Medicine's PubMed system that contains over 11 million journal citations from the MEDLINE database and additional life science journals important to health researchers, practitioners and consumers. CAM on PubMed also displays links to publisher web sites offering full text of articles.

How Can I Find a Practitioner in My Area?

To find a qualified complementary and alternative medical health care practitioner, you may want to contact medical regulatory and licensing agencies in your state. These agencies may be able to provide information about a specific practitioner's credentials and background. Many states license practitioners who provide alternative therapies such as acupuncture, chiropractic services, naturopathy, herbal medicine, homeopathy, and massage therapy.

You may also locate practitioners by asking your health care provider, or by contacting a professional association or organization. These organizations can provide names of local practitioners, and provide information about how to determine the quality of a specific practitioner's services.

Also, you may find complementary and alternative health care practitioners by asking people you trust, like friends and family members, who may have experience with practitioners of complementary and alternative medicine.

Can I Receive an Alternative Treatment at the National Center for Complementary and Alternative Medicine (NCCAM)?

The NCCAM is not a treatment facility and cannot answer specific medical questions. The NCCAM cannot make referrals to individual practitioners or recommend particular therapies for patients.

Will My Experience Help in the Evaluation of Complementary and Alternative Medical Therapies?

Many people write to the NCCAM with their own testimony about a successful treatment or a particular healer or health care practitioner. To have this information reviewed, people may ask their practitioners whether he/she is collecting information on the success of their treatments. A practitioner can collect and organize the information and present it to the NCCAM once there is sufficient data to make a case for the effectiveness of a particular treatment.

Will the NCCAM Evaluate My Own Invention or Treatment?

Many people contact the NCCAM with ideas for alternative medical cures. To have a method or cure tested, one must formulate a research protocol. This entails collaborating with individuals who have expertise in research and evaluation, if one does not possess this expertise.

The NCCAM supports rigorous research into a range of alternative medical treatments either by awarding grants or by setting up studies.

Can Complementary and Alternative Medicine Be Investigated Using the Same Methods Used in Conventional Medicine?

People sometimes ask whether the NCCAM uses the same standard of science as conventional medicine. Complementary and alternative medicine needs to be investigated using the same scientific methods used in conventional medicine. The NCCAM encourages valid information about complementary and alternative medicine, applying at least as rigorous, and, in some cases, even more rigorous research methods than the current standard in conventional medicine. This is because the research often involves novel concepts and claims, and uses complex systems of practice that need systematic, explicit, and comprehensive knowledge and skills to investigate.

Assess the Safety and Effectiveness of the Therapy

Generally, safety means that the benefits outweigh the risks of a treatment or therapy. A safe product or practice is one that does no harm when used under defined conditions and as intended. Effectiveness is the likelihood of benefit from a practice, treatment, or technology applied under typical conditions by the average practitioner for the typical patient.

Many people find that specific information about an alternative and complementary therapy's safety and effectiveness may be less readily available than information about conventional medical treatments. Research on these therapies is ongoing, and continues to grow.

You may want to ask a healthcare practitioner, whether a physician or a practitioner of complementary and alternative healthcare, about the safety and effectiveness of the therapy or treatment he or she uses. Tell the practitioner about any alternative or conventional treatments or therapies you may already be receiving, as this information may be used to consider the safety and effectiveness of the entire treatment plan.

The practitioner may have literature with information about the safety and effectiveness of the therapy. Credible information may be found in scientific research literature obtained through public libraries, university libraries, medical libraries, and online computer services, such as CAM on PubMed and the U.S. National Library of Medicine at the National Institutes of Health.

For general, nonscientific information, thousands of articles on health issues and complementary and alternative medicine are published in books, journals, and magazines every year. Articles that appear in popular magazines and journals may be located by using the *Reader's Guide to Periodical Literature* available in most libraries. For articles published in more than 3,000 health science journals, consult the *Index Medicus*, found in medical and university libraries and some public libraries.

Be an informed health consumer and continue gathering information even after a practitioner has been selected. Ask the practitioner about specific new research that may support or not support the safety and effectiveness of the treatment or therapy. Ask about the advantages and disadvantages, risks, side effects, expected results, and length of treatment that you can expect. Speak with people who have undergone the treatment, preferably both those who were treated recently and those treated in the past. Optimally, find people with the same health condition that you have and who have received the treatment.

Remember that patient testimonials used alone do not adequately assess the safety and effectiveness of an alternative therapy, and should not be the exclusive criterion for selecting a therapy. Controlled scientific trials usually provide the best information about a therapy's effectiveness and should be sought whenever possible.

Examine the Practitioner's Expertise

Health consumers may want to take a close look into the background, qualifications, and competence of any potential healthcare practitioner, whether a physician or a practitioner of alternative and complementary healthcare.

First, contact a state or local regulatory agency with authority over practitioners who practice the therapy or treatment you seek. The practice of complementary and alternative medicine usually is not as regulated as the practice of conventional medicine. Licensing, accreditation, and regulatory laws, however, are increasingly being implemented.

Local and state medical boards, other health regulatory boards or agencies, and consumer affairs departments provide information about a specific practitioner's license, education, and accreditation, and whether there are any complaints lodged against the practitioner. Check to see if the practitioner is licensed to deliver the services the practitioner says he or she delivers.

Appropriate state licensing of education and practice is the only way to ensure that the practitioner is competent and provides quality services. Most types of complementary and alternative practices have national organizations of practitioners that are familiar with legislation, state licensing, certification, or registration laws.

Some organizations will direct medical consumers to the appropriate regulatory agencies in their state. These organizations also may provide referrals and information about specific practitioners. The organizations usually do not function as regulatory authorities, but promote the services of their members.

Second, talk with those who have had experience with this practitioner, both health practitioners and other patients. Find out about the confidence and competence of the practitioner in question, and whether there have ever been any complaints from patients.

Third, talk with the practitioner in person. Ask about the practitioner's education, additional training, licenses, and certifications, both unconventional and conventional. Ask about the practitioner's approach to treatment and patients. Find out how open the practitioner is to communicating with patients about technical aspects of methods, possible side effects, and potential problems.

When selecting a healthcare practitioner, many medical consumers seek someone knowledgeable in a wide variety of disciplines. Look for a practitioner who is easy to talk to. You should feel comfortable asking questions. After you select a practitioner, the education process and dialogue between you and your practitioner should become an ongoing aspect of complementary healthcare.

Consider the Service Delivery

The quality of the service delivery, or how the treatment or therapy is given and under what conditions, is an important issue. However, quality of service is not necessarily related to the effectiveness or safety of a treatment or practice.

Visit the practitioner's office, clinic, or hospital. Ask the practitioner how many patients he or she typically sees in a day or week, and how much time the practitioner spends with the patient. Look at the conditions of the office or clinic.

Many issues surround quality of service delivery, and each one individually does not provide conclusive and complete information. For example, are the costs of the service excessive for what is delivered? Can the service be obtained only in one place, requiring travel to that place? These issues may serve as warning signs of poor service.

The primary issue to consider is whether the service delivery adheres to regulated standards for medical safety and care.

Consider the Costs

Costs are an important factor to consider as many complementary and alternative treatments are not currently reimbursed by health insurance. Many patients pay directly for these services. Ask your practitioner and your health insurer which treatments or therapies are reimbursable.

Find out what several practitioners charge for the same treatment to better assess the appropriateness of costs. Regulatory agencies and professional associations also may provide cost information.

Consult Your Healthcare Provider

Most importantly, discuss all issues concerning treatments and therapies with your healthcare provider whether a physician or practitioner of complementary and alternative medicine. Competent healthcare management requires knowledge of both conventional and alternative therapies for the practitioner to have a complete picture of your treatment plan.

Chapter 2

Selecting the Best Alternative Medicine Program

Learn Your Options

Add to your M.D.'s recommendations by researching the latest resources to get all your treatment options.

Knowledge is power. Whether you are looking for information to enhance your health or searching for the answer to reverse a terminal illness, you'll want all the credible information you can find about your condition. And you can do just that when you learn all your options.

In order to do that, you'll need "The Seven Key Sources to Good Health Care Information." They are:

1. Your doctor and other health care providers

2. Other patients and their friends

3. Libraries

4. The Internet

5. Medical and Health Information Service Organizations

6. Advocacy Organizations and Support Groups

7. Professional Organizations and Trade Associations

Further, when gathering health care information, it important to use "The Three Question Test for Complete and Dependable Health Care Information." They are:

1. What are the best treatments available in the world today for my health care condition/diagnosis?

2. Are those treatment proven effective?

3. How do I know if the information is reliable?

By using this test you can gain access to all the accurate and dependable health care information you need to make informed choice about your treatment options. By getting informed you become a savvy health care consumer no longer bound to one doctor's opinion or one medical system's answers to meet yours and your family's health care needs. Remember, by learning all of your options, you increase your chances of getting the health care results you want.

Get Good Referrals

Find referrals through various sources and verify that these referrals have the capability to really help you.

An effective selection process is the key to locating a good health care professional. Getting high quality referrals of good candidates is the best way to start that process. The following information provides you with the information and knowledge you need to get those high quality referrals and to begin a selection strategy which can be used in hiring almost any alternative health care provider. Remember—they work for you!

Relying just on family and friends may not give you the selection choice you may need to find the alternative health professional that is right for you. You may need to rely on more than one referral source.

Here are the seven key sources for getting good referrals:

1. Family, friends and colleagues

2. Local alternative practitioners

3. Local health-food stores

4. Support groups

5. Professional associations

12

6. Alternative health care schools and colleges

7. Referrals services and advertisements

When getting a referral, you'll want to get as much information from your source as possible. Many times, with just a little extra information, you'll know immediately whether this referral has possibility for you or not. For this reason it is important to know the right questions to ask.

With a list of good referrals, you can feel confident that you have tipped the scales in your favor and you are now just a few steps away from finding a health care provider who you'll want to work with.

Screening the Candidate

Make use of an alternative practitioner's staff to get reliable information about the provider and how they work.

The alternative health care provider's office staff is an invaluable information source to you. Without spending a penny in fees, you can get a more in-depth picture about a provider's personality, his or her expertise, his or her educational training, and which associations or professional organizations he or she belongs to. From this information, as well as additional information you will garner from asking some very specific, well-targeted questions, you will gain greater certainty as to whether this candidate could be your health care provider.

In order to do that, you need to know what those questions are as well some other important information that can assist you in getting the answers you need to make an informed and educated health care decision about the practitioner.

Here are some examples:

* Can you provide me with literature about the health care provider's educational background and philosophy of treatment?

* What success has this alternative doctor had in treating patients with physical problems similar to mine?

* How long has this practitioner/doctor been in practice?

* What is the practitioner's fee structure and your policy with insurance?

* How much can I expect to pay on my first visit, including tests, supplements, and prescriptions?

13

By using this information you can narrow your list of practitioner candidates to a select few whom you would like to meet personally. By doing this, you are only one step away from the alternative health care practitioner with whom you will want to develop a health care partnership.

Interviewing the Provider

Ask the provider all the pertinent questions to know if you can confidently work with this professional.

To successfully interview a health care provider, you must ask the right questions and use your own gut instincts to get a feel of who this person is and if they are right for you. A well-conducted interview will provide you with the valuable data to determine if this is the health care professional you will want to work with.

In order to do, it is best to first ask yourself, "What kind of personality do I need in a health care provider?" Superbly trained health care providers come in a wide range of personalities. Some have nurturing bedside manners and are compassionate and sensitive with their patient/clients. Some are cold rationalist who don't really care about the thoughts and feelings of their patients. Others are somewhere in the middle.

You need to determine which type of personality is best for you and your current health care needs. Knowing this will assist you during your interview process in determining if a particular health care provider is right for you.

Also, you need to know the key strategies to make the most of your meeting. Here are some examples:

- Be courteous, comfortable and frank during your meeting.

- Describe clearly what you know about your condition.

- Share what you have learned about treatment options.

- Respond honestly yet courteously to the provider's recommendations, especially if you disagree.

- Pace the interview and remember to listen.

- Keep the details straight. Taking notes or bringing a tape recorder can help.

- Use your intuition as well as you mind when sizing up this professional.

This step requires that you make the effort and take the time to visit a health care provider. Sometimes you will also have to pay a small fee for the provider's time. You'll find, however, that the effort, time and money in a productive interview is a good investment in your health.

Forming a Partnership

Maximize your healing potential by developing an active alliance with your alternative health care provider. A health care professional as a "partner" may be a new concept for you. As a result, you may feel like your are making up the rules as you go along. For the most part you will be.

In order to have the best results from such a partnership, it is important to bring "The Four Cornerstones to All Good Health Care Relationships" into this special relationship. These cornerstones will help you form a relationship that will benefit both you and your health care provider. They are:

1. Mutual respect and caring

2. Honest communication

3. A shared commitment to healing

4. A treatment contract

To ensure that your health care partnership produces the results you want, use "The Four Action Steps for Forming a Successful Health Care Partnership." They are:

1. Be responsible for agreeing to, monitoring, and evaluating the treatments you receive

2. Negotiate a "health care contract" with your provider

3. Support your healing physically, emotionally, mentally, and spiritually

4. Practice balancing flexibility with inflexibility

By forming a health care partnership you join an ever growing number of health care consumers who have empowered themselves by taking control of their health care destiny. Keep in mind that your goal is to have a beneficial alliance with a health care professional so you can get healthy. Remember to keep the concept of getting health as your main objective.

Chapter 3

Physicians' Attitudes toward Alternative Medicine

What is the state of the gap between patients' utilization of complementary and alternative medicine (CAM) and physicians' attitudes toward these therapies in the United States? Until recently, little was known about the prevalence of alternative medicine use in the US. In 1993, Eisenberg et al.[1] published a landmark study ... in the *New England Journal of Medicine*, stunning many in the medical community. According to this study, Americans made an estimated 425 million visits to alternative healthcare providers in 1990, more than to all primary care physicians combined. Total amount spent on unconventional therapy was estimated at 13.7 billion, 10.3 billion of which was out of pocket. A more recent survey of family practice patients in Oregon,[2] and the attention unconventional medicine receives from the popular media indicate the public's appetite for alternatives to allopathic treatment has not waned since Eisenberg's data was collected in 1990.

Some proponents of alternative medicine claim these therapies are already considered mainstream within the healthcare system of the US.[3] The opening of the Office of Alternative Medicine in the National Institutes of Health in 1992, and the reimbursement by some third-party payers for selected alternative therapies are evidence of the integration of CAM. In addition, a sizeable number of US medical schools and residency training programs have started to offer instruction in a variety of CAM therapies.[4,5] However, the motivations behind these changes are diverse, and care must be taken not to confuse acceptance of the popularity of CAM with validation of its effectiveness.

Do physicians believe CAM therapies are useful or effective? A recent meta-analysis by Ernst et al. attempted to answer this question.[6] In general, physicians viewed complementary medicine as moderately effective, with younger physicians more optimistic about these therapies than their older counterparts. None of the 12 studies sited in this meta-analysis asked the views of American physicians. Two surveys of primary care physicians in the US found a high level of acceptance of less controversial complementary therapies such as diet and exercise, behavioral medicine, and biofeedback.[7,8] However, a more skeptical eye was cast upon such therapies as acupuncture, chiropractic, and homeopathy.

In our study, we surveyed physicians representing a broad variety of specialties in a mid-sized southeastern US city. The following issues were addressed: (1) physicians' attitudes toward complementary and alternative medicine, and (2) patterns of physician utilization of complementary and alternative medicine.

Methods

The survey instrument was a questionnaire distributed to physicians representing a broad variety of specialties. The questionnaire was designed to assess the attitudes of physicians toward alternative therapies. Questions were asked concerning the respondents' opinions about the legitimacy of alternative therapies as medical treatments, patterns of prescribing alternative therapies for their patients, levels of personal utilization, and training in alternative medicine. The 17 alternative medicine therapies included in the questionnaire were:

1. Acupuncture

2. Chiropractic

3. Herbal medicine

4. Hypnosis

5. Homeopathic medicine

6. Megavitamin therapy

7. Massage

8. Prayer

9. Biofeedback

10. Energy healing (e.g., therapeutic touch, psychic healing, sound therapy, reflexology, etc.)

11. Relaxation techniques (e.g., meditation, breathing exercises, etc.)

12. Imagery

13. Spiritual healing

14. Lifestyle diets (e.g. macrobiotics, vegetarian, allergy elimination, etc.)

15. Self-help groups

16. Folk remedies

17. Lifestyle exercise (e.g. Tai Chi, Yoga, etc.)

Respondents were asked to rank the therapies on a 9-point Likert-type scale, from 1 (not legitimate) to 9 (very legitimate) for use in medical practice. A response of 5 was rated as somewhat legitimate.

Additionally, respondents were surveyed regarding the types of evidence they consider when utilizing a complementary therapy for their patients. They were asked to rate the following areas on a 5-point Likert-type scale ranging from 1 (very important) to 5 (not at all important): proven mechanism, proposed mechanism, clinical trials, epidemiological data, published case studies, success in own practice, colleague recommendation, personal use, or patient report.

Demographic variables assessed included age, race, gender, medical specialty, geographic location of training, and years in practice. The number of years in practice was assessed separately from age, as there is not an absolute relationship between the two variables.

Results

Questionnaires were mailed to 380 physicians. One hundred thirty-eight completed questionnaires were returned, for a 38% response rate. The respondents consisted of 108 men, 22 women, and 8 who did not state their sex. One hundred fifteen of the respondents were white, 5 were African-American, one was Asian, and 14 did not state their race. Ages ranged from 29 to 76 years, with the median age being 44 years. Nine respondents did not state their age. Slightly less than one-half of the respondents had been in practice for 10 years or

Table 3.1. Percentage of responding physicians considering various alternative medicines legitimate

Type of alternative medicine	Legitimate medical practice	In practice less than 10 years	In practice more than 10 years	p
Prayer	64.5	73.0	57.3	NS
Lifestyle exercise	60.9	71.4	52.0	p = .020
Self-help groups	56.5	61.9	52.0	NS
Relaxation techniques	52.9	66.7	41.3	p = .003
Biofeedback	49.3	58.7	41.3	p = .042
Lifestyle diets	47.8	57.1	40.0	p = .045
Massage therapy	45.7	57.1	36.0	p = .013
Chiropractic	30.4	38.1	24.0	p = .073
Acupuncture	29.7	41.3	20.0	p = .006
Spiritual healing	25.4	30.2	21.3	NS
Hypnosis	23.9	34.9	14.7	p = .005
Herbal medicine	19.6	27.0	13.3	p = .044
Homeopathic medicine	16.7	22.0	12.0	NS
Megavitamin therapy	13.0	15.9	10.7	NS
Folk remedies	9.4	14.3	5.3	p = .073
Energy healing	9.4	15.9	4.0	p = .017

NS, not significant.

Therapies are listed in order of acceptance as a legitimate medical practice.

less, whereas 54.3% had been in practice more than 10 years. The greatest number of years in practice was 57 years. Thirty specialties were represented. However, for comparison, the specialties were collapsed into two categories: (1) primary care, which included family medicine, internal medicine, and general pediatrics; and (2) specialty care, which included all other areas of specialization. Under this grouping, 61 of the respondents were classified as being in primary care and 77 in specialty care.

Attitudes toward Complementary and Alternative Therapies

More than 50% of the surveyed physicians viewed prayer, lifestyle exercise, self-help groups, and relaxation techniques as legitimate medical practice (see Table 3.1). Legitimate medical practice was defined as a ranking of 5 (somewhat legitimate) to 9 (very legitimate). More than 45% viewed massage, lifestyle diets, and biofeedback as legitimate medical practice. Less than a third of the surveyed physicians had favorable opinions about chiropractic and acupuncture. The remainder of the CAM therapies were considered legitimate medical practice by 25% or fewer of the respondents.

A statistically significant degree of greater acceptance of CAM therapies was noted among those physicians who had been in practice less than 10 years (Table 3.1). All 17 CAM therapies had a higher level of acceptance among more recently trained physicians, with statistical significance seen in the difference of opinion for all therapies except prayer, self-help groups, spiritual healing, homeopathy, and megavitamin therapy. With regard to training in CAM, approximately one-fifth of respondents had received training, and expressed interest in receiving training in the area.

No significant difference in attitude toward CAM was noted between primary care physicians and specialists. Also, no differences were observed for age, race, or gender. However, our sample consisted primarily of white men, with a mean age of 44 years.

Patterns of Utilization of Complementary and Alternative Therapy

Responding physicians were asked if they had utilized an alternative therapy in their practice, with utilization defined as prescribing or referring patients for the therapies in question. Nearly two-thirds of the physicians surveyed had utilized at least one complementary therapy. The most commonly utilized modalities are listed in Table 3.2. Only energy and spiritual healing are not represented. Most referrals were to nonphysician providers (62.3%); 17% referred patients to physicians, and 20.8% referred to both physicians and nonphysicians. The most common condition for referral was management of pain. Other conditions mentioned included migraine headaches, anxiety, stress, depression, and insomnia.

Personal use of CAM modalities was not uncommon, with 48 of the 138 respondents (34.8%) having tried at least one alternative therapy. Those physicians who personally utilized alternative therapies were more likely than their colleagues to consider alternative therapies

Table 3.2. Percentage of responding physicians who have prescribed alternative treatments for their patients.

Type of alternative medicine	Prescribing physicians
Chiropractic	21.0
Biofeedback	16.7
Massage	13.8
Relaxation techniques	13.0
Acupuncture	10.9
Lifestyle exercise	10.9
Prayer	7.2
Self-help groups	7.2
Lifestyle diet	7.2
Megavitamin therapy	5.1
Herbal medicine	3.6
Imagery	2.2
Homeopathic medicine	1.4
Folk remedies	1.4
Hypnosis	0.7

Therapies are listed in descending order of prescribing by physicians. Energy healing and spiritual healing were not prescribed by any physicians.

legitimate, but no significant difference was noted in their prescription or referral for unconventional therapies. No significant differences in prescribing or referring for CAM were noted for any other variable, including years in practice, prior training in CAM, age, race, or gender.

There were no differences noted among physicians in the types of evidence they considered prior to referring or prescribing CAM. Table 3.3 lists the modal responses for those physicians in practice less than 10 years, and their more experienced colleagues.

Discussion

Physician attitudes in this survey appear consistent with previous studies. A modest degree of usefulness was perceived for some of the unconventional therapies, which agrees with the conclusions of Ernst et al.[6] A more positive attitude toward CAM was consistently noted among more recently trained physicians. Previous studies by Reilly and Perkin[9,10,11] support this finding.

These surveys showed a greater degree of optimism about CAM therapies among trainees and medical students. It would appear that the higher degree of acceptance by more recently trained physicians

Table 3.3. Evidentiary rules valued by responding physicians for CAM therapies (modal responses are reported).

Evidence	Less than 10 years in practice	More than 10 years in practice
Proven mechanism	1	1
Proposed mechanism	2	2
Clinical trials	1	1
Epidemiology	2	2
Case studies	2	2
Success in practice	2	2
Colleague recommendation	2	2
Personal use	2	3
Patient report	2	2

Scoring: 1=Very important; 5=Not important at all.

in our study was not the result of demanding different standards of evidence.

Furthermore, attitudes were not influenced by the age of the practitioner or specialization. There has been a rapid development of medical school and training program education in CAM over the past several years.[12] Therefore, the positive attitude toward CAM in more recently trained physicians is possibly the result of increased exposure to unconventional healing methods. Fifty-six percent of more recently trained physicians reported having some training in CAM therapies compared with 44% of their counterparts; however, this difference did not reach statistical significance. Interestingly, although recently trained physicians were more optimistic about the usefulness of most of CAM, no significant differences were noted in prescribing or referring patterns. We have no data regarding reasons for not utilizing CAM therapies.

Our survey did find a relatively high rate of usage of CAM. More than 65% of the physicians surveyed had utilized some form of alternative therapy in their practices. We do not find this rate of utilization alarming. The empirical use of a therapy has traditionally preceded the documentation of its efficacy, as long as safety has been assured. For example, few physicians would view the use of massage or relaxation techniques as an adjunct in the treatment of chronic pain or anxiety as harmful, but many may withhold judgment concerning their effectiveness. Additionally, it should be recognized that few of our current allopathic treatments have been proven efficacious through extensive clinical research.[13]

Should CAM therapies, then, be held to a higher standard than their allopathic counterparts? Some of the therapies in question (e.g., homeopathy and energy medicine) have no recognized physiological basis for effectiveness, at least in our western culture. The absence of a recognized scientific foundation demands documentation of safety and some efficacy before widespread integration of individual therapies into mainstream medicine. Conversely, therapies such as biofeedback and relaxation techniques have demonstrated efficacy through clinical trials.[14,15,16]

Unfortunately, it appears many physicians are not aware of the research that exists in this area. In our study population, approximately one-half of the physicians surveyed recognized biofeedback or relaxation techniques as legitimate medical practice, and less than 20% had prescribed these effective therapies for their patients.

For the purposes of this study, we adopted the definition of unconventional medicine used by Eisenberg.[1] This definition is based on what the typical physician or hospital in the U.S. offers as medical practice. It has little to do with what has been proven effective or safe as a medical therapy. For example, relaxation techniques are considered CAM because few physicians are taught or practice them. However, an abundance of research supports their beneficial effects and use as medical therapy. Therefore, we suggest for future studies that the definition of unconventional medicine refer to therapies for which there is no recognized scientific basis and little or no evidence of efficacy.

Of concern is the fact that two-thirds to one-half of patients who utilize CAM do not share this information with their allopathic physicians.[1,2] Unsupervised use of CAM therapies is potentially harmful,[17] and this lack of open communication reflects a deficiency in the doctor-patient relationship. Ignorance about CAM makes open discussion with patients extremely difficult for physicians and contributes to the lack of communication. Physician awareness of alternative therapies has likely increased since Eisenberg's survey in 1990. However, our study found only 19.7% of surveyed physicians had received any training in CAM therapies, and only 29% expressed an interest in further training. In this age of consumerism and patient autonomy, physicians need to be conversant in the area of CAM to garner the trust of patients who are using these therapies. The importance of trust and communication in the doctor-patient relationship makes the physician's level of knowledge of CAM an important area for further research.

Limitations of this study include the small sample size as well as the single geographic location. Despite the locale and small sample size, the results obtained are similar to those reported in other studies. Demographically, the sample was composed predominantly of white males and therefore may not represent the attitudes and behaviors of all physicians. Selection bias is also a concern. Other authors have found that a high response rate was indicative of a more favorable view of alternative medicine.[6] Our response rate was only 38%, and, therefore, may not be representative of the attitude toward or the utilization of CAM by the average physician. In retrospect, we recognize that we did not define training in our survey. Therefore, in future studies, we suggest asking respondents if they have any significant knowledge of individual therapies as a marker of familiarity with CAM.

Although certainly incomplete, an extensive body of literature does exist in a number of areas of alternative medicine,[18] and publication of peer-reviewed articles related to alternative medicine is growing at a rate of 12% a year. This degree of research is encouraging and should be continued. Additionally, the University of Arizona has established a postgraduate training program in CAM, and this program should provide a cadre of knowledgeable physicians who can provide leadership in this area. It is imperative that physicians educate themselves in the field of alternative medicine in order to give sound advice to, and fully participate with, patients in their treatment.

References

1. D.M. Eisenberg, R.C. Kessler, C. Foster, F.E. Norlock, D.R. Calkins and T.L. Delbanco, Unconventional medicine use in the United States: Prevalence, costs and patterns of use. *N Engl J Med* 328 (1993), pp. 246-252.

2. N.C. Elder, A. Gillcrist and R. Minz, Use of alternative health care by family practice patients. *Arch Fam Med* 6 (1997), pp. 181-184.

3. E.F. Hughes, Alternative medicine in family practice: It's already mainstream. *Fam Prac Recert* 19 10 (1997), pp. 22-44.

4. M. Carlston, M.R. Stuart and W. Jonas, Alternative medicine instruction in medical schools and family practice residency programs. *Fam Med* 29 (1997), pp. 559-562.

5. D. Daly, Alternative medicine courses taught at US medical schools: An ongoing listing. *J Altern Complement Med* 1 (1995), pp. 205-207.

6. E. Ernst, K. Resch and A.R. White, Complementary medicine, what physicians think of it: A meta-analysis. *Arch Intern Med* 155 (1995), pp. 2405-2408.

7. B.M. Berman, B.K. Singh, L. Lao, B.B. Singh, K.S. Ferentz and S.M. Hartnoll, Physicians' attitudes toward complementary or alternative medicine: A regional survey. *J Am Board Fam Pract* 8 (1995), pp. 361-366.

8. D.L. Blumberg, W.D. Grant, S.R. Hendricks, C.A. Kamps and M.J. Dewan, The physician and unconventional medicine. *Altern Ther Health Med* 1 3 (1995), pp. 31-35.

9. D.T. Reilly, Young doctors' views on alternative medicine. *BMJ* 287 (1983), pp. 337-339.

10. M.R. Perkin, R.M. Pearcy and J.S. Fraser, A comparison of the attitudes shown by general practitioners, hospital doctors and medical students toward alternative medicine. *J R Soc Med* 87 (1994), pp. 523-525.

11. D.T. Reilly and M. Taylor, Developing integrated medicine. *Comp Ther Med* 1 suppl 1 (1993), pp. 9-10.

12. M.S. Wetzel, D.M. Eisenberg and T. Kaptchuk, Courses involving complementary and alternative medicine at US medical schools. *JAMA* 280 (1998), pp. 784-787.

13. R. Smith, Where is the wisdom?: The poverty of medical evidence. *BMJ* 303 (1991), pp. 798-799.

14. H. Benson, The relaxation response. William Morrow & Co, New York (1975).

15. D.L. Chambless, Empirically validated treatments. In: J.C. Norcross Editor, *Psychologists' desk reference* Oxford University Press, New York (1998).

16. E.B. Blanchard and L.D. Young, Clinical applications of biofeedback training: A review of the evidence. *Arch Gen Psychiatry* 30 (1974), pp. 573-589.

17. D.M. Eisenberg, Advising patients who seek alternative medical therapies. *Ann Intern Med* 127 (1997), pp. 61-69.

18. National Institutes of Health, Office of Alternative Medicine Alternative medicine: Expanding medical horizons. A report to the National Institutes of Health on alternative medical systems and practices in the United States (NIH Publication 94-066) National Institutes of Health, Bethesda, MD (1994).

Part Two

Alternative Medical Systems

Chapter 4

Major Domains of Complementary and Alternative Medicine (CAM)

Complementary and alternative healthcare and medical practices (CAM) are those healthcare and medical practices that are not currently an integral part of conventional medicine.[1] The list of practices that are considered CAM changes continually as CAM practices and therapies that are proven safe and effective become accepted as "mainstream" healthcare practices. Today, CAM practices may be grouped within five major domains:[2] (1) alternative medical systems, (2) mind-body interventions, (3) biologically-based treatments, (4) manipulative and body-based methods, and (5) energy therapies. The individual systems and treatments comprising these categories are too numerous to list in this document. Thus, only limited examples are provided within each.

Alternative Medical Systems

Alternative medical systems involve complete systems of theory and practice that have evolved independent of and often prior to the conventional biomedical approach. Many are traditional systems of medicine that are practiced by individual cultures throughout the world, including a number of venerable Asian approaches.

Traditional oriental medicine emphasizes the proper balance or disturbances of qi (pronounced chi), or vital energy, in health and disease,

"Major Domains of Complementary and Alternative Medicine," an undated fact sheet produced by the National Center for Complementary and Alternative Medicine (NCCAM), cited December 2001.

31

respectively. Traditional oriental medicine consists of a group of techniques and methods, including acupuncture, herbal medicine, oriental massage, and qi gong (a form of energy therapy described more fully below). Acupuncture involves stimulating specific anatomic points in the body for therapeutic purposes, usually by puncturing the skin with a needle.

Ayurveda is India's traditional system of medicine. Ayurvedic medicine (meaning "science of life") is a comprehensive system of medicine that places equal emphasis on body, mind, and spirit, and strives to restore the innate harmony of the individual. Some of the primary Ayurvedic treatments include diet, exercise, meditation, herbs, massage, exposure to sunlight, and controlled breathing.

Other traditional medical systems have been developed by Native American, Aboriginal, African, Middle-Eastern, Tibetan, Central and South American cultures.

Homeopathic and naturopathic medicine are also examples of complete alternative medical systems. Homeopathic medicine is an unconventional Western system that is based on the principle that "like cures like," i.e., that the same substance that in large doses produces the symptoms of an illness, in very minute doses cures it. Homeopathic physicians believe that the more dilute the remedy, the greater its potency. Therefore, they use small doses of specially prepared plant extracts and minerals to stimulate the body's defense mechanisms and healing processes in order to treat illness.

Naturopathic medicine views disease as a manifestation of alterations in the processes by which the body naturally heals itself and emphasizes health restoration rather than disease treatment. Naturopathic physicians employ an array of healing practices, including diet and clinical nutrition; homeopathy; acupuncture; herbal medicine; hydrotherapy (the use of water in a range of temperatures and methods of applications); spinal and soft-tissue manipulation; physical therapies involving electric currents, ultrasound and light therapy; therapeutic counseling; and pharmacology.

Mind-Body Interventions

Mind-body interventions employ a variety of techniques designed to facilitate the mind's capacity to affect bodily function and symptoms. Only a subset of mind-body interventions are considered CAM. Many that have a well-documented theoretical basis, for example, patient education and cognitive-behavioral approaches are now considered "mainstream." On the other hand, meditation, certain uses of hypnosis, dance, music, and art therapy, and prayer and mental healing are categorized as complementary and alternative.

Biological-Based Therapies

This category of CAM includes natural and biologically-based practices, interventions, and products, many of which overlap with conventional medicine's use of dietary supplements. Included are herbal, special dietary, orthomolecular, and individual biological therapies.

Herbal therapies employ individual or mixtures of herbs for therapeutic value. An herb is a plant or plant part that produces and contains chemical substances that act upon the body. Special diet therapies, such as those proposed by Drs. Atkins, Ornish, Pritikin, and Weil, are believed to prevent and or control illness as well as promote health. Orthomolecular therapies aim to treat disease with varying concentrations of chemicals, such as, magnesium, melatonin, and mega-doses of vitamins. Biological therapies include, for example, the use of laetrile and shark cartilage to treat cancer and bee pollen to treat autoimmune and inflammatory diseases.

Manipulative and Body-Based Methods

This category includes methods that are based on manipulation and/or movement of the body. For example, chiropractors focus on the relationship between structure (primarily the spine) and function, and how that relationship affects the preservation and restoration of health, using manipulative therapy as an integral treatment tool. Some osteopaths, who place particular emphasis on the musculoskelatal system, believing that all of the body's systems work together and that disturbances in one system may have an impact upon function elsewhere in the body, practice osteopathic manipulation. Massage therapists manipulate the soft tissues of the body to normalize those tissues.

Energy Therapies

Energy therapies focus either on energy fields originating within the body (biofields) or those from other sources (electromagnetic fields).

Biofield therapies are intended to affect the energy fields, whose existence is not yet experimentally proven, that surround and penetrate the human body. Some forms of energy therapy manipulate biofields by applying pressure and/or manipulating the body by placing the hands in, or through, these fields. Examples include Qi gong, Reiki and Therapeutic Touch. Qi gong is a component of traditional oriental medicine that combines movement, meditation, and regulation of breathing to enhance the flow of vital energy (qi) in the body, to improve blood circulation, and to enhance immune function. Reiki, the Japanese word representing Universal Life Energy, is based on the belief that by channeling spiritual energy through the practitioner the spirit is healed, and it in turn heals the physical body. Therapeutic Touch is derived from the ancient technique of "laying-on of hands" and is based on the premise that it is the healing force of the therapist that affects the patient's recovery and that healing is promoted when the body's energies are in balance. By passing their hands over the patient, these healers identify energy imbalances.

Bioelectromagnetic-based therapies involve the unconventional use of electromagnetic fields, such as pulsed fields, magnetic fields, or alternating current or direct current fields, to, for example, treat asthma or cancer, or manage pain and migraine headaches.

Notes

1. The term conventional medicine refers to medicine as practiced by holders of M.D. (medical doctor) or D.O. (doctor of osteopathy) degrees, some of whom may also practice complementary and alternative medicine. Other terms for conventional medicine are allopathy, Western, regular, and mainstream medicine, and biomedicine.

2. These are the categories within which NCCAM has chosen to group the numerous CAM practices; others employ different, broad groupings.

Chapter 5

Acupuncture

Acupuncture is one of the oldest, most commonly used medical procedures in the world. Originating in China more than 2,000 years ago, acupuncture became widely known in the United States in 1971 when *New York Times* reporter James Reston wrote about how doctors in Beijing, China, used needles to ease his abdominal pain after surgery. Research shows that acupuncture is beneficial in treating a variety of health conditions.

In the past two decades, acupuncture has grown in popularity in the United States. In 1993, the U.S. Food and Drug Administration (FDA) estimated that Americans made 9 to 12 million visits per year to acupuncture practitioners and spent as much as $500 million on acupuncture treatments.[1] In 1995, an estimated 10,000 nationally certified acupuncturists were practicing in the United States. By the year 2000, that number is expected to double. Currently, an estimated one-third of certified acupuncturists in the United States are medical doctors.[2]

The National Institutes of Health (NIH) has funded a variety of research projects on acupuncture that have been awarded by its National

This chapter includes text from "Acupuncture Information and Resources," an undated fact sheet produced by the National Center for Complementary and Alternative Medicine (NCCAM), cited December 2001. The sections titled "Disorders Treated with Acupuncture," "Complications of Acupuncture," and "Patient Selection and Treatment," are reprinted from *Integrative Medicine*, Volume 1, Number 3, 1998, pp.107-115, Robin Leake, MA, and Joan E. Broderick, PhD, originally titled "Treatment Efficacy of Acupuncture: A Review of the Research Literature," with permission from Elsevier Science.

Center for Complementary and Alternative Medicine (NCCAM), National Institute on Alcohol Abuse and Alcoholism, National Institute of Dental Research, National Institute of Neurological Disorders and Stroke, and National Institute on Drug Abuse.

Acupuncture Theories

Traditional Chinese medicine theorizes that the more than 2,000 acupuncture points on the human body connect with 12 main and 8 secondary pathways, called meridians. Chinese medicine practitioners believe these meridians conduct energy, or qi, between the surface of the body and internal organs.

Qi regulates spiritual, emotional, mental, and physical balance. Qi is influenced by the opposing forces of yin and yang. According to traditional Chinese medicine, when yin and yang are balanced, they work together with the natural flow of qi to help the body achieve and maintain health. Acupuncture is believed to balance yin and yang, keep the normal flow of energy unblocked, and restore health to the body and mind.

Traditional Chinese medicine practices (including acupuncture, herbs, diet, massage, and meditative physical exercises) all are intended to improve the flow of qi.[3]

Western scientists have found meridians hard to identify because meridians do not directly correspond to nerve or blood circulation pathways. Some researchers believe that meridians are located throughout the body's connective tissue;[4] others do not believe that qi exists at all.[5,6] Such differences of opinion have made acupuncture a source of scientific controversy.

Preclinical Studies

Preclinical studies have documented acupuncture's effects, but they have not been able to fully explain how acupuncture works within the framework of the Western system of medicine.[7,8,9,10,11,12]

Mechanisms of Action

Several processes have been proposed to explain acupuncture's effects, primarily those on pain. Acupuncture points are believed to stimulate the central nervous system (the brain and spinal cord) to release chemicals into the muscles, spinal cord, and brain. These chemicals either change the experience of pain or release other chemicals, such as hormones, that influence the body's self-regulating systems. The biochemical changes may stimulate the body's natural healing abilities and promote physical and emotional well-being.[13] There are three main mechanisms:

1. Conduction of electromagnetic signals: Western scientists have found evidence that acupuncture points are strategic conductors of electromagnetic signals. Stimulating points along these pathways through acupuncture enables electromagnetic signals to be relayed at a greater rate than under normal conditions. These signals may start the flow of pain-killing biochemicals, such as endorphins, and of immune system cells to specific sites in the body that are injured or vulnerable to disease.[14,15]

2. Activation of opioid systems: Research has found that several types of opioids may be released into the central nervous system during acupuncture treatment, thereby reducing pain.[16]

3. Changes in brain chemistry, sensation, and involuntary body functions: Studies have shown that acupuncture may alter brain chemistry by changing the release of neurotransmitters and neurohormones in a good way. Acupuncture also has been documented to affect the parts of the central nervous system related to sensation and involuntary body functions, such as immune reactions and processes whereby a person's blood pressure, blood flow, and body temperature are regulated.[3,17,18]

Clinical Studies

According to an NIH consensus panel of scientists, researchers, and practitioners who convened in November 1997, clinical studies have shown that acupuncture is an effective treatment for nausea caused by surgical anesthesia and cancer chemotherapy as well as for dental pain experienced after surgery. The panel also found that acupuncture is useful by itself or combined with conventional therapies to treat addiction, headaches, menstrual cramps, tennis elbow, fibromyalgia, myofascial pain, osteoarthritis, lower back pain, carpal tunnel syndrome, and asthma; and to assist in stroke rehabilitation.[19]

Increasingly, acupuncture is complementing conventional therapies. For example, doctors may combine acupuncture and drugs to control surgery-related pain in their patients.[20] By providing both acupuncture and certain conventional anesthetic drugs, doctors have found it possible to achieve a state of complete pain relief for some patients.[16] They also have found that using acupuncture lowers the need for conventional pain-killing drugs and thus reduces the risk of side effects for patients who take the drugs.[21,22]

Table 5.1. Conditions Appropriate for Acupuncture Therapy

Digestive
Abdominal pain
Constipation
Diarrhea
Hyperacidity
Indigestion

Emotional
Anxiety
Depression
Insomnia
Nervousness
Neurosis

Eye-Ear-Nose-Throat
Cataracts
Gingivitis
Poor vision
Tinnitis
Toothache

Gynecological
Infertility
Menopausal symptoms
Premenstrual syndrome

Miscellaneous
Addiction control
Athletic performance
Blood pressure regulation
Chronic fatigue
Immune system tonification
Stress reduction

Musculoskeletal
Arthritis
Back pain
Muscle cramping
Muscle pain/weakness
Neck pain
Sciatica

Neurological
Headaches
Migraines
Neurogenic bladder dysfunction
Parkinson's disease
Postoperative pain
Stroke

Respiratory
Asthma
Bronchitis
Common cold
Sinusitis
Smoking cessation
Tonsillitis

Source: World Health Organization, United Nations. "Viewpoint on Acupuncture." 1979 (revised).[23]

Outside the United States, the World Health Organization (WHO), the health branch of the United Nations, lists more than 40 conditions for which acupuncture may be used.[23] Table 5.1 lists these conditions.

Currently, one of the main reasons Americans seek acupuncture treatment is to relieve chronic pain, especially from conditions such as arthritis or lower back disorders.[24,25] Some clinical studies show that acupuncture is effective in relieving both chronic (long-lasting) and acute or sudden pain, but other research indicates that it provides no relief from chronic pain.[27] Additional research is needed to provide definitive answers.

Disorders Treated with Acupuncture

Pain Management

Perhaps the most common use of acupuncture is for treatment of pain, usually chronic or post-surgical pain. One of the earliest comprehensive reviews of the clinical effects of acupuncture in treating chronic pain concluded that acupuncture effectively relieved pain in 60-75% of patients, while sham acupuncture reduced pain in 50% and placebo (control) in 30% of patients. A recent meta-analysis of acupuncture effectiveness for the treatment of chronic pain yielded similar results.

When the fourteen random control studies included in the analysis were pooled, results indicated that acupuncture was significantly more effective than placebo or sham acupuncture in treating chronic pain, particularly headaches and neck pain.

Headaches and Neck Pain

The NIH consensus statement identified 16 randomized controlled studies for acupuncture of tension and migraine headaches. Based upon their review, they concluded that acupuncture should be considered an effective treatment for tension and migraine headaches. This independent review yielded similar findings. One study on tension headaches found that acupuncture and sham treatment (placing acupuncture needles at neighboring points, but not directly on actual, meridian acupuncture points) were equally effective in reducing the frequency, pain index, and medication dosage.

Two other studies found that acupuncture was significantly more effective in reducing headache pain than placebo and sham treatment. Moreover, other studies found acupuncture to be just as effective as standard treatment. One recent, well-designed study examining tension and migraine headaches found that acupuncture treatment was more effective than placebo treatment and just as effective, with fewer side effects, as standard treatment.

Evidence supporting acupuncture for neck pain is beginning to emerge but, to date, there are relatively few controlled studies in this area. One research group found that acupuncture was significantly more effective than sham and placebo treatments in a pilot sample, but not in a later follow-up study. Another study found that acupuncture was significantly more effective than placebo-diazepam in the treatment of osteoarthritic pain, and just as effective as sham acupuncture or diazepam treatment.

Musculoskeletal Pain

Electroacupuncture was found to be more effective than sham in the treatment of fibromyalgia, a disorder that causes musculoskeletal pain, fatigue, and abdominal discomfort. In this randomized clinical study, patients who received electroacupuncture treatment for 6 weeks showed improved pain threshold, took less medication, and reported better sleep than patients who received sham treatment. A randomized, controlled trial of the effects of acupuncture on osteoarthritic patients found that patients who received acupuncture around the knee for 3 weeks reported less pain and increased functioning than no-treatment controls. Since there was no sham treatment, however, placebo effects were not controlled. Another study compared the success of diazepam, placebo diazepam, acupuncture and sham acupuncture in alleviating pain in patients with chronic cervical osteoarthritis. Results indicated that diazepam, acupuncture, and placebo acupuncture were all equally effective in reducing pain, suggesting that acupuncture may be used as an alternative treatment to benzodiazepines in the treatment of osteoarthritis pain.

Postoperative Pain

Acupuncture is often used to treat post-operative pain, either in lieu of or combined with standard medication. The few randomized, controlled studies examining the effectiveness of acupuncture in relieving dental pain are promising. An early study found that patients who received the combined treatment of acupuncture and codeine after a wisdom tooth extraction reported less post-operative pain than patients who received only either acupuncture, medication, or placebo treatment. While a later study found no differences in pain immediately post-operative, patients receiving acupuncture and standard medication treatments reported significantly less pain and medication consumption during the 10-day follow-up compared with patients receiving only medication. In a recent study, Lao et al. found that acupuncture was more effective than placebo (in which a needle was taped to the body to elicit minor sensation) in reducing the duration and intensity of pain after surgical extraction of molars.

Randomized, controlled trials for other types of postoperative pain have yielded promising findings. For example, in a study of postoperative pain after hysterectomy, Christensen and colleagues found that women who received electroacupuncture while still anaesthetized reported less pain and self-administered 40% less pain medication than women in the no-treatment control condition. The pain relief from electroacupuncture treatment lasted approximately 2 hours.

However, a similar study of electroacupuncture administered before and during hysterectomy surgery found no differences in postoperative pain ratings between treatment and control patients.

Back Pain and Tennis Elbow

Several studies have found that acupuncture treatment may provide relief from lower back pain and tennis elbow. Macdonald and colleagues conducted a random placebo-controlled study on patients with low back pain. Those who received acupuncture reported less pain and showed greater reductions in visual analog scale (VAS) assessed pain than patients receiving placebo treatments with inactive electrodes. Another study comparing standard medical care with standard care plus acupuncture treatment, found that low back pain was significantly reduced when acupuncture was given in conjunction with physiotherapy.

Finally, one study examining whether acupuncture relieves acute pain due to tennis elbow found that acupuncture treatment had an immediate analgesic effect on the duration and level of pain for the acupuncture patients compared with patients receiving placebo treatment. A unique aspect of this study was the use of suggestive placebo rather than sham treatment, where the patients were led to believe that acupuncture needles were placed in their backs. This design prevented any inadvertent analgesic effects from needling non-specific acupuncture points.

Asthma

An estimated 13 million people in the United States suffer from asthma, and the incidence, especially among children, is increasing.

Although asthma is treated with medication, non-pharmacological treatment options are desirable to avoid side effects and increased risks associated with long-term steroid inhalation.

Several random controlled studies indicate that a single acupuncture treatment reduces asthmatic symptoms, including airway resistance, forced expiratory flow volume, and thoracic gas volume significantly more than sham, or no-treatment controls. Another study found that asthmatic patients who received several acupuncture treatments showed significantly better bronchodilation of the lungs than control patients. In a similar, single-treatment study with exercise-induced asthma, acupuncture administered 20 minutes prior to exercise reduced asthma attacks significantly more than sham treatment.

While these studies find that acupuncture leads to immediate and short-term relief of asthma symptoms, attempts to assess the efficacy of acupuncture as a long-term therapeutic treatment for bronchial asthma have yielded contradictory results. Specifically, two recent reviews of 13 and 15 random clinical studies determined that the evidence supporting acupuncture as treatment for asthma was inconclusive. The first review by Kleijnen and colleagues in 1991 concluded that the quality of the studies was "mediocre" and the results were contradictory. A second, more recent review stated that there is still insufficient data to determine the efficacy of acupuncture in asthma treatment. However, the authors assert that acupuncture may be a potentially beneficial and safe treatment for bronchial asthma, and there is no reason to withhold such treatment until empirical evidence indicates otherwise.

Nausea and Vomiting

Post-Operative

Debilitating post-operative nausea and vomiting occur in 60-70% of surgical patients. Unfortunately, standard antiemetics frequently are ineffective or accompanied by severe side effects. A number of studies indicate that acupuncture and acupressure administered to sites on the wrist may be a viable alternative to antiemetic drugs. Two recent, random controlled trials found that acupuncture and acupressure significantly reduced post-operative nausea and vomiting in hospital patients compared to a placebo control group. In another randomized, controlled study, Ho and colleagues demonstrated that acupressure effectively reduced nausea and eliminated vomiting in women receiving epidural morphine for pain relief during a caesarian-section. The antiemetic action of acupuncture and acupressure is strongest when administered before opioid premedication and is blocked by local anesthesia at the acupuncture point.

Acupuncture for the treatment of post-operative nausea has been studied in pediatric populations as well, with very different results. In several studies with children undergoing corrective eye surgery and tonsillectomy, acupuncture or acupressure has not been effective in reducing postoperative vomiting and nausea.

Pregnancy-Induced

Over 70% of pregnant women experience nausea and/or vomiting, especially during the first trimester of pregnancy. The causes of pregnancy-induced nausea remain unclear, and there are few available pharmacological treatments that have been shown to be safe for the fetus. In the search for safe and effective remedies, some clinicians recommend acupressure, in which wristbands ("sea bands") apply constant pressure to the wrist. Few controlled studies, however, have examined whether acupressure effectively relieves nausea and vomiting, and the results are not compelling. A 1994 study reported that acupressure was found to be somewhat effective in relieving nausea, but not vomiting, when compared to a sham therapy. One of the largest random controlled studies found no differences between a group of pregnant women who wore acupressure wrist bands for 7 days and those in the control or placebo groups. Another randomized, controlled study did find that pregnant women who wore a device over the wrist that delivered an electric current reported significantly less nausea and vomiting than women wearing a sham device. However, this study has been criticized because the women in the experimental group were probably able to feel the current from the device, suggesting that results may be due to placebo effects. In an extensive review of the literature, Murphy concluded that there is little scientific evidence to support acupressure as an effective remedy for pregnancy-induced nausea and vomiting.

Chemotherapy-Induced

The majority of evidence suggesting that acupuncture and acupressure effectively relieve the emetic side effects of cancer chemotherapy comes from research conducted by Dundee and his colleagues at the Northern Ireland Radiotherapy Centre. Although they did not conduct controlled, randomized studies, these investigators observed that over 100 cancer patients who were unresponsive to standard anti-emetic medications after chemotherapy responded well to electrical stimulation of the wrist. They further noted that the optimal reduction of nausea and vomiting occurs when acupuncture stimulation is used in conjunction with standard antiemetic medication. A placebo-controlled study by another group of researchers confirmed these effects by finding that electroacupuncture was more effective than sham acupuncture and antiemetic medication in reducing chemotherapy-induced nausea and vomiting.

In summary, evidence suggests that acupuncture and acupressure are effective for postoperative nausea and vomiting (except in children), but is less effective for treating nausea due to pregnancy. More evidence is needed before conclusions can be reached about acupuncture as an antiemetic treatment for chemotherapy-induced side effects.

Drug and Alcohol Abuse

Treating drug addiction is notoriously difficult as well as expensive, and relapse rates remain high. Currently, more than 300 facilities in 20 states in the United States provide acupuncture-assisted detoxification. However, both clinical research and opinion concerning acupuncture for the treatment of substance dependency is contradictory and controversial. In Hong Kong during the early 1970s, practitioners observed that patients who received acupuncture to points on the ears (auricular acupuncture) reported fewer symptoms of opium withdrawal, specifically pain, nausea, and vomiting. Acupuncture was thought to ease withdrawal by causing the release of endogenous hormones, which mimicked exogenous opiates such as heroin.

The goal of acupuncture treatment during detoxification is to reduce the primary symptoms of withdrawal as well as associated aches and pains. During the next stage, rehabilitation, the goal shifts to relieving depression and anxiety by promoting relaxation. Acupuncture treatment is also administered to prevent relapse, primarily by reducing the symptoms associated with craving as well as encouraging relaxation.

Evidence concerning the efficacy of acupuncture as a treatment for substance abuse is contradictory. One random controlled study found that severe recidivist alcoholics receiving acupuncture experienced fewer withdrawal symptoms and better rehabilitation than those in the sham or placebo conditions. These effects were maintained through the 6-month follow-up assessment. A later study, however, failed to replicate these results. A 1994 review concluded that opiate addicts in detoxification programs receiving acupuncture treatment had better program attendance than those patients receiving sham treatment. Another study found that acupuncture in conjunction with methadone maintenance was more successful in mitigating withdrawal symptoms than methadone without acupuncture.

Thus, there is suggestive evidence that acupuncture may have an important role in the challenging field of substance abuse treatment. A 1991 meta-analysis of 21 studies examining the efficacy of acupuncture in treating addiction concluded that most of the clinical research was of poor methodological quality. However, the compelling need for improvement of current substance abuse treatment and the evidence of the studies reported to date argue for further consideration of acupuncture. Methodologically rigorous research is clearly needed before firm conclusions may by drawn.

Carpal Tunnel Syndrome

Carpal Tunnel Syndrome (CTS) is compression of the median nerve in the wrist by the tendons in the wrist bones, resulting in pain, numbness, tingling, and weakness in the hand and forearm. CTS affects approximately 15% of workers whose jobs involve repetitive hand movements, resulting in millions of diagnosed cases. Several randomized, controlled studies indicate that acupuncture and laser acupuncture may be an effective, painless, and cost-effective alternative to surgical treatment of CTS. One study in particular found that laser stimulation of acupuncture points significantly reduced pain more than sham acupuncture. Other studies indicate that laser acupuncture may have therapeutic anti-inflammatory effects and increase serotonin levels.

Dysmenorrhea

Approximately 30-75% of women suffer from primary dysmenorrhea, the most common of all gynecological complaints. At least half of these women manage their symptoms, including painful abdominal cramping, nausea, headache and backache, with pharmacological treatment. Although there have been few clinical studies in the area; acupuncture has been recommended for the treatment and management of primary dysmenorrhea, or painful menstruation. Some practitioners suggest that acupuncture administered in the pelvic region influences the release of hormones that may decrease pain, but no research has been conducted to examine this assertion. One controlled study comparing the efficacy of acupuncture administered for 3 months with sham acupuncture treatment and no-treatment controls, found that acupuncture significantly reduced pain associated with dysmenorrhea more effectively than sham or control treatments.

Stroke Rehabilitation

Currently, stroke is the leading cause of disability in the United States. Studies have shown that stroke victims who receive acupuncture in addition to their standard treatment show greater recovery from paralysis than those patients receiving only standard therapy. However, few of these studies use sham or placebo controls. One study comparing acupuncture to a sham control in stroke patients with arm or leg paralysis found that acupuncture increased range of motion while sham acupuncture did not. Several studies have found that acupuncture is most effective if treatment is given within 36 hours post-onset of the stroke, particularly when severe paralysis results. A study examining the long-term effects of acupuncture on stroke recovery found that patients receiving acupuncture treatment showed significantly greater improvements in motor skills functioning both during the treatment and during the following year.

It is unclear why acupuncture is more effective when administered in the early stages of post-stroke, or what the mechanism is for improving motor functioning in paralysis. Researchers speculate that acupuncture increases cerebral blood flow and promotes vasorestriction. Acupuncture may also reduce swelling in the brain, decreasing the extent of brain injury.

Cerebral Palsy and Paralysis

Another area with limited research but promising possibilities is the use of acupuncture to treat cerebral palsy in infants and children. Two studies found that acupuncture was more effective than control treatments (either limb massage or vitamins) in improving motor functioning and reducing spasticity. Preliminary studies have found that acupuncture or laser acupuncture may be effective in treating paralysis due to spinal cord injuries and peripheral facial paralysis. However, at the present time, no controlled studies have been conducted in either area.

Complications of Acupuncture

Although complications due to acupuncture are few and comparatively minor in nature, there are some risks associated with the procedure. Technical problems that can occur with acupuncture treatment include bent or broken needles, and the inability to remove a needle due to muscle spasm. However, the commercial availability and government regulation of stronger needles has reduced these complications. "Stuck" needles can usually be removed by relaxing the patient, or placing another needle in a nearby site. In one study, 197 acupuncturists and 1135 physicians were asked to recall if they had encountered any patients who had had any negative reactions to acupuncture.

Thirty-one percent of acupuncturists and 12% of physicians reported at least one adverse effect. A 1996 literature review estimated that there have been less than 300 total adverse reactions to acupuncture reported in the last 10 years. However, these authors suspect that many complications, particularly minor ones, are underreported. The most common serious complication is pneumothorax due to improper needling. Other organ puncture injuries, though rare, have been reported in case studies. For example, one case study described a woman who died when an acupuncture needle was inserted into her heart. Fainting, local infection, and increased pain are the most commonly reported minor complaints. Less common complaints included hepatitis, arthritis, osteomyelitis, and endocarditis. Unsterile acupuncture needles carry the risk of infection, although there are few documented cases. One hundred and twenty-six cases of hepatitis B have been directly linked to single practitioners using unsterilized needles, and one case of bacterial endocarditis was reported in a woman with a prosthetic heart valve who was already at high risk for endocarditis. Theoretically, unsterile needling could lead to HIV infection, although there is no empirical evidence that HIV has ever been transmitted through acupuncture needling.

Patient Selection and Treatment

Ample empirical evidence suggests that acupuncture can be integrated into mainstream clinical medicine as a complementary or primary treatment for a variety of disorders. However, in the United States, acupuncture is frequently considered a last-resort option for intractable conditions, if at all. Given the empirical support, health practitioners should consider recommending acupuncture to patients with pain disorders, asthma, post-operative nausea, dysmenorrhea, and stroke.

Acupuncture is a particularly appealing option for those patients, especially children, the elderly, and pregnant women, who cannot tolerate typical medical interventions. In addition, there are increasing numbers of patients who are seeking less invasive, more "natural" forms of interventions. Working within patients' preferences and expectations for optimal care can improve treatment compliance, patient satisfaction and, ultimately, treatment outcome.

As acupuncture has gained both greater public awareness and acceptance within the medical community, the demand for strict regulations and guidelines for the safe practice of acupuncture has increased. For example, in March of 1996, The Food and Drug Administration (FDA) reclassified acupuncture needles from the class 3 category of "experimental devices" to class 2 status of "medical tools." This ruling indicates acceptance of acupuncture by the FDA as a safe and effective medical treatment.

FDA's Role

The FDA approved acupuncture needles for use by licensed practitioners in 1996. The FDA requires manufacturers of acupuncture needles to label them for single use only.[28] Relatively few complications from the use of acupuncture have been reported to the FDA when one considers the millions of people treated each year and the number of acupuncture needles used. Still, complications have resulted from inadequate sterilization of needles and from improper delivery of treatments. When not delivered properly, acupuncture can cause serious adverse effects, including infections and puncturing of organs.[1]

NCCAM-Sponsored Clinical Research

Originally founded in 1992 as the Office of Alternative Medicine (OAM), the NCCAM facilitates the research and evaluation of unconventional medical practices and disseminates this information to the public. The NCCAM, established in 1998, supports nine Centers, where researchers conduct studies on complementary and alternative medicine for specific health conditions and diseases. Scientists at several Centers are investigating acupuncture therapy.

Researchers at the NCCAM Center at the University of Maryland in Baltimore conducted a randomized controlled clinical trial and found that patients treated with acupuncture after dental surgery had less intense pain than patients who received a placebo.[20] Other scientists at the Center found that older people with osteoarthritis experienced significantly more pain relief after using conventional drugs and acupuncture together than those using conventional therapy alone.[29]

Researchers at the Minneapolis Medical Research Foundation in Minnesota are studying the use of acupuncture to treat alcoholism and addiction to benzodiazepines, nicotine, and cocaine. Scientists at the Kessler Institute for Rehabilitation in New Jersey studied acupuncture to treat a stroke-related swallowing disorder and the pain associated with spinal cord injuries.

The OAM, now the NCCAM, also funded several individual researchers in 1993 and 1994 to conduct preliminary studies on acupuncture. In one small randomized controlled clinical trial, more than half of the 11 women with a major depressive episode who were treated with acupuncture improved significantly.[30]

In another controlled clinical trial, nearly half of the seven children with attention deficit hyperactivity disorder who underwent acupuncture treatment showed some improvement in their symptoms. Researchers concluded that acupuncture was a useful alternative to standard medication for some children with this condition.[31]

In a third small controlled study, eight pregnant women were given a type of acupuncture treatment, called moxibustion, to reduce the rate of breech births, in which the fetus is positioned for birth feet-first instead of the normal position of head-first. Researchers found the treatment to be safe, but they were uncertain whether it was effective.[32] Then, researchers reporting in the November 11, 1998, issue of the *Journal of the American Medical Association* conducted a larger randomized controlled clinical trial using moxibustion. They found that moxibustion applied to 130 pregnant women presenting breech significantly increased the number of normal head-first births.[33]

Acupuncture and You

The use of acupuncture, like many other complementary and alternative treatments, has produced a good deal of anecdotal evidence. Much of this evidence comes from people who report their own successful use of the treatment. If a treatment appears to be safe and patients report recovery from their illness or condition after using it, others may decide to use the treatment. However, scientific research may not substantiate the anecdotal reports.

Lifestyle, age, physiology, and other factors combine to make every person different. A treatment that works for one person may not work for another who has the very same condition. You, as a health care consumer (especially if you have a preexisting medical condition);

should discuss acupuncture with your doctor. Do not rely on a diagnosis of disease by an acupuncturist who does not have substantial conventional medical training. If you have received a diagnosis from a doctor and have had little or no success using conventional medicine, you may wish to ask your doctor whether acupuncture might help.

Finding a Licensed Acupuncture Practitioner

Doctors are a good resource for referrals to acupuncturists. Increasingly, doctors are familiar with acupuncture and may know of a certified practitioner. In addition, more medical doctors, including neurologists, anesthesiologists, and specialists in physical medicine, are becoming trained in acupuncture, traditional Chinese medicine, and other alternative and complementary therapies. Friends and family members may be a source of referrals as well. In addition, national referral organizations provide the names of practitioners, although these organizations may be advocacy groups for the practitioners to whom they refer.

Check a practitioner's credentials.

A practitioner who is licensed and credentialed may provide better care than one who is not. About 30 states have established training standards for certification to practice acupuncture, but not all states require acupuncturists to obtain a license to practice. Although proper credentials do not ensure competency, they do indicate that the practitioner has met certain standards to treat patients with acupuncture.

The American Academy of Medical Acupuncture can give you a referral list of doctors who practice acupuncture. The National Acupuncture and Oriental Medicine Alliance lists thousands of acupuncturists on its Web site and provides the list to callers to their information and referral line. The Alliance requires documentation of state license or national board certification from its listed acupuncturists. The American Association of Oriental Medicine can tell you the state licensing status of acupuncture practitioners across the United States as well.

Check treatment cost and insurance coverage.

Reflecting public demand, an estimated 70 to 80 percent of the nation's insurers covered some acupuncture treatments in 1996. An

50

acupuncturist may provide information about the number of treatments needed and how much each will cost. Generally, treatment may take place over a few days or several weeks. The cost per treatment typically ranges between $30 and $100, but it may be appreciably more. Physician acupuncturists may charge more than nonphysician practitioners.[13]

Check treatment procedures.

To find out about the treatment procedures that will be used and their likelihood of success. You also should make certain that the practitioner uses a new set of disposable needles in a sealed package every time. The FDA requires the use of sterile, nontoxic needles that bear a labeling statement restricting their use to qualified practitioners. The practitioner also should swab the puncture site with alcohol or another disinfectant before inserting the needle.

Some practitioners may use electroacupuncture; others may use moxibustion. These approaches are part of traditional Chinese medicine, and Western researchers are beginning to study whether they enhance acupuncture's effects.

During your first office visit, the practitioner may ask you at length about your health condition, lifestyle, and behavior. The practitioner will want to obtain a complete picture of your treatment needs and behaviors that may contribute to the condition. This holistic approach is typical of traditional Chinese medicine and many other alternative and complementary therapies.

Let the acupuncturist, or any doctor for that matter, know about all treatments or medications you are taking and whether you have a pacemaker, are pregnant, or have breast or other implants. Acupuncture may be risky to your health if you fail to tell the practitioner about any of these matters.

The Sensation of Acupuncture

Acupuncture needles are metallic, solid, and hair-thin, unlike the thicker, hollow hypodermic needles used in Western medicine to administer treatments or take blood samples. People experience acupuncture differently, but most feel minimal pain as the needles are inserted. Some people are energized by treatment, while others feel relaxed.[34] Some patients may fear acupuncture because they are afraid of needles. Improper needle placement, movement of the patient, or a defect in the needle can cause soreness and pain during treatment.[35] This is why it is so important to seek treatment from a qualified acupuncture practitioner.

As important research advances continue to be made on acupuncture worldwide, practitioners and doctors increasingly will work together to give you the best care available.

References

1. Lytle, C.D. *An Overview of Acupuncture.* 1993. Washington, DC: United States Department of Health and Human Services, Health Sciences Branch, Division of Life Sciences, Office of Science and Technology, Center for Devices and Radiological Health, Food and Drug Administration.

2. Culliton, P.D. "Current Utilization of Acupuncture by United States Patients." *National Institutes of Health Consensus Development Conference on Acupuncture, Program & Abstracts* (Bethesda, MD, November 3-5, 1997). Sponsors: Office of Alternative Medicine and Office of Medical Applications Research. Bethesda, MD: National Institutes of Health, 1997.

3. Beinfield, H. and Korngold, E.L. *Between Heaven and Earth: A Guide to Chinese Medicine.* New York, NY: Ballantine Books, 1991.

4. Brown, D. "Three Generations of Alternative Medicine: Behavioral Medicine, Integrated Medicine, and Energy Medicine." *Boston University School of Medicine Alumni Report.* Fall 1996.

5. Senior, K. "Acupuncture: Can It Take the Pain Away? " *Molecular Medicine Today.* 1996. 2(4):150-3.

6. Raso, J. *Alternative Health Care: A Comprehensive Guide.* Buffalo, NY: Prometheus Books, 1994.

7. Eskinazi, D.P. "National Institutes of Health Technology Assessment Workshop on Alternative Medicine: Acupuncture." *Journal of Alternative and Complementary Medicine.* 1996. 2(1):1-253.

8. Tang, N.M., Dong, H.W., Wang, X.M., Tsui, Z.C., and Han, J.S. "Cholecystokinin Antisense RNA Increases the Analgesic Effect Induced by Electroacupuncture or Low Dose Morphine: Conversion of Low Responder Rats into High Responders." *Pain.* 1997. 71(1):71-80.

9. Cheng, X.D., Wu, G.C., He, Q.Z., and Cao, X.D. "Effect of Electroacupuncture on the Activities of Tyrosine Protein Kinase in Subcellular Fractions of Activated T Lymphocytes from the Traumatized Rats." *Acupuncture and Electro-Therapeutics Research.* 1998. 23(3-4):161-170.

10. Chen, L.B. and Li, S.X. "The Effects of Electrical Acupuncture of Neiguan on the PO2 of the Border Zone Between Ischemic and Non-Ischemic Myocardium in Dogs." *Journal of Traditional Chinese Medicine.* 1983. 3(2):83-8.

11. Lee, H.S. and Kim, J.Y. "Effects of Acupuncture on Blood Pressure and Plasma Renin Activity in Two-Kidney One Clip Goldblatt Hypertensive Rats." *American Journal of Chinese Medicine.* 1994. 22(3-4):215-9.

12. Okada, K., Oshima, M., and Kawakita, K. "Examination of the Afferent Fiber Responsible for the Suppression of Jaw-Opening Reflex in Heat, Cold and Manual Acupuncture Stimulation in Anesthetized Rats." *Brain Research.* 1996. 740(1-2):201-7.

13. National Institutes of Health. *Frequently Asked Questions About Acupuncture.* Bethesda, MD: National Institutes of Health, 1997.

14. Dale, R.A. "Demythologizing Acupuncture. Part 1. The Scientific Mechanisms and the Clinical Uses." *Alternative & Complementary Therapies Journal.* April 1997. 3(2):125-31.

15. Takeshige, C. "Mechanism of Acupuncture Analgesia Based on Animal Experiments." *Scientific Bases of Acupuncture.* Berlin, Germany: Springer-Verlag, 1989.

16. Han, J. S. "Acupuncture Activates Endogenous Systems of Analgesia." *National Institutes of Health Consensus Conference on Acupuncture, Program & Abstracts* (Bethesda, MD, November 3-5, 1997). Sponsors: Office of Alternative Medicine and Office of Medical Applications of Research. Bethesda, MD: National Institutes of Health, 1997.

17. Wu, B., Zhou, R.X., and Zhou, M.S. "Effect of Acupuncture on Interleukin-2 Level and NK Cell Immunoactivity of Peripheral Blood of Malignant Tumor Patients." *Chung Kuo Chung Hsi I Chieh Ho Tsa Chich.* 1994. 14(9):537-9.

18. Wu, B. "Effect of Acupuncture on the Regulation of Cell-
     Mediated Immunity in Patients With Malignant Tumors."
     Chen Tzu Yen Chiu. 1995. 20(3):67-71.

19. National Institutes of Health Consensus Panel. "Acupuncture."
     *National Institutes of Health Consensus Development State-
     ment* (Bethesda, MD, November 3-5, 1997). Sponsors: Office of
     Alternative Medicine and Office of Medical Applications of Re-
     search. Bethesda, MD: National Institutes of Health, 1997.

20. Lao, L., Bergman, S., Langenberg, P., Wong, R., and Berman,
     B. "Efficacy of Chinese Acupuncture on Postoperative Oral
     Surgery Pain." *Oral Surgery, Oral Medicine, Oral Pathology.*
     1995. 79(4):423-8.

21. Lewith, G.T. and Vincent, C. "On the Evaluation of the Clini-
     cal Effects of Acupuncture: A Problem Reassessed and a
     Framework for Future Research." *Journal of Alternative and
     Complementary Medicine.* 1996. 2(1):79-90.

22. Tsibuliak, V.N., Alisov, A.P., and Shatrova, V.P. "Acupuncture
     Analgesia and Analgesic Transcutaneous Electroneurostimu-
     lation in the Early Postoperative Period." *Anesthesiology and
     Reanimatology.* 1995. 2:93-8.

23. World Health Organization. *Viewpoint on Acupuncture.*
     Geneva, Switzerland: World Health Organization, 1979.

24. Bullock, M.L., Pheley, A.M., Kiresuk, T.J., Lenz, S.K., and
     Culliton, P.D. "Characteristics and Complaints of Patients
     Seeking Therapy at a Hospital-Based Alternative Medicine
     Clinic." *Journal of Alternative and Complementary Medicine.*
     1997. 3(1):31-7.

25. Diehl, D.L., Kaplan, G., Coulter, I., Glik, D., and Hurwitz,
     E.L. "Use of Acupuncture by American Physicians." *Journal of
     Alternative and Complementary Medicine.* 1997. 3(2):119-26.

26. Levine, J.D., Gormley, J., and Fields, H.L. "Observations on
     the Analgesic Effects of Needle Puncture (Acupuncture)."
     Pain. 1976. 2(2):149-59.

27. Ter Reit, G., Kleijnen, J., and Knipschild, P. "Acupuncture and
     Chronic Pain: A Criteria-Based Meta-Analysis." *Clinical Epi-
     demiology.* 1990. 43:1191-9.

28. U.S. Food and Drug Administration. "Acupuncture Needles No Longer Investigational." *FDA Consumer Magazine.* June 1996. 30(5).

29. Berman, B., Lao, L., Bergman, S., Langenberg, P., Wong, R., Loangenberg, P., and Hochberg, M. "Efficacy of Traditional Chinese Acupuncture in the Treatment of Osteoarthritis: A Pilot Study." *Osteoarthritis and Cartilage.* 1995. (3):139-42.

30. Allen, John J.B. "An Acupuncture Treatment Study for Unipolar Depression." *Psychological Science.* 1998. 9:397-401.

31. Sonenklar, N. *Acupuncture and Attention Deficit Hyperactivity Disorder.* National Institutes of Health, Office of Alternative Medicine Research Grant #R21 RR09463. 1993.

32. Milligan, R. *Breech Version by Acumoxa.* National Institutes of Health, Office of Alternative Medicine Research Grant #R21 RR09527. 1993.

33. Cardini, F. and Weixin, H. "Moxibustion for Correction of Breech Presentation: A Randomized Controlled Trial." *Journal of the American Medical Association.* 1998. 280:1580-4.

34. American Academy of Medical Acupuncture. Doctor, *What's This Acupuncture All About? A Brief Explanation for Patients.* Los Angeles, CA: American Academy of Medical Acupuncture, 1996.

35. Lao, L. "Safety Issues in Acupuncture." *Journal of Alternative and Complementary Medicine.* 1996. 2(1):27-9.

Chapter 6

Ayurveda

Ayurveda is a Sanskrit word, derived from two roots: ayur, which means life, and veda, knowledge. Knowledge arranged systematically with logic becomes science. During the due course of time, Ayurveda became the science of life. It has its root in ancient vedic literature and encompasses our entire life, the body, mind and spirit.

Purusha/Prakruti

According to Ayurveda, every human being is a creation of the cosmos, the pure cosmic consciousness, as two energies: male energy, called Purusha and female energy, Prakruti. Purusha is choiceless passive awareness, while Prakruti is choiceful active consciousness. Prakruti is the divine creative will. Purusha doesn't take part in creation, but Prakruti does the divine dance of creation called leela. In creation, Prakruti is first evolved or manifested as supreme intelligence, called mahat. Mahat is the buddhi principal (individual intellect), which further manifests as self identity, called ahamkara, which is ego. Ahamkara is influenced by three basic universal qualities: satva, rajas and tamas. Satva is responsible for clarity of perception. Rajas cause movement, sensations, feelings and emotions. Tamas is

"An Introduction to Ayurveda," ©1994, 2001, Dr. Vasant Lad and The Ayurvedic Institute. All rights reserved. Originally published in *Ayurveda Today*, Volume 6, Number 4, Spring 1994. For more information on Ayurveda or The Ayurvedic Institute, contact The Ayurvedic Institute, P.O. Box 23445, Albuquerque, NM 87192-1445, 505-291-9698, http://www.ayurveda.com.

the tendency towards inertia, darkness, heaviness, and is responsible for periods of confusion and deep sleep.

Manifestation of Creation

From the essence of satva the five senses are created: the ears to hear, skin to perceive touch, eyes to see, the tongue to taste, and the nose, to smell. The essence of rajas is manifested as the five motor organs: speech, hands, feet, genitals and the organs of excretion. The mind is derived from satva, while rajas is manifested as prana, the life force. The tamasic quality is also responsible for the creation of tan matra, the subtle elements, and from whom the five basic elements are manifested. They are space, air, fire, water and earth. It is from pure consciousness that space is manifested.

Space

Expansion of consciousness is space and space is all enclosive. We need space to live, and our bodily cells contain spaces. The synaptic, cellular and visceral spaces give freedom to the tissues to perform their normal physiological functions. (A change in tissue space, however, may lead to pathological conditions.) The space in between two conjunctive nerve cells aids communication, while the space in the mind encompasses love and compassion.

Air

The movement of consciousness determines the direction along which change of position in space takes place. This course of action causes subtle activities and movements within space. According to the Ayurvedic perspective, this is the air principle. There is a cosmic magnetic field responsible for the movement of the earth, wind and water. Its representative in the body is the biological air, responsible for movement of afferent and efferent, sensory and motor-neuron impulses. When someone touches the skin, that tactile skin sensation is carried to the brain by the principal of movement, which is the sensory impulse. Then there is a reaction to the impulse, which is the motor response, which is carried from the brain to the periphery. This is a very important function of air. Our breathing is due to the movement of the diaphragm. Movements of the intestines and subtle cell movements are also governed by the biological principal of air. The movement of thought, desire and will are also governed by the air principal.

Fire

Where there is movement, there is friction, which creates heat, so the third manifestation of consciousness is fire, the principal of heat. There are many different representations of fire in the body. The solar plexus is the seat of fire, and this fire principle regulates body temperature. Fire is also responsible for digestion, absorption and assimilation. It is present in the eyes, therefore we perceive light, and the luster in the eyes is a result of the fire principal. There is a fire in the brain as the grey matter, which governs understanding, comprehension and appreciation. Fire is necessary for transformation, comprehension, appreciation, recognition and total understanding. In our small universe, the sun is a burning ball of consciousness and the sun gives us light and heat. In the body, the representative of the sun is the biological fire: the solar plexus, which gives us heat, digestion, and liver function.

Water

Because of the heat of the fire, consciousness melts into water. According to chemistry, water is H2O, but according to Ayurveda water is liquefaction of consciousness. Water exists in the body in many different forms, such as: plasma, cytoplasm, serum, saliva, nasal secretion, orbital secretion and cerebrospinal fluid. Excess water, which we eliminate in the form of urine and sweat is water. Water is necessary for nutrition and to maintain the water/electrolyte balance in the body. Without water, the cells cannot live.

Earth

The next manifestation of consciousness is the earth element. Because of the heat of the fire and water, there is crystallization. According to Ayurveda, earth molecules are nothing but crystallization of consciousness. In the human body, all solid structures, hard, firm and compact tissues are derived from the earth element (e.g. bones, cartilage, nails, hair, teeth and skin). Even in a single cell, the cell membrane is earth, cellular vacuoles are space, cytoplasm is water, nucleic acid and all chemical components of the cell are fire, and movement of the cell is air. All of these five elements are present in every human cell. According to Ayurveda, man is a creation of universal consciousness. What is present in the cosmos, the macrocosm, the same thing is present in the body, the microcosm. Man is a miniature of nature.

Mental Constitution

Vedic philosophy classifies human temperaments into three basic qualities: satvic, rajasic and tamasic. These individual differences in psychological and moral dispositions and their reactions to socio-cultural and physical environments are described in all the classic texts of Ayurveda. Satvic qualities imply essence, reality, conscious-ness, purity and clarity of perception which are responsible for good-ness and happiness. All movements and activities are due to rajas. It leads to the life of sensual enjoyment, pleasure and pain, effort and restlessness. Tamas is darkness, inertia, heaviness and materialis-tic attitudes. There is a constant interplay of these three gunas (quali-ties) in the individual consciousness, but the relative predominance of either satva, rajas, or tamas is responsible for individual psycho-logical constitution.

Satvic Mental Constitutions

The people in whom satvic qualities predominate are religious, lov-ing, compassionate and pure minded. Following truth and righteous-ness, they have good manners, behavior and conduct. They do not get easily upset or angry. Although they work hard mentally, they do not get mental fatigue, so they need only several hours of sleep each night. They look fresh, alert, aware, and full of luster, wisdom, joy and hap-piness. They are creative, humble and respectful of their teachers.

Worshipping God and humanity, they love all. They care for people, animals, trees, and are respectful of all life and existence. They have balanced intuition and intelligence.

Rajasic Mental Constitutions

The people in whom rajasic qualities predominate are egoistic, am-bitious, aggressive, proud, competitive, and have a tendency to con-trol others. They like power, prestige, position, and are perfectionists. They are hard working people, but are lacking in proper planning and direction. They are ungrounded, active and restless. Emotionally, they are angry, jealous, ambitious, and have few moments of joy due to success. They have a fear of failure, are subject to stress, and soon lose their mental energy. They require about eight hours of sleep. They are loving, calm and patient only as long as their self interests are served. They are good, loving, friendly and faithful only to those who are helpful to them. They are not honest to their inner consciousness. Their activities are self-centered and egotistical.

Tamasic Mental Constitutions

The people in whom tamasic qualities predominate are less intelligent. They tend towards depression, laziness, and excess sleep, even during the day. A little mental work tires them easily. They like jobs of less responsibility, and they love to eat, drink, sleep and have sex. They are greedy, possessive, attached, irritable, and do not care for others. They may harm others through their own self interest. It is difficult for them to focus their minds during meditation.

Vata, Pitta and Kapha: The Three Doshas

The structural aspect of the body is made up of five elements, but the functional aspect of the body is governed by three biological humors. Ether and air together constitute vata; fire and water, pitta; and water and earth, kapha. Vata, pitta and kapha are the three biological humors that are the three biological components of the organism. They govern psycho-biological changes in the body and physio-pathological changes too. Vata-pitta-kapha are present in every cell, tissue and organ. In every person they differ in permutations and combinations.

The sperm is the male seed, and the ovum is the female egg. They also contain vata-pitta-kapha (VPK). Bodily vata-pitta-kapha changes according to diet, life style and emotions. The sperm gets influenced by the father's lifestyle, diet and emotions, and the ovum by the mother's. At the time of fertilization, when a single sperm enters a single ovum, individual constitution is determined.

According to Ayurveda, there are seven body types: mono-types (vata, pitta or kapha predominant), dual types (vata-pitta, pitta-kapha or, kapha-vata), and equal types, (vata, pitta and kapha in equal proportions). Every individual has a unique combination of these three doshas. To understand individuality is the foundation of healing according to Ayurveda, "The Science of Life."

Vata Qualities

Vata, pitta and kapha are distinctly present in every individual and express in each human being differently according to the predominance of the different qualities (gunas). For example vata is dry, light, cold, mobile, active, clear, astringent, and it is dispersing. All of these qualities can manifest in an individual. For example, if a person has excess vata in his or her constitution, because of the dry quality, he or she will have dry hair, dry skin, dry colon and a tendency towards constipation. Because of the light quality, which is opposite of heavy, the vata person will have a light body frame, light muscles, and light fat, and so will be thin and underweight, or "skinny-minny." Because of the cold quality, the vata person will have cold hands, cold feet and poor circulation. They hate the cold season and love summer. Because of the mobile quality, vata people are very active. They like jogging and jumping and don't like sitting in one place. Vata is subtle, and this subtle quality is responsible for the emotions of fear, anxiety, insecurity and nervousness.

Vata is clear, therefore vata people can be clairvoyant; they have clear understanding and perception. They understand things immediately, but forget things immediately. Vata is astringent, which is a drying and choking quality of taste, therefore the vata person, while eating feels a drying choking sensation in the throat. These qualities are all expressed in a vata individual to some degree.

Pitta Qualities

Pitta is a biological combination of fire and water elements. It has hot, sharp, light, liquid, sour, oily and spreading qualities. Pitta has a strong smell, like a fleshy smell, and has a sour or bitter taste. If an individual has excess pitta in the body, these qualities will be manifested. Because of the hot quality, the pitta person has a strong appetite and warm skin. The body temperature is a little higher than the vata person. The pitta person can perspire at a fifty degree temperature, but the vata person cannot perspire even at a much higher temperature. This difference is very important. Pitta is hot, therefore the pitta person has a strong appetite. If hungry, he has to eat otherwise he will become irritable and hypoglycemic.

The second quality of pitta is sharp, therefore the pitta person has a sharp nose, teeth, eyes, mind and while talking uses sharp words. They also have very sharp memory. Because of the oily quality, they have soft warm oily skin, straight oily hair, and the feces are oily and liquid. Because of the hot, sharp, and oily qualities, pitta people have a tendency to grey prematurely, a sign of early maturity. Pitta girls get earlier menstruation and reach puberty earlier. They can even start their menstruation at the age of ten. Pitta is light, which is the opposite of both heaviness and darkness. Because of this light quality, pitta people are moderate in body frame, and they do not like bright light. They like to read before they go to bed, and sometimes the pitta person sleeps with a book on the chest. Because of too much heat in the body, the pitta person tends to lose his hair in the full bloom of youth. The pitta person can get a receding hair line, or a big, beautiful, bald head.

The next quality of pitta is strong smell. When the pitta person perspires, under the arm pit there is a typical sulphur smell, and if he doesn't wash his socks, they will have a strong smell. That's why a pitta person loves perfumes. Pitta people are lovers of knowledge and have a great capacity of organization and leadership. They are often wise, brilliant people, but can have a controlling, dominating personality. Pitta people have a tendency towards comparison, competition, ambition, and they have a quality of aggressiveness, so naturally they criticize. If there is no one to criticize, pitta people will criticize themselves. They are perfectionists. Pitta people tend to get pittagenic inflammatory diseases, while vata predominant people tend to get neurological, muscular and rheumatic problems.

Kapha Qualities

The next dosha is kapha. Subjects having more kapha in their body, will have heavy, slow, cool, oily, liquid, dense, thick, static and cloudy qualities. These are the important qualities of kapha, and kapha is sweet and salty. Because of the heavy quality, kapha people have heavy bones, muscles and fat. They will have a tendency to put on weight. A kapha person may even do a water fast and will put on weight. Kapha is slow, therefore a kapha person has slow metabolism and digestion. The kapha person can work without food, while it is very difficult for a pitta person to concentrate without food. Kapha is cool hence kapha people have cool, clammy skin. The skin is cool, but within the G.I. tract the digestive fire is high therefore they have a strong appetite.

Kapha people have other qualities, thick wavy hair, and big, attractive eyes. They have slow but prolonged, steady memory. Kapha people are forgiving, loving and compassionate. Because of the slow quality, kapha people walk slowly and talk slowly. They don't like jogging and jumping. They love eating, sitting and doing nothing.

Because of the cloudy quality, their mind is heavy and foggy and after a full meal they feel lethargic and sleepy. Unless they have a cup of coffee or strong stimulant in the morning they cannot move. Finally, the kapha person has a sweet tooth and loves candy, cookies and chocolate.

Prakruti, Individual Constitution

Individual constitution is determined at conception by the particular combination of the three doshas: vata, pitta and kapha. Every human being is a unique entity with its own individual constitution. The constitution, the psycho-somatic temperament of a person, is primarily genetic in origin. The male seed, sperm, and female egg, ovum, carry within them the constitution of both the parents. At the time of conjugation, the dominant factor of prakruti in the sperm (predominance of vata, pitta or kapha) can either neutralize a weaker or exaggerate the similar attributes of the prakruti of the ovum. For example, a sperm of strong vata constitution can inhibit some of the characteristics in the ovum of kapha constitution. The dry, light, rough, mobile qualities of vata will suppress the oily, heavy, smooth, and stable qualities of kapha. Vata and kapha are both cold, so the cold quality will be exaggerated in the prakruti of the foetus and the baby will be sensitive to the cold. The baby in this case will inherit a vata-kapha constitution. If both parents, i.e. the sperm and ovum, are of vata constitution, the offspring will inherit a vata predominant constitution. The constitution of the parents and therefore of the foetus is influenced by diet, lifestyle, country, climate, age and emotions.

Samprapti, the Disease Process

According to Ayurveda, health is a state of balance between the body, mind and consciousness. Within the body, Ayurveda recognizes the three doshas, or bodily humors vata, pitta and kapha; seven dhatus, or tissues, plasma, blood, muscle, fat, bone, nerve, and reproductive; three malas, or wastes; feces, urine and sweat; and agni, the energy of metabolism. Disease is a condition of disharmony in any of these factors. The root cause of imbalance, or disease, is an aggravation of dosha, vata-pitta-kapha, caused by a wide variety of internal and external factors. According to the attributes of these different etiological factors the bodily humors become aggravated and start to accumulate at their respective sites. Vata tends to accumulate in the colon, pitta in the intestines and kapha in the stomach. If the provocation continues, the accumulated dosha reaches a state of overflowing the original site and spreads throughout the body. The aggravated dosha then enters and creates a lesion in a specific weak tissue where pathological changes are manifested in the organ or system.

Causes of Disease

There are many factors that affect the doshas. Disease can result from imbalanced emotions. If a person has deep seated unresolved anger, fear, anxiety, grief or sadness that also effects the doshas.

Ayurveda classifies seven major causative factors in disease: hereditary, congenital, internal, external trauma, seasonal, natural tendencies or habits and supernatural factors. Disease can also result from misuse, overuse and under-use of the senses: hearing, touch, sight, taste, and smell. The disease itself can be described by the number of doshas involved, the specific tissues effected, the quality or combination of qualities that aggravated the dosha, whether the disease is primary or secondary, strength, and the length of time of the disease.

There are many recognized hereditary pathologies. These can take the form of tendencies or dispositions towards a specific problem or manifest as actual abnormalities. A mother's lifestyle, diet, habits, activities, emotions and relationships can also affect the foetus.

Internal conditions such as ulcers or a damaged liver, may be caused by overuse of taste, e.g. too much hot spicy food or alcohol. External traumas are violent actions, such as automobile accidents, gunshots, etc.

Seasonal causes usually are more indirect. A person has a tendency to take his or her own primary dosha (vata, pitta or kapha) to an imbalanced state. There are four seasons. Summer season, bright light and too much heat, that is the pitta season. The autumn season is cold, windy and dry, it is a vata season. The winter season is cold, windy, snowing and raining, a kapha season.

The spring season is both kapha and pitta. Early spring is cooler, with beautiful flowers and new leaves and is gorgeous and extremely beautiful, so earlier spring is kapha, and later spring is pitta. So these four seasons, have vata, pitta and kapha qualities. Apart from the lifestyle, diet, and all these changes, the vata person has a tendency for their vata to go out of balance. Vata people have a tendency towards constipation, sciatica, arthritis and rheumatism. Pitta people in the summer season aggravate their pitta and may get hives, rash, acne, biliary disorders, diarrhea or conjunctivitis. The kapha person, during spring season, has a tendency to get colds, hay fever, cough, congestion, sneezing and kapha type of sinus disorders.

Natural tendencies can also be a problem, such as overeating and smoking. Supernatural causes are those such as sunburns, lightning, and the influence of planetary bodies.

Clinical Barometers of Ayurveda

Ayurveda is an ancient clinical art of diagnosing the disease process through questioning (inquiring about the past, present and family history), observation (inspection), tactile experience (palpation), percussion, and listening to the heart, lungs and intestines (auscultation). In this art, Ayurveda talks much about interpreting the pulse, tongue, eyes and nails in the clinical examination, and also a specific examination of functional systems separately.

Ayurveda describes the basic three types of pulses (vata, pitta and kapha) and their characteristics. There are twelve different radial pulses; six on the right side, three superficial and three deep; and similarly, six on the left side. There is a relationship between the superficial and deep pulses and the internal organs. One can sensitively feel the strength, vitality, and normal physiological tone of the respective organs separately under each finger.

An ancient art of tongue diagnosis also describes quite characteristic patterns which can reveal the functional status of respective internal organs merely by observing the surface of the tongue. The tongue is the mirror of the viscera and reflects many pathological conditions.

A discoloration and/or sensitivity of a particular area of the tongue indicates a disorder in the organ corresponding to that area. A whitish tongue indicates a kapha derangement and mucus accumulation; a red or yellow-green tongue indicates a pitta derangement; and a black to brown coloration indicates a vata derangement. A dehydrated tongue is symptomatic of a decrease in the rasa dhatu (plasma), while a pale tongue indicates a decrease in the rakta dhatu (red blood cells).

Ayurvedic physicians also do urine examinations as one of the diagnostic tools to understand the doshic imbalance in the body. The body fluids, such as blood (rakta) and lymph (rasa), serve to carry wastes (malas) away from the tissues that produce them. The urinary system removes water (kleda), salt (kshar) and nitrogenous wastes (dhatu malas). The urinary system also helps to maintain the normal concentration of water (apa dhatu) and electrolytes within body fluids. It helps to regulate the volume of body fluid and thus the urine helps to maintain the balance of the three humors vata, pitta and kapha, and water (kleda).

For clinical examination of urine, take a clean vessel and collect the early morning urine in midstream. Observe the color. If the color is blackish-brown, this indicates a vata disorder. If the color is dark yellow, a pitta disorder. Also when there is constipation or the body has less intake of water, the urine will be dark yellow. If the urine is cloudy, there is a kapha disorder. Red color of urine indicates a rakta (blood) disorder. Next there is the oil drop test. With a dropper, place one drop of sesame oil into the same sample of urine. If the drop spreads immediately, the physical disorder is probably easy to cure.

If the drop sinks to the middle of the urine sample the illness is more difficult to cure. If the drop sinks to the bottom, the illness may be very difficult to cure. If the drop spreads on the surface in wave like movements, this indicates a vata disorder. If the drop spreads on the surface with multiple colors visible like a rainbow, this indicates a pitta disorder. If the drop breaks up into pearl like droplets on the surface of the urine, this indicates a kapha disorder. Normal urine has a typical uremic smell. However, if the urine has a foul odor this indicates ama dosha (toxins) in the system. Acidic urine which creates a burning sensation indicates excess pitta. A sweet smell to the urine indicates a diabetic condition. In this condition, the individual may experience goose bumps on the skin surface while passing urine. Gravel in the urine indicates stones in the urinary tract.

Chikitsa, Disease Management

Ayurveda says that to restore health we must understand the exact quality, nature and structure of disease, disorder, or imbalance. The body has its own intelligence to create balance and we are helping in that process. There are four main classifications of management of disease in Ayurveda: shodan, or cleansing; shaman or palliation; rasayana, or rejuvenation; and satvajaya, or mental hygiene.

Shodan, Cleansing

The purpose of shodan, is to remove excess doshas and ama from the body. Shodan includes purvakarma (initial procedures), pradhanakarma (the main procedures), and pashchatkarma (post-operative procedures). Purvakarma procedures move the aggravated doshas and ama from sites deeper in the body to locations in preparation for elimination. Panchakarma (five actions), which belongs to pradhanakarma, then removes these doshas and ama. It includes vaman (vomiting), virechan (purgation), basti (medicinal enema), rakta-moksha (blood cleansing) and nasya (nasal insufflation, administration).

Vaman is vomiting therapy for removing excess kapha impurities out of the body. Virechan is for removing pitta by giving purgation therapy. Basti is to remove excess vata from the body by enema therapy. Nasya is administration of certain herbal powders, medicated oils and medicated concoctions, and ghee into the nose for purification of prana, mind and consciousness. Rakta-moksha includes blood letting by application of leaches or removing blood or donating blood to the blood bank, and using certain cleansing and blood thinning herbs.

Ayurveda says toxins are produced when the aggravated dosha, vata-pitta-kapha, effects the biological fire, agni, which in turn effects digestion, metabolism and assimilation. So undigested, un-absorbed, unassimilated food products remain in the body as a morbid substance. Ama, then, is a toxic, morbid, raw, undigested, unabsorbed, unassimilated, non-homogeneous, sticky substance in the body that adheres to the tissues, clogs the channels and creates toxicity in the body. It enters the blood and creates toxemia, which is a root cause of disease. The root cause of ama is the aggravated dosha attacking agni (fire) and producing low digestion and metabolism. So Ayurveda says that one should remove these aggravated doshas by panchakarma.

Shaman, Palliation

According to Ayurveda shaman, or palliation is the balancing and pacification of bodily doshas (as opposed to elimination). Shaman is of seven types: dipan, kindling the fire (agni); pachan, burning the toxic ama; ksud-nigraha, fasting; trut-nigraha, observing thirst, (not drinking water); vyayama, yoga stretching; atap-seva, lying in the sunlight [Sometimes they make a fire during the daytime or evening and that heat of the fire does cleansing of the astral body, physical body, subtle body and causal body. Lying in the sun, which is also used for kindling the fire in the solar plexus.]; marut-seva, sitting and doing pranayama, meditation.

Shaman is a very spiritual cleansing method of purification. People with insufficient strength to undergo panchakarma, who are emotionally weak and not strong enough to face panchakarma are good candidates for shaman. Any pitta disorder, vata disorder, and chronic kapha disorder which effects the immune system of an individual and affects the agni or fire of the individual, is a very good subject for shaman. Shaman can be done in the healthy person also, because shaman has both curative and preventative aspects. Prevention is better than curing. If we prevent the future ailment through shaman we can attain success in healing the soul.

The first method in shaman is dipan, kindling the fire. Kindling the bodily fire is absolutely necessary in kapha and vata disorders, where the person has low gastric fire. That can be accomplished by using certain herbs like pippili, ginger, cinnamon, black pepper, and chitrak. These different herbs are used in certain proportions with honey internally, which does kindling of the fire. You can do the fire ceremony, by burning certain special woods, making an agnikunda, like a yagyakunda, or fireplace, arranging the woods in a certain pyramidal, square fashion, putting camphor and cotton at the center, and kindling the fire while chanting special mantras. By doing these mantras, you can increase the internal fire. While watching the external fire, you are meditating and chanting certain mantras for agni, the internal fire. Concentrating at the solar plexus, you can also kindle the agni, and that will burn the toxins in the physical body, subtle body, and causal body. This kind of ceremony is very effective for kapha and vata people, but for pitta people it should be done with great caution.

Pachan, burning the toxins is done with certain herbs in certain proportions, because kindling the gastric fire is necessary to improve the digestive capacity. For pachan, Ayurveda uses trikatu, chitrak, cinnamon, ginger, cumin, coriander and fennel. All of these herbal teas are used after meals to improve the digestive capacity of agni. Pachan can be improved through concentration, meditation and contemplation so that the person's digestive capacity will improve and there will be proper assimilation and nutrition of the bodily tissue.

Ksud-nigraha is fasting, or eating a mono-diet. In acute fever, acute indigestion, acute dysentery and diarrhea, Ayurveda suggests fasting. A person may only eat cooked apple with ghee or basmati rice with mung dal and ghee, or just yogurt and rice, and in small quantity. But in acute fever, acute diarrhea and dysentery it is better not to eat anything for a couple of days, so that the bodily fire will kindle and burn the internal toxins. For this, observing a fast is very important.

Trut-nigraha, observing thirst (not drinking water) is very important when water disorders take place, kapha disorders. For example, kidney disorders like edema, or ascites where there is accumulated water in the peritoneal cavity, or certain other kapha urinary disorders where too much water is retained in the system, there Ayurveda says not to give water. Observing thirst means not to drink water. It is not a water fast, a water fast is different. If you drink too much water, it will retain in the body. Trut-nigraha means observing thirst, which is very effective in certain kapha types of disorders.

The next important shaman is vyayam, exercise, yoga stretching. Exercise is defined here as stretching of the muscles in a particular direction with a goal so that you can reach the goal with effort and in that effort you are creating physical stress. Physical stress kindles the fire, like hiking in the mountains, walking, jogging and jumping. Ayurveda says exercise has such a quality that it improves circulation, accelerates the heart rate, enhances the combustion of calories and also stimulates metabolism, regulates body temperature and maintains body weight. Exercise makes your senses alert and attentive and your mind becomes very sharp and develops keen perception. These qualities of exercise are very important, but again, exercise varies from person to person.

Ayurveda suggests certain exercises according to individual constitution. The vata person should do certain yoga postures. The important seat of vata in the body is the pelvic cavity, so any exercise which will help the stretching of the pelvic muscles is good. Therefore the forward bend, backward bend, spinal twist, cobra pose, camel pose, shoulder stand and plow pose help to move the vata in a particular direction and that helps to calm down vata.

The important seat of pitta is the solar plexus, so any exercise that will stretch the muscles of the solar plexus will be very effective for the pitta person. So the fish pose, boat pose, camel pose as well as locust pose and bow pose will help to calm down pitta.

The important seat of kapha is the chest, therefore exercises which will stretch the chest are very effective. Ayurveda says that you can do the shoulder stand, plow pose, locust pose, cat pose, cow pose and bow pose. These different poses improve the circulation of kapha in the pulmonary cavity. Jogging is not good for vata, it is good for kapha, but kapha people don't like jogging. Swimming is good exercise for the pitta person. Swimming is also good for the vata person. Mountain climbing and hiking are good for kapha people, but they don't like hiking. So this is a very interesting thing, that proper exercise is a wonderful art of shaman.

Atap-seva, lying in the sun, is another ancient shaman. The sun is the source of heat and light. The sun is the source of higher consciousness. Pitta predominant people can lie in the sun and apply certain oils (sun blockers) so that they will reduce their exposure. The pitta person should not lie in the sun more than half an hour. The vata person can lie in the sun for about an hour. The kapha person can lie in the sun for more than an hour. If the proper care is taken, lying in the sun and meditating upon the solar plexus, is a wonderful shaman for kapha and vata. It improves circulation, the absorption of vitamin D, and strengthens the bones.

Today, however, lying in the sunlight is becoming very bad because the ionosphere and ozone are damaged and the unwanted radiation (ultraviolet rays) comes to the earth and that aggravates brajak-pitta under the skin which can result in skin cancer. The person that has multiple moles should not lie in the sun. Lying in the moon light is also an ancient art of shaman for reducing pitta.

Lastly, there is breathing. Respiration is partly conscious and partly unconscious. One should do proper breathing through both nostrils by doing alternate nostril pranayama. There are different types of pranayama, the breathing exercise, and there is a totally different science of breath one can study from an experienced teacher. But if you sit quietly, inhale deeply through one nostril, hold the breath into the lower abdomen, and slowly exhale through the opposite nostril, repeating alternately, this kind of pranayama helps to bring balance to prana, apana and udana (subtypes of prana). Out of that balance, one can attain the highest state of tranquility.

Shaman as a whole does bring balance between the body, mind and consciousness and balance to the three bodily humors, vata-pitta-kapha. It cleanses the physical body, subtle body and causal body. According to Ayurveda, every soul is immortal, every soul is sacred, and to understand the individual, to understand oneself, is the foundation of life. Without this self knowing, life has no meaning. So by understanding the basic principals of life, by understanding one's own constitution as explained in the Ayurvedic literature, and by understanding the exact nature and structure of doshic aggravation, one can follow the proper guidelines of shodan, cleansing, and shaman, palliation and pacification.

Rasayana, Rejuvenation

Rasayana has three sub categories: restoration of tissues through herbs, minerals and exercises; re-virilization, which is restoring vitality to the system; and longevity, slowing or stopping of the aging process.

Satvajaya, Mental Hygiene and Spiritual Healing

The categories of satvajaya include: mantra, (sounds), yantra (physical devices), tantra (directing energies in the body), meditation, and gems, metals and crystals, specifically given for the imbalance or disease.

Ayurveda and Relationships

According to Ayurveda, our life is a relationship; the relationship between you and your spouse, girlfriend and boyfriend, and parents and children. Equally important is the relationship with yourself, your relationship between the body, mind and consciousness, and the inner relationship between vata-pitta-kapha. These relationships are life, and Ayurveda is a healing art which helps bring clarity in relationships. Clarity in relationships brings compassion, and compassion is love, therefore love is clarity. Without this clarity, there is no insight. Ayurveda is an art of insight which brings harmony, happiness, joy and bliss in our daily life, in our relationships, and in our daily living. Ayurveda can definitely bring longevity to life. It can bring a quality of consciousness, such that one can get insight to deal with one's inner life, one's inner emotions, one's inner hurt, grief and sadness. Ayurveda is a total healing art.

Chapter 7

Chinese Traditional Medicine

Yin and Yang

The theory of yin and yang is a kind of world outlook. It holds that all things have two opposite aspects, yin and yang, which are both opposite and at the same time interdependent. This is a universal law of the material world. These two aspects are in opposition to each other but because one end of the spectrum cannot exist without the other they are interdependent.

The ancient Chinese used water and fire to symbolize yin and yang; anything moving, hot, bright and hyperactive is yang, and anything quiescent, cold, dim and hypoactive is yin.

The yin and yang properties of things are not absolute but relative. As an object or person changes so the yin and yang components change at a gradual rate. Each of the yin and yang properties of the object is a condition for the existence of the other; neither can exist in isolation. These two opposites are not stationary but in constant motion. If we imagine the circadian rhythm, night is yin and day is yang; as night (yin) fades it becomes day (yang), and as yang fades it becomes yin. Yin and yang are therefore changing into each other as well as balancing each other.

"The Basic Principles of Chinese Traditional Medicine," © George T. Lewith, M.A., D.M., FRCP, MRCGP. Excerpted from *Modern Chinese Acupuncture*, 2nd ed. (Thorsons Publishing, 1984). Reprinted with permission. Despite the age of this document, readers interested in understanding the principles underlying Chinese traditional medicine will still find the information useful.

The Application of Yin and Yang to Chinese Medicine

Each organ has an element of yin and yang within it. The histological structures and nutrients are yin, and the functional activities are yang. Some organs are predominantly yang in their functions, such as the gan-liver, while others are predominantly yin, such as the shen-kidney. Even though one organ may be predominantly yin (or yang) in nature, the balance of yin and yang is maintained in the whole healthy body because the sum total of the yin and yang will be in a fluctuating balance.

If a condition of prolonged excess or deficiency of either yin or yang occurs then disease results. In an excess of yin the yang qi would be damaged, and a disease of cold of shi nature would develop. Excess of yang will consume yin and a disease of heat of shi nature would develop. In a deficiency of yin, diseases of heat of xu nature develop, while a deficiency of yang causes diseases of cold of xu nature.

The Channels and Collaterals

The channels and collaterals are the representation of the organs of the body. They are also a functional system in their own right and they are responsible for conducting the flow of qi and blood through the body. The flow of qi can be disrupted by direct damage to the channels, such as trauma, or by an internal imbalance of yin and yang within the body.

The central principle of traditional Chinese medicine is to diagnose the cause of the internal disease, or yin yang imbalance within the body, and, by using the relevant acupuncture points, to correct the flow of qi in the channels and thus correct the internal disease. The acupuncture points that are on the channels have a direct influence on the flow of qi through the channels, and also on the internal organs. The zang channels are yin in nature and the fu channels are yang in nature. Qi circulates through the channels of the body in a well-defined circadian rhythm.

Zang and Fu Organs

The zang and fu organs are the internal visible organs of the body. The xin-heart, gan-liver, pi-spleen, fei-lung, shen-kidney and pericardium are the zang organs. The small intestine, large intestine, stomach, gall-bladder, urinary bladder and sanjiao are the fu organs.

The zang organs have a Chinese prefix because a direct translation from the Chinese might be misleading. The Chinese xin has functions rather different from the concept of the heart in Western medicine, so if we call the heart "xin-heart," or the liver "gan-liver," we are able to understand that we are referring to the organ of the heart or the liver, but it is really rather different from our concept of those organs.

The zang organs are of paramount importance in the body. They co-ordinate with the fu organs and connect with the five tissues (channels, jin[1] muscles, skin-hair, bones), and the nine openings (eyes, nose, ears, mouth, tongue, anus and external genitalia), to form the system of the Five Zang. The pericardium is not considered to be an important zang organ.

Qi, Blood and Body Fluid

Qi, blood and body fluid are important substances and structures in the body. They sustain the vital activities and they nourish the body, thereby keeping the functions of the tissues, organs and channels in good order. The production and circulation of qi and blood also depends on the health of the tissues and organs that are nourished by these substances.

Qi

Qi is a complex concept; it relates to both substance and function. Clean qi (oxygen), waste qi (carbon dioxide) and qi (nutrients) are generally known as material qi, and the existence of material qi is shown by the functional activity of various organs. The function of an organ depends on the functional qi of that organ; for instance, qi of xin-heart or qi of pi-spleen is the vital energy and functional activity of the xin-heart or pi-spleen. The function of an organ, or its functional qi, cannot exist without material qi, and vice versa.

Zhong Qi

Zhong qi is found mainly in the chest. It nourishes the structures and functions of the xin-heart and fei-lung.

Nourishing Qi

Nourishing qi circulates in the channels and collaterals, mainly in the viscera.

75

Defensive Qi

Defensive qi is in the muscles and skin. It circulates outside the channels, in the subcutaneous tissues, and it defends the body against invasion by pathogens.

The original qi is nourished and maintained by qi derived after birth. These combine to form genuine qi, i.e. the total sum of qi in the healthy body. This contrasts with pathogenic factors that are known as pathogenic qi.

Blood

The nutrients from food are digested by the pi-spleen and stomach and they are then transported to the xin-heart and fei-lung and turned into red (oxygenated) blood by qi. The essence of shen-kidney produces bone marrow, and bone marrow uses the digested food to produce blood. Qi of shen-kidney promotes digestion by pi-spleen, which in turn strengthens the xin-heart and fei-lung. This interaction therefore promotes haemopoesis.

There is a close relationship between qi and blood. The formation and circulation of blood depends on qi, whereas the formation and distribution of qi, as well as the health of the various organs of the body, is dependent on adequate nourishment from the blood. If the flow of blood "stagnates" the circulation of qi is "retarded" and, conversely, if the circulation of qi is "retarded" then the blood flow "stagnates."

Body Fluid

Body fluid is formed from food and drink. It exists in the blood, the tissues, and all the body openings and cavities.

The Pathogenesis of Disease

In traditional Chinese Medicine various elements and other factors cause disease. These are known as pathogenic factors or pathogens. Normally the human body is able to resist pathogens and maintain a healthy balance between the body and the environment. This ability is a function of normal qi, especially the defensive qi.

Disease develops because normal qi is unable to resist the onslaught of the pathogenic qi; if pathogenic qi overwhelms normal qi then a functional disturbance of the body results. The major principle of treating a disease in Chinese medicine is to strengthen and protect normal qi and maintain a healthy body. In ancient China a physician was only paid while his patient was healthy, not while his patient was ill!

Pathogenic Factors

These are divided into three main groups, exogenous pathogens, mental pathogens and various miscellaneous pathogens. "Phlegm and humour" and "stagnant blood" are pathological products; once they are formed new pathological changes will ensue so they are considered to be secondary pathogens.

Pathological factors serve as a generalization of clinical symptoms and signs, reflecting the struggle of normal qi and pathogenic qi. By differentiating the clinical symptoms and signs the cause of the disease can be traced, and then treatment can be determined. In order to do this the diseased organs must be defined and the pathogen causing that disease must also be diagnosed. This is called the "determination of treatment on the basis of the differentiation of a syndrome," and it is the basis of diagnosis and treatment in Chinese medicine.

The Exogenous Pathogens

These refer to six relatively abnormal meteorological conditions; wind, cold, summer heat, damp, dryness and heat (fire, warmth). The diseases caused by these pathogens include most viral, bacterial and protozoal diseases and some "allergic" conditions such as urticaria.

Mental Pathogens

These are overjoy, anger, anxiety, overthinking, grief, fear and fright.

Excessive fear and fright, or overjoy, injures the xin-heart. This causes palpitations, insomnia, irritability, anxiety and mental abnormality.

Excessive anger causes dysfunction of the gan-liver. This impairs the function of freeing, and causes pain and distention in the costal and hypochondriac region, abnormal menstruation, depression and irritability. If the function of storing blood is disturbed then menorrhagia and hemorrhage can result.

Excessive grief, anxiety and overthinking cause dysfunction of the pi-spleen and stomach. This causes anorexia and a feeling of fullness or distension after meals.

Excessive grief, anxiety and anger cause poor circulation of qi and blood. If there is retardation of qi and stagnation of blood then this can cause a tumor.

Appendix

Stagnant blood and phlegm and humour are pathogenic products that may cause further pathological change if they are not eliminated. They have substantive and non-substantive meanings. Substantively they could be described as a blood clot or sputum, the non-substantive meaning is a generalization of a clinical syndrome, for instance, the stertorous breathing that may occur after a severe stroke is described as "phlegm covering the orifice of the xin-heart."

Stagnant Blood

Stagnant blood can cause pain. The painful area is fixed and has a stabbing, boring or colicky nature. Stagnant blood causes hemorrhage. This produces deep purple blood, often with clots. Stagnant blood causes ecchymosis or petechia. Stagnant blood can cause a mass. This can be any sort of mass, tumor, splenomegaly or hepatomegaly.

Phlegm and Humour

Phlegm and humour are formed when water metabolism is disordered; an accumulation of excess water then turns into phlegm or humour. Phlegm and humour in the lung causes cough, dyspnoca and excessive sputum.

Phlegm and humour in the stomach causes abdominal distension and a succussion sound. Phlegm covering the heart orifice causes coma and a rattling sound from the sputum in the throat, such as in a stroke. Phlegm blocking the channels and collaterals causes hemiplegia, numbness of the extremities and difficulty in speech, such as in a stroke. Phlegm accumulating subcutaneously occurs when there is a subcutaneous lymph node.

Differentiation of Disease According to the Eight Principles

This is the diagnostic system of Chinese traditional medicine. The notes in the ensuing section explain the broad principles of diagnosis, using the history and examination of the patient as a basis.

Diseases are either exterior or interior. If a pathogen such as cold invades the body then it may be superficial or exterior in its damaging effect, such as the common cold, or it may be deep or interior, such as septicaemia. Usually diseases of the exterior show mild fever, headache, generalized aches and pains, and a superficial pulse. Diseases of the interior are characterized by a high fever, thirst, restlessness, delirium, vomiting, diarrhea, a purplish-red tongue proper, with a white or yellow coating and a deep pulse.

Disease may be hot or cold. This means they may be due to the pathogen factors cold or heat. Diseases of heat show the signs of an acute infection or intestinal obstruction, whereas diseases of cold are more chronic in nature. Diseases of cold are characterized by a dislike of cold, pallor, loose stool, polyuria, a large flabby white tongue with a white coating, and a slow or deep and thready pulse. Diseases of heat show fever, dislike of heat, thirst, a red face, constipation, red scanty urine, and a red tongue proper with a yellow coating, associated with a rapid pulse.

Diseases may be xu or shi: Diseases of xu are usually more chronic in nature and are due to a deficiency of either the yin or the yang within the body. The patient is in low spirits, pale, emaciated, has palpitations and the tongue proper is light or red with a white or yellow coating, and there is a xu pulse. A shi disease is often more acute and is due to an excess of the yin or the yang within the body. This presents with irritability, distension and fullness of the chest and abdomen, scanty urine and dysuria, a red or white tongue proper with a yellow or white coating, and a shi or forceful pulse. There is a great deal of reference to xu and shi and it is important to realize that xu really means a deficiency, and shi really means an excess.

Methods Of Diagnosis

Facial Complexion

A red face occurs with febrile diseases, a pale wizened face is due to anaemia or xu diseases, a yellow face occurs in jaundice and a purple face occurs in anoxia, severe pain or stagnation of blood.

Body Build, Posture and Motion

In an obese person there is a chronic deficiency of qi with invasion of phlegm and damp, while in an emaciated person there is hyperactivity of fire due to a deficiency of yin. Paralysis of the limbs indicates insufficiency of qi and blood with blocked channels and collaterals. Convulsions and muscle spasm are often due to an invasion of the channels by wind, due to an insufficiency of yin.

Examination of the Tongue

This is a most important diagnostic tool; the tongue is divided into the tongue proper and the tongue coating. A normal tongue has a pink tongue proper with a white clear coating over the tongue.

The Tongue Proper

A light coloured tongue proper: A light tongue proper indicates insufficiency of qi and blood, invasion of cold, and xu of yang.

A red tongue proper: A red tongue proper indicates diseases due to heat, or internal diseases of heat due to xu of yin.

A purplish-red tongue proper: This occurs in acute diseases of heat when heat has been transmitted from the exterior of the body to the interior, for instance septicaemia. It can also be seen in diseases that exhaust the body fluid, causing hyperactivity of yang due to an insufficiency of yin, for instance terminal carcinoma.

A purplish tongue proper: A purple or bluish-purple tongue proper indicates retardation of qi and stagnation of blood, causing internal cold due to xu of yang, for instance ischaemic heart disease or heart failure.

A large flabby tongue proper: A large and flabby tongue proper with teeth marks indicates xu of qi and xu of yang, for instance chronic enteritis. If there are purplish-red spots on the tongue then this means that there is an invasion of heat.

A streaked tongue proper: Some people have a congenital streaked tongue (this is called a geographical tongue in Western medicine) and it must be ignored. Streaks or red prickles on the tongue normally indicate hyperactivity of fire causing consumption of the body fluid and this is often found after infectious diseases.

Stiff and tremulous tongue proper: The tongue shows fasciculation and it may curl up. This is often accompanied by indistinct speech and mental disorders and indicates disturbance of the mind by phlegm and heat, or deficiency of yin of the gan-liver.

The Tongue Coating

A white coating: A thick white coating indicates stagnation of food, for instance dyspepsia. A white greasy coating indicates invasion by the pathogen cold and damp, or phlegm, for instance chronic bronchitis.

2

A white powder-like coating indicates invasion by plague, for instance typhoid.

A yellow coating: A thick yellow coating indicates chronic indigestion.

A thin yellow coating indicates invasion of fei-lung by wind and heat, for instance a cold.

A greasy yellow coating indicates internal damp and heat, or phlegm and heat, for instance bacillary dysentry or a lung abscess.

A charring yellow coating indicates the accumulation of heat in the intestines which damages the yin, for instance infectious diseases of the intestine.

A yellow tongue coating may also be caused by smoking.

A greyish-black coating: A grayish-black slippery coating indicates excessive cold due to xu of yang, and this occurs in certain types of dyspepsia.

A grayish-black dry coating indicates exhaustion of the body fluids due to excessive heat, for instance dehydration.

A peeling coating: When the tongue coating is partially or completely peeled off the tongue proper can be seen. This indicates severe damage of the normal qi and an extreme deficiency of yin, for instance the late stages of terminal cancer.

Auscultation

Listening to the Speech

Speaking in a low feeble voice indicates diseases of xu nature and sonorous speech indicates shi diseases. A partial loss of consciousness means that heat and phlegm are covering the heart orifice. Talking to oneself means that there is a derangement of the mind, and indistinct speech often means that the channels are blocked by wind and phlegm.

Listening to the Respiration

Feeble respiration with dyspnoea and excessive sweating indicates xu of qi of the xin-heart and fei-lung. Heavy respiration, with a productive cough, indicates a shi disease of fei-lung due to an accumulation of phlegm and heat, or phlegm and humour, in fei-lung.

Listening to the Cough

A heavy unclear cough is caused by invasion of fei-lung with wind and cold, or accumulation of cold and humour in fei-lung. A loud clear cough often indicates wind and heat, or phlegm and heat, in fei-lung. A dry cough with minimal sputum is often caused by a chronic xu of yin of fei-lung, for instance tuberculosis.

Smell

A rank foul smell of any discharge or secretion indicates a disease of shi nature (infection). A light smell indicates a disease of xu nature, for instance scanty red urine with a foul smell indicates a hot shi-disease, like cystitis, while clear profuse urine indicates a cold xu disease, like diabetes insipidus.

Interrogation

This is best summed up by the translation of an old Chinese text called the ten askings: One ask chill and fever, two perspiration, three ask head and trunk, four stool and urine, five food intake and six chest. Deafness and thirst are seven and eight, nine past history and ten causes. Besides this you should ask about the drugs taken, and for women patients you should ask their menstrual and obstetric history. Finally, for infants, ask about the normal childhood diseases.

Palpation

Palpation of the Pulse

The pulse provides a great deal of the information gained from palpation, although a mass or trauma will obviously have to be examined on a more Westernized basis. In classical Chinese medicine there are six pulses at each wrist. These pulses occupy three positions at each wrist over the radial artery, and each position has a deep and superficial pulse. Each of these pulses represents a different organ and in this way all twelve of the zang fu organs are represented by a wrist pulse. The character of the pulse indicates the state of health of each organ and also the balance between each organ. Although traditional pulse diagnosis is still used in China we were taught a much simpler form of pulse "generalization" rather than the traditional pulse diagnosis, and it is this purse "generalization" that will be discussed in the following section.

A superficial pulse: This pulse responds to the finger when pressed lightly and becomes weak on heavy pressure. It is often seen in the early stages of diseases caused by exogenous pathogens, such as infections.

A deep pulse: This pulse is not clear on superficial palpation but it is felt on deep pressure. It is often seen in interior diseases such as glomerulonephritis.

A slow pulse: This pulse is less than sixty beats per minute; it may be normal or it may be seen in atrio-venticular block, i.e. diseases of cold.

A rapid pulse: This pulse is greater than sixty beats per minute; it is often seen in diseases of heat.

A xu pulse: The pulse is weak and forceless and goes on heavy pressure. This is seen in diseases of xu nature, such as malnutrition or diseases of pi-spleen.

A shi pulse. The pulse is forceful and will not go on deep palpation; it is seen in shi diseases. A large pulse: This is an abundant pulse; it is like a surging wave and is seen in diseases of shi nature and heat.

A thready pulse: This is like a thready flow of water and it is often seen in xu diseases.

A bowstring pulse. The pulse is hard and forceful and gives the sensation of pressing on the string of a bent bow. It may be normal or it may be seen in diseases where there is hyperactivity of the yang of the gan-liver.

A gliding pulse: This is round and forceful, like beads rolling on a plate. It is often seen in cases of indigestion or obstruction of phlegm. Sometimes a gliding pulse may be seen in a healthy person, especially in pregnancy.

An intermittent pulse. The pulse is irregular. This occurs in retardation of qi and stagnation of blood, causing a deficiency of qi in the xin-heart, such as atrial fibrillation. Palpation for all other pathology, such as mass or trauma, follows the same rules as in Western medicine.

The Differentiation of Syndromes

The Chinese described symptom pictures which allow the differentiation of specific zang fu syndromes. The major syndromes are described below and provide further useful information which will enable the acupuncturist to reach a clear zang fu diagnosis.

Syndromes of the Xin-Heart

Weakness of the Qi of the Xin-Heart

Clinical Manifestations: Palpitations, dyspnoea aggravated by exertion, a pale tongue and a thready xu or irregular pulse. If there is evidence of a deficiency of the yang of the xin-heart then cold limbs, pallor, and purplish lips can be found. Exhaustion of the yang of the xin-heart may manifest itself as profuse sweating, mental confusion and a fading, thready pulse.

Etiology and pathology: This syndrome is usually caused by general malaise after anxiety or a long illness, which injures the qi of the xin-heart. When the qi of the xin-heart is weak it fails to pump blood normally resulting in palpitations, dyspnoea and a thready irregular or xu pulse. Alternatively, a prolonged weakness of the qi of the xin-heart may lead to weakness of the yang of the xin-heart. When the body lacks yang it lacks energy and heat, therefore symptoms such as chills, cold limbs and pallor occur. If the yang of the xin-heart is exhausted, the defensive qi of the body surface can no longer protect the essential qi and lets it dissipate, this results in profuse sweating and a fading, thready pulse.

Insufficiency of the Yin of the Xin-Heart

Clinical Manifestations: Palpitations, insomnia, dream disturbed sleep, anxiety and possible malar flush with a low grade fever. A red tongue proper and a thready and rapid pulse will also be found.

Etiology and pathology: This syndrome is usually due to damage of the yin by a febrile disease or anxiety, which consumes the yin of the xin-heart. Insufficiency of the yin of the xin-heart often leads to hyperactivity of the fibber of the xin-heart, resulting in the above symptoms. Insufficiency of the yin of the xin-heart may also cause insufficiency of the blood of the xin-heart. If this happens then there is not enough yin and blood to nourish the xin-heart, and the xin-heart fails in its function of keeping the mind. The symptoms of insomnia, poor memory and dream-disturbed sleep will therefore appear.

Stagnation of the Blood of the Heart

Clinical Manifestations: Palpitations, cardiac retardation and pain (paroxysms of pricking pain, or in more severe cases colicky pain often referred to the shoulders and the back), peripheral and central cyanosis and a thready or irregular pulse.

Etiology and pathology: This syndrome is due to anxiety leading to stagnation of qi and stagnation of blood. It may also be due to insufficiency of the qi of the xin-heart after a chronic illness; if the qi of the xin-heart is too weak to sustain the cardiac circulation then stagnation of blood of the xin-heart and obstruction of the blood vessels results. Stagnation of the blood often impedes the distribution of yang qi in the chest causing discomfort in the chest (angina) and peripheral cyanosis. A dark purplish tongue proper, or purple spots on the tongue, and a thready or irregular pulse are manifestations of stagnation of blood and confinement of the yang qi.

Hyperactivity of the Fire of the Xin-Heart

Clinical Manifestations: Ulceration, swelling and pain in the mouth and tongue, insomnia accompanied by fever, a flushed face, a bitter taste in the mouth, hot, dark and yellow urine, a red tongue proper and a rapid pulse.

Etiology and pathology: This syndrome is often due to mental irritation which causes depression of qi. The depressed qi may turn into endogenous fire and disturb the mind, causing the symptoms of insomnia and fever to appear. As the xin-heart has the tongue as its orifice, and its function is reflected in the face, a disorder of the fire of the xin-heart may cause many of the above symptoms.

Derangement of the Mind

Clinical Manifestations: Depression, dullness, muttering to oneself, anxiety, incoherent speech, mania and in severe cases coma.

Etiology and pathology: This syndrome is often due to mental irritation which causes depression of qi. The body fluid stagnates to form damp and/or phlegm which causes blurring of the xin-heart and mind, resulting in dullness and depression. If the depressed qi turns into fire and the phlegm and fire disturb the xin-heart, anxiety, incoherent speech and mania result. Blurring of the mind by phlegm and/or damp, or phlegm and/or fire causes coma. A high fever, coma and delirium resulting from invasion of the pericardium by heat, are due to pathogenic heat invading deep into the interior of the body and disturbing the mind.

Syndromes of the Gan-liver

Depression of the Qi of the Gan-Liver

Clinical manifestations: Hypochondrial and lower-abdominal pain and distension, a distended sensation in the breasts, discomfort in the chest and belching, sighing, or a sensation of a foreign body in the throat. Women may experience irregular periods.

Etiology and pathology: This syndrome is usually due to mental irritation causing depression of the qi of the gan-liver and stagnation of the qi in the liver channel. This leads to hypochondrial and lower abdominal pain and distension, a distended sensation in the breasts and discomfort in the chest. Stagnation of the qi of the gan-liver may affect the stomach, causing failure of the qi of the stomach to descend and resulting in belching. The sensation of a foreign body in the throat is due to stagnation of the qi of the liver channel, which with the phlegm forms a lump in the throat.

Depression of the qi of the gan-liver and the subsequent lack of freeing may further impair the gan-liver's function of blood storage. Stagnation of qi leads to stagnation of blood, the cause of irregular periods.

Flare-up of the Fire of the Gan-Liver

Clinical manifestations: Dizziness, a distended sensation in the head, headache, red eyes, a bitter taste in the mouth, a flushed face, irritability and sometimes haematemesis and epistaxis can occur. The tongue proper is red with a yellow coating and the pulse is wiry and rapid.

Etiology and pathology: This syndrome is often due to a long-standing depression of the qi of the gan-liver which can turn into fire. It may also be due to over-indulgence in alcohol and tobacco causing an accumulation of heat which turns into fire. The upward disturbance of the fire of the gan-liver causes dizziness, a distended sensation in the head, headache, red eyes, a bitter taste in the mouth and a flushed face. Fire injures the gan-liver, causing impairment of its function in promoting the free flow of qi and this causes irritability. When the fire of the gan-liver injures the blood vessels it causes extravasation of blood and haematemesis and epistaxis can occur.

Stagnation of Cold in the Liver Channel

Clinical manifestations: Lower-abdominal pain, swelling and distension in the testis with tenesmus. The scrotum may be cold and contracted and these symptoms can be alleviated by warmth. The tongue proper is pale with a white coating and the pulse deep and wiry or slow.

Etiology and pathology: The liver channel curves around the external genitalia and passes through the lower abdomen. When cold, which is characterized by contraction and stagnation, stays in the liver channel, stagnation of the qi and blood may occur and cause lower-abdominal pain, swelling and distension of the testis with tenesmus. Cold and contraction of the scrotum are also due to the pathogen cold.

Insufficiency of the Blood of the Gan-Liver

Clinical manifestations: Dizziness, blurred vision, dry eyes, pallor, spasm of the tendons and muscles, numb limbs and a scanty light coloured menstrual flow with a prolonged cycle.

Etiology and pathology: This syndrome often occurs after a hemorrhage or another chronic disease in which blood is destroyed, and the reserves of the gan-liver are depleted, thereby resulting in a failure of the gan-liver to nourish the channels. A xu (deficiency) of blood may cause endogenous wind so that the symptoms of muscle spasticity and numb limbs appear. An upward disturbance of endogenous wind (xu type) can cause dizziness and blurred vision. Insufficiency of the blood of the gan-liver and disruption of its blood storage function results in emptiness of the chong channel which will cause menstrual abnormalities.

Stirring of the Wind of the Gan-Liver by Heat

Clinical manifestations: High fever, convulsions, neck rigidity (Opisthotonos) and coma. A deep-red tongue proper and a wiry, rapid pulse are also found.

Etiology and pathology: This syndrome is due to transmission of the pathogen heat from the exterior to the interior, which burns the yin of the gan-liver and deprives the tendons and blood vessels of nourishment. Furthermore, pathogenic heat in the interior stirs up endogenous wind causing fever, convulsions and neck rigidity. Coma is due to pathogenic heat affecting the pericardium and disturbing the mind.

Syndromes of the Pi-Spleen

Weakness of the Qi of the Pi-Spleen

Clinical manifestations: Sallow complexion, anorexia, loose stools, oedema, and lassitude. There may be distension and a bearing-down sensation in the abdomen, a prolapse of the rectum and/or uterus, or a chronic blood disorder such as purpura, bloody stools or uterine bleeding. A pale tongue proper and a thready xu pulse will be found on examination. If there is evidence of xu (deficiency) of the yang of the pi-spleen, symptoms of cold such as cold limbs will occur.

Etiology and pathology: This syndrome is often caused by irregular food intake, excessive mental strain or chronic disease. These problems result in weakness of the qi of the pi-spleen and impair its function of transportation and transformation, which consequently results in a poor appetite and loose stools. Accumulation of fluid in the interior is the cause of the oedema. The general malaise is due to a lack of food failing to provide a nourishing basis for blood formation.

When the qi of the pi-spleen is weak, it loses its ability to uplift tissues so that there is distension, a bearing-down sensation in the abdomen and a prolapse of the rectum and/or uterus. Weakness of the qi of the pi-spleen also causes the blood disorders. Xu (deficiency) of the yen of the pi-spleen causes cold limbs.

Invasion of the Pi-Spleen by Cold and Damp

Clinical manifestations: Fullness and distension in the chest and epigastrium, a poor appetite, a heavy feeling in the head, malaise, borborygmii, abdominal pain and loose stools. A white sticky tongue coating and a thready pulse will be found.

Etiology and pathology: This syndrome usually occurs after rain, or it may be due to over-indulgence of raw or cold food. In both cases the pathogen cold and damp injure the pi-spleen impairing its function of transportation and transformation and resulting in a poor appetite, borborygmii, abdominal pain and loose stools. As pathogenic damp is sticky and stagnant, it is liable to block the flow of qi causing a sensation of epigastric fullness and distension.

Syndromes of the Fei-Lung

Invasion of the Fei-Lung by the Pathogen Wind

Clinical manifestations: An itchy throat and cough associated with fever and chills. If the wind is accompanied by cold then the patient usually feels cold and presents with nasal obstruction, a watery nasal discharge and mucoid sputum. The tongue coating is thin and white. If the wind is associated with heat, fever will be the most prominent symptom and will be associated with a red, swollen throat, a purulent nasal discharge and purulent sputum. The tongue coating will be yellow.

Etiology and pathology: Invasion of the fei-lung by the pathogen wind disturbs its function of dispersal and descent. Normal respiration is affected producing the symptoms of cough and nasal obstruction. Cold is a yin pathogen and therefore liable to damage the yang qi. Consequently when wind is associated with cold, the sensation of cold will be more severe than that of fever and will be accompanied by a watery nasal discharge and white mucoid sputum. Heat is a yang pathogen, and if wind is accompanied by heat, fever will become the most prominent symptom and will be associated with a purulent nasal discharge and purulent sputum.

Retention of Damp and/or Phlegm in the Fei-Lung

Clinical manifestations: Cough, dyspnoea and white frothy sputum The onset is generally precipitated by cold, and the tongue coating is white and sometimes sticky.

Etiology and pathology: This syndrome is due to the disturbance of the normal circulation of body fluid, the body fluid accumulates and precipitates the formation of damp/or phlegm. When damp and phlegm remain in the fei-lung the passage of qi is blocked and the functions of the fei-lung are impaired, this results in the above symptoms.

Retention of Phlegm and/or Heat in the Fei-Lung

Clinical manifestations: Cough, dyspnoea, wheezing and thick yellow and/or green sputum (occasionally pus). This can be associated with rigors and a fever; the tongue proper is red with a yellow coating and there is a rapid pulse.

Etiology and pathology: This syndrome is caused by invasion of exogenous wind and/or heat, or wind and/or cold, which later develops into heat. The heat mixes with phlegm, which remains in the fei-lung and blocks the circulation of qi; this impairs the functions of the fei-lung and causes cough, dyspnoea and wheeze. Heat exhausts body fluid causing purulent sputum. When phlegm and heat are found in the fei-lung, stagnation of blood results which in turn leads to purulent, bloody sputum.

Insufficiency of the Yin of the Fei-Lung

Clinical manifestations: A dry, unproductive cough associated with sticky, scant, blood-stained sputum, fever, a malar flush, a feverish sensation in the palms and soles, a dry mouth and night sweats. A red tongue proper and a thready and rapid pulse will be found.

Etiology and pathology: Such symptoms are usually caused by chronic disease of the fei-lung, which consumes the yin and results in insufficiency of body fluid. The fei-lung is deprived of nourishment, its functions are impaired and this produces a dry mouth. Xu (deficiency) of yin causes endogenous heat which drives out body fluid and injures blood vessels, this results in a fever, a malar flush, a feverish sensation in the palms and soles, night sweats and bloody sputum.

Syndromes of the Shen-Kidney

Weakness of the Qi of the Shen-Kidney

Clinical manifestations: A sore and weak sensation in the lumbar region and knee joints, urinary frequency, polyuria, dribbling, enuresis, urinary incontinence, dyspnoea, wheezing, and occasionally infertility. The pulse will be thready.

Etiology and pathology: This syndrome is often caused by malaise after a prolonged chronic illness, or may be the result of senility or congenital deficiency. Weakness of the qi of the shen-kidney results in an inability of the urinary bladder to control urination; this causes enuresis, incontinence, frequency and urgency. Shen-kidney stores essence (shen), but when the qi of the shen-kidney is deficient, infertility can result. When the qi of the shen-kidney is weak, it fails to help the fei-lung perform its function of descent, qi therefore attacks the fei-lung resulting in dyspnoca and wheezing.

Insufficiency of the Yang of the Shen-Kidney

Clinical manifestations: These are broadly similar to the syndrome described as "Weakness of qi of the shen-kidney." The major symptoms are a dull ache in the lumbar region and knee joints, cold, pallor, impotence, oliguria and oedema of the lower limbs. A pale, tooth-marked tongue and a deep thready pulse will be found.

Etiology and pathology: This syndrome usually occurs after a prolonged chronic illness in which the yang of the shen-kidney is injured, it may occasionally be due to an excess of sexual activity which also injures the yang of the shen-kidney. In either instance, the yang of the shen-kidney fails to warm the body which results in cold aching sensations in the low back and knee joints, and impotence. Then shen-kidney controls water metabolism, and an insufficiency of the yang of the shen-kidney results in oliguria; the subsequent fluid excess presents with the symptom of oedema.

Insufficiency of the Yin of the Shen-Kidney

Clinical manifestations: Blurred vision, tinnitus, amnesia, feverish sensation in the palms and soles, a malar flush, night sweats, hot yellow urine and constipation. The tongue proper will be red and the pulse thready and rapid.

Etiology and pathology: This usually occurs after a prolonged chronic illness in which the yin of the shen-kidney is impaired, it may also be due to an over-indulgence in sexual activity, which consumes the shen-kidney. Either of these factors can result in the shen-kidney failing to produce marrow and maintaining normal cerebral function. The symptoms that result are dizziness, blurred of nourishment. Furthermore, pathogenic heat in the interior stirs up endogenous wind causing fever, convulsions and neck rigidity. Coma is due to pathogenic heat affecting the pericardium and disturbing the mind.

Syndromes of the Pericardium

The syndromes of the pericardium are seen clinically as the invasion of the pericardium by heat. The symptoms are a high fever, coma and delirium, these result from heat invading the interior of the belly, which in turn disturbs the mind.

Syndromes of the Small Intestine

Disturbance of the function of the small intestine is included in the syndromes of the pi-spleen, particularly with respect to its main function (transformation and transportation).

Syndromes of the Gall Bladder

Damp and Heat in the Gall Bladder

Clinical manifestations: Yellow sclera and skin, pain in the costal and hypochondrial region, pain in the right upper abdominal quadrant and a bitter taste in the mouth. Some patients may vomit sour and/or bitter fluid. The tongue coating is yellow and sticky.

Etiology and pathology: The function of the gall bladder is to store and excrete bile, and this depends on the normal function of the gan-liver. Exogenous damp and/or heat (heat caused by depression of the gan-liver, damp and heat caused by overindulgence in alcohol and rich food) may accumulate in the gan-liver and gall bladder, thereby impairing the free flow of qi. Bile cannot therefore be secreted and freely excreted, and the subsequent biliary overflow causes jaundice, a bitter taste in the mouth and vomiting. Stagnation of the qi of the gan-liver and gall bladder also leads to stagnation of blood, causing right hypochondrial pain. This syndrome is closely related to the gan-liver, and is also known as "damp and heat in the gan-liver and gall bladder."

Syndromes of the Stomach

Retention of Food in the Stomach

Clinical manifestations: Distension and pain in the epigastric region, anorexia, belching, heartburn and vomiting. The tongue has a thick sticky coating.

Etiology and pathology: This syndrome is usually caused by overeating, which leads to the retention of undigested food in the stomach; the qi of the stomach ascends rather than descending.

Retention of Fluid in the Stomach Due to Cold

Clinical manifestations: The sensation of fullness associated with a dull epigastric pain, aggravated by cold and alleviated by warmth. The tongue coating will be white and sticky and the pulse thready or slow.

Etiology and pathology: This syndrome usually follows a cold after rain, or may be precipitated by the excessive ingestion of raw or cold food. Either of these factors result in cold in the stomach which causes stagnation of qi and pain. Prolonged damage injures the yang qi of the pi-spleen and stomach so that body fluid is retained in the stomach instead of being transported and transformed, this results in vomiting.

Hyperactivity of the Fire of the Stomach

Clinical manifestations: A burning in the epigastrium, thirst, a preference for cold drinks, vomiting of undigested food or sour fluid, gingival swelling pain and ulceration, halitosis. The tongue proper will be red with a dry yellow coating.

Etiology and pathology: This syndrome is usually due to overeating rich food, which causes heat to accumulate in the stomach. The heat consumes body fluid and causes the qi of the stomach to ascend. This results in a burning epigastric pain, thirst, a preference for cold drinks and vomiting. Halitosis and gingival ulceration are due to the fire element in the stomach.

Syndromes of the Large Intestine

Damp and Heat in the Large Intestine

Clinical manifestations: Fever, abdominal pain, loose dark smelly stools, frequent bowel movements. White or red mucus may be present in the stool, and can be associated with perineal pain and tenesmus. The tongue proper is red with a yellow coating, and the pulse rolling and rapid.

Etiology and pathology: This syndrome is usually caused by eating too much raw, cold or contaminated food. It may also be due to invasion of summer heat and damp. Damp and heat accumulate in the large intestine, blocking the passage of qi and disturbing its function of transmission and transformation; this produces diarrhea, abdominal pain and dark smelly stool.

Damp and heat may also injure the blood vessels of the large intestine producing bloody mucus in the stool. The downward pressure of the damp and heat causes perineal pain and tenesmus.

Stasis of the Large Intestine

Clinical manifestations: A distended full abdomen, abdominal pain (intensified with pressure), constipation, nausea and vomiting. The tongue coating is white and sticky and the pulse shi and deep.

Etiology and pathology: This syndrome may be due to food retention, gastro-intestinal parasites, or blood stagnation; all these factors cause obstruction of the qi and functional derangement of the large intestine. This results in constipation, abdominal distension and pain. The nausea and vomiting are caused by the qi of the large intestine impeding the descending qi of the stomach.

Stagnation of Blood and Heat in the Large Intestine

Clinical manifestations: A severe boring or fixed pain in the lower abdomen, which is made worse by pressure, constipation and/or mild diarrhea, fever and vomiting. The tongue proper is red with a yellow sticky coating.

Etiology and pathology: This syndrome is usually due to the individual's failure to adapt to changes in the weather, or may be caused by over-eating and/or excessive exercise. These factors result in stagnation of heat and blood and retardation of qi; heat injures the vessels of the large intestine, causing local inflammation and pain in the lower abdomen. If the qi of the stomach is affected then this can result in nausea and vomiting.

Syndromes of the Urinary Bladder

Damp and Heat in the Urinary Bladder

Clinical manifestations. Frequency, urgency, dysuria, bloodstained urine and the presence of clots or stones in the urine. The tongue proper will be red with a yellow coating, and the pulse rapid.

Etiology and pathology. Damp and heat injures the urinary bladder and disturbs its function of storing urine, this results in frequency and urgency. When damp and heat injure the blood vessels of the urinary bladder, stagnation of blood and heat occur leading to haematuria and blood clots in the urine. Prolonged retention of damp and heat in the bladder results in stone formation.

Disturbance in the Function of the Urinary Bladder

Clinical manifestations: Dribbling, weak stream, urinary retention, a lumbar ache associated with pain in the knee joints and a dislike of cold. The tongue proper is pale with a white coating, and the pulse thready and deep (xu).

Etiology and pathology: This syndrome is due to an insufficiency of the yang of the shen-kidney and impairment of its function of urinary filtration. The symptoms of cold therefore result, such as a dislike of cold, cold extremities and weakness and pain in the lumbar region and knee joints.

Syndromes of the Sanjiao

The syndromes of the sanjiao relate to the organs present in the upper, middle and lower jiao. Obstruction of the upper jiao usually refers to confinement of the qi of the fei-lung, insufficiency of the qi of the middle jiao refers to weakness of the pi spleen and stomach and damp and heat in the lower jiao refers to damp and heat in the urinary bladder. The Sanjiao cannot be explained as a single entity.

Conclusion

The principles that are outlined in this chapter enable the acupuncturist to use traditional medicine to find out which organ is diseased, and what pathogen is causing that disease. This allows the classical differentiation of syndromes, and the subsequent determination of treatment based on the differentiation of the symptoms and signs. In essence this represents a simplified form of the pure traditional Chinese medicine. It is a fairly swift method to understand and it is also accurate. Because there are so many different concepts to absorb it is very difficult to explain each one as it occurs in the text, but ultimately the text fits together as a system. We therefore suggest that the reader goes through it initially without trying to understand it all at once; it should be much clearer on a second reading.

Furthermore, we wish to stress that this information will only tell the acupuncturist what the problem is. Point selection, and the rules that govern this, are discussed in the next section, but it is essential to understand this initial theory before the rules of point selection will make sense.

Note

1. Jin is a tissue that is composed of nerves, ligaments, tendons and some parts of the muscle. It is roughly equivalent to connective tissue.

Chapter 8

Chiropractic

What Is Chiropractic?

Chiropractic is a branch of the healing arts which is concerned with human health and disease processes. Doctors of Chiropractic are physicians who consider man as an integrated being and give special attention to the physiological and biochemical aspects including structural, spinal, musculoskeletal, neurological, vascular, nutritional, emotional and environmental relationships.

The practice and procedures which may be employed by Doctors of Chiropractic are based on the academic and clinical training received in and through accredited chiropractic colleges and include, but are not limited to, the use of current diagnostic and therapeutic procedures. Such procedures specifically include the adjustment and manipulation of the articulations and adjacent tissues of the human body, particularly of the spinal column. Included is the treatment of intersegmental aberrations for alleviation of related functional disorders.

Chiropractic is a drug-free, non-surgical science and, as such, does not include pharmaceuticals or incisive surgery. Due regard shall be given to the fact that state laws, as well as the nation's antitrust laws, may allow Doctors of Chiropractic to utilize ancillary health care procedures commonly referred to as being in the common domain.

From "About Chiropractic," ©1999 American Chiropractic Association, available online at http://www.amerchiro.org; reprinted with permission.

Benefits of Chiropractic

Thirty-one million Americans have low back pain at any given time.[1] One half of all working Americans admit to having back symptoms each year.[2] One third of all Americans over age 18 had a back problem in the past five years severe enough for them to seek professional help.[3] And the cost of this care is estimated to be a staggering $50 billion yearly—and that's just for the more easily identified costs.[4]

These are just some of the astounding facts about Americans and their miserable backs. Is there any wonder why some experts estimate that as many as 80% of all of us will experience a back problem at some time in our lives?[5]

Because back problems are this common it's probably going to happen to you too. Shouldn't you find out what to do about it before it happens rather than after? Why wait until you're hurting to learn about your treatment options?

When you're hurting you may not give this important decision the time and attention it needs to make the best choice. Manipulation is one of several established forms of treatment used for back problems. Used primarily by Doctors of Chiropractic (DCs) for the last century, manipulation has been largely ignored by most others in the health care community until recently. Now, with today's growing emphasis on treatment and cost effectiveness, manipulation is receiving much more widespread attention. In fact, after an extensive study of all currently available care for low back problems, the Agency for Health Care Policy and Research—a federal government research organization—recommended that low back pain suffers choose the most conservative care first. And it recommended spinal manipulation as the only safe and effective, drugless form of initial professional treatment for acute low back problems in adults.[6] Chiropractic manipulation, also frequently called the chiropractic adjustment, is the form of manipulation that has been most extensively used by Americans for the last one hundred years.[7] Satisfied chiropractic patients already know that DCs are uniquely trained and experienced in diagnosing back problems and are the doctors most skilled in using manipulation for the treatment of back pain and related disorders.[8]

As a public service, the American Chiropractic Association (ACA) urges you to make an informed choice about your back care.

What Is a DC?

Chiropractors are first-contact physicians who possess the diagnostic skills to differentiate health conditions that are amenable to their management from those conditions that require referral or co-management. Chiropractors provide conservative management of neuro-musculoskeletal disorders and related functional clinical conditions including, but not limited to, back pain, neck pain and headaches.

Chiropractors are expert providers of spinal and other therapeutic manipulation/adjustments. They also utilize a variety of manual, mechanical and electrical therapeutic modalities.

Chiropractors also provide patient evaluation and instructions regarding disease prevention and health promotion through proper nutrition, exercise and lifestyle modification among others.

History/Evolution

Chiropractic is a natural form of health care with a rich history. Spinal manipulation, chiropractic's primary treatment, is used instead of drugs or surgery to promote the body's natural healing process. One of the earliest indications of soft tissue manipulation is demonstrated by the ancient Chinese Kong Fou Document written about 2700 B.C., which was brought to the Western World by missionaries. Chiropractic became more recognized about 100 years ago when Daniel David Palmer gave an "adjustment" to what was felt to be a misplaced vertebra in the upper spine of a deaf janitor. The janitor then observed that his hearing improved.

The word "chiropractic" is derived from the Greek words "cheir" and "praktkos" meaning "done by hand." From these simple beginnings, chiropractic became more sophisticated as a formal educational program evolved, requirements by the schools were developed, and state and governing laws were established.

Frequently Asked Questions

How many DCs practice in the U.S.?

This number is difficult to determine. In 1998, FCLB reported 79,674 active DC licenses in the U.S.; however, not all of these DCs are practicing and some may be duplicates (i.e., the same DC may have active licenses in multiple states). A query of a well-known *U.S. Yellow Pages* CDROM counted over 55,000 ads; consequently, the range is probably between 55,000 and 70,000 practicing DCs in the U.S.

How many Americans visit DCs per year?

A 1991 Gallup Poll commissioned by the ACA found that, 10.1% of adults (18 and over) had used chiropractic services within the last year. According to the U.S. Census Bureau, today there are approximately 273 million people in the U.S. Assuming the 10% annual figure has remained unchanged, the number of people who visit a chiropractor every year is now approximately 27 million. This number can also be calculated by multiplying the number of individual patients the average DC sees per year (approximately 375) by the number of DCs in the country. This produces a range between 21 and 28 million people.

References

1. Jensen M, Brant-Zawadzki M, Obuchowski N, et al. Magnetic Resonance Imaging of the Lumbar Spine in People Without Back Pain. *N Engl J Med* 1994; 331: 69-116.

2. Vallfors B. Acute, Subacute and Chronic Low Back Pain: Clinical Symptoms, Absenteeism and Working Environment. *Scan J Rehab Med Suppl* 1985; 11: 1-98.

3. Finding from a national study conducted for the American Chiropractic Association. Risher P. *Americans' Perception of Practitioners and Treatments for Back Problems.* Louis Harris and Associates, Inc. New York: August, 1994.

4. This total represents only the more readily identifiable costs for medical care, workers compensation payments and time lost from work. It does not include costs associated with lost personal income due to acquired physical limitation resulting from a back problem and lost employer productivity due to employee medical absence. In Project Briefs: Back Pain Patient Outcomes Assessment Team (BOAT). In *MEDTEP Update,* Vol. 1 Issue 1, Agency for Health Care Policy and Research, Rockville, MD, Summer 1994.

5. In Vallfors B, previously cited.

6. Bigos S, Bowyer O, Braen G, et al. *Acute Low Back Problems in Adults.* Clinical Practice Guideline No. 14. AHCPR Publication No. 95-0642. Rockville, MD: Agency for Health Care Policy and Research, Public Health Service, U.S. Department of Health and Human Services, December, 1994.

7. The RAND Corporation reported from its analysis of spinal manipulation research literature that 94% of all spinal manipulation is performed by chiropractors, 4% by osteopaths, and the remainder by medical doctors.

8. In Risher P, previously cited.

Chapter 9

Herbal Medicine

Medicinal herbs are some of our oldest medicines and their increasing use in recent years is evidence of a public interest in having alternatives to conventional medicine. Herbal medicines continue to be a major market in U.S. pharmacies and constitute a multi-billion dollar industry. Although approximately 1500 botanicals are sold as dietary supplements or ethnic traditional medicines, herbal formulations are not subject to FDA premarket toxicity testing to assure their safety or efficacy.

In response to concerns regarding the use and efficacy of medicinal herbs and to recent nominations of these products for study by the National Toxicology Program (NTP), a workshop on herbal medicines was held in 1998. Recommendations from the workshop included a call for more research on herbals, the identification and standardization of product ingredients by industry, and increased consumer education through package inserts.

In follow-up to this workshop, the NTP staff is working with the NIH Office of Dietary Supplements, the U.S. Food and Drug Administration, the academic community, and others to further define and implement research that addresses deficiencies in our knowledge about herbal medicines and their potential toxicities. Herbs and active or toxic ingredients found in some herbs, continue to be nominated and selected for study by the NTP. Studies have been designed

A fact sheet produced by the National Toxicology Program, National Institute of Environmental Health Sciences (NIEHS), 2001.

101

for many of these herbal products and several studies are in progress. These studies focus on characterization of potential adverse health effects including reproductive toxicity, neurotoxicity, and immunotoxicity as well as those associated with acute high dose exposure and chronic exposure to lower doses. In addition, special attention is being given to the potential for herb/herb and herb/drug interactions and the responses of sensitive subpopulations (e.g. pregnant women, the young, the developing fetus, the elderly, etc). NTP studies include both traditional toxicological research and molecular mechanistic considerations. Comments from the public and others regarding NTP research

Table 9.1. Herbs and Active or Toxic Ingredients for Study by the NTP (continued on next page)

Herb or Ingredient	Information
Aloe Vera Gel	Seventh most widely used herb; used as both a dietary supplement and component of cosmetics. The gel has been used for centuries as a treatment for minor burns and is increasingly being used in products for internal consumption (e.g., "health" drinks).
Black Walnut Extract	Black walnut extract is found in hair dye formulations and walnut oil stain. It is used both internally and externally as herbal remedy for a variety of conditions. Juglone is a major constituent of black walnut extract.
Comfrey	Herb consumed in teas and as fresh leaves for salads; however, it contains pyrrolizidine alkaloids (e.g., symphatine), which are known to be toxic. Used externally as an anti-inflammatory agent in the treatment of bruises, sprains, and other external wounds. No toxicity studies on comfrey are planned. Based in part on NTP chemistry studies of the alkaloid components of comfrey, the FDA has asked makers of dietary supplements containing the herb to remove them from the market.
Echinacea purpurea Extract	One of the most commonly used medicinal herbs in the United States. Used as an immunostimulant to treat colds, sore throat, and flu.

102

in this area are welcome and should be forwarded to the NTP Liaison and Scientific Review Office.

For further information, contact:

Dr. Tom Burka
NIEHS
P.O. Box 12233, MD B3-10
Research Triangle Park, NC 27709
Phone: (919) 541-4667
e-mail: burka@niehs.nih.gov

Table 9.1. Herbs and Active or Toxic Ingredients for Study by the NTP (continued on next page)

Herb or Ingredient	Information
Ginkgo biloba Extract	Among the five or six most frequently used medicinal herbs. Ginkgo fruits and seeds have been used medicinally for thousands for years. The extract of green-picked leaves has increasing popularity in the United States. Ginkgo biloba extract promotes vasodilatation and improved blood flow and appears beneficial, particularly for short-term memory loss, headache, and depression.
Ginseng and Ginsenosides	Fourth most widely used medicinal herb; ginsenosides are thought to be the active ingredients. Ginseng has used as a treatment for a variety of conditions: hypertension, diabetes, and depression, and been associated with various adverse health effects.
Goldenseal	Second or third most popular medicinal herb used in this country; traditionally used to treat wounds, digestive problems, and infections. Current uses include as a laxative, tonic, and diuretic.
Grape Seed Extract	US grape seed extract market is estimated to be $40-$50 million per year. The extract contains phenolic antioxidants and is used to promote health of the cardiovascular system. A similar product, pine bark extract, is also being considered for study.

Table 9.1. Herbs and Active or Toxic Ingredients for Study by the NTP (continued from previous page)

Herb or Ingredient	Information
Kava Kava	Reported to be the fifth most widely used medicinal herb, has psychoactive properties, and is sold as a calmative and antidepressant.
Milk Thistle Extract	Used to treat depression and several liver conditions including cirrhosis and hepatitis and to increase breast milk production.
Pulegone	Pulegone is a major terpenoid constituent of the herb Pennyroyal and is found in lesser concentrations in other mints. Pennyroyal has been used as a carminative insect repellent, emmenagogue, and abortifacient. Pulegone has well-recognized toxicity to the liver, kidney, and central nervous system
Thujone	Terpenoid found in a variety of herbs, including sage and tansy, and in high concentrations in wormwood. Suspected as the causative toxic agent associated with drinking absinthe, a liqueur flavored with wormwood extract.

Chapter 10

Homeopathy

Some of the medicines of homeopathy evoke positive images—chamomile, marigold, daisy, onion. But even some of Mother Nature's cruelest creations—poison ivy, mercury, arsenic, pit viper venom, hemlock—are part of homeopathic care.

Homeopathy is a medical theory and practice that developed in reaction to the bloodletting, blistering, purging, and other harsh procedures of conventional medicine as it was practiced more than 200 years ago. Remedies made from many sources—including plants, minerals or animals—are prescribed based on both a person's symptoms and personality. Patients receiving homeopathic care frequently feel worse before they get better because homeopathic medicines often stimulate, rather than suppress, symptoms. This seeming reversal of logic is a relevant part of homeopathy because symptoms are viewed as the body's effort to restore health.

The Food and Drug Administration regulates homeopathic remedies under provisions of the Food, Drug, and Cosmetic Act.

Kinder, Gentler Medicine

In the late 1700s, the most popular therapy for most ailments was bloodletting. Some doctors had so much faith in bleeding that they were willing to remove up to four-fifths of the patient's blood. Other

"Homeopathy: Real Medicine or Empty Promises?" by Isadora Stehlin, *FDA Consumer*, U.S. Food and Drug Administration, December 1996.

therapies of choice included blistering—placing caustic or hot substances on the skin to draw out infections—and administering dangerous chemicals to induce vomiting or purge the bowels. Massive doses of a mercury-containing drug called calomel cleansed the bowels, but at the same time caused teeth to loosen, hair to fall out, and other symptoms of acute mercury poisoning.

Samuel Hahnemann, a German physician disenchanted with these methods, began to develop a theory based on three principles: the law of similars, the minimum dose, and the single remedy.

The word homeopathy is derived from the Greek words for like (homoios) and suffering (pathos). With the law of similars, Hahnemann theorized that if a large amount of a substance causes certain symptoms in a healthy person, smaller amounts of the same substance can treat those symptoms in someone who is ill. The basis of his theory took shape after a strong dose of the malaria treatment quinine caused his healthy body to develop symptoms similar to ones caused by the disease. He continued to test his theory on himself as well as family and friends with different herbs, minerals and other substances. He called these experiments "provings."

But, as might be expected, the intensity of the symptoms caused by the original proving was harrowing. So Hahnemann began decreasing the doses to see how little of a substance could still produce signs of healing.

With the minimum dose, or law of infinitesimals, Hahnemann believed that a substance's strength and effectiveness increased the more it was diluted. Minuscule doses were prepared by repeatedly diluting the active ingredient by factors of 10. A "6X" preparation (the X is the Roman numeral for 10) is a 1-to-10 dilution repeated six times, leaving the active ingredient as one part per million. Essential to the process of increasing potency while decreasing the actual amount of the active ingredient is vigorous shaking after each dilution.

Some homeopathic remedies are so dilute, no molecules of the healing substance remain. Even with sophisticated technology now available, analytical chemists may find it difficult or impossible to identify any active ingredient. But the homeopathic belief is that the substance has left its imprint or a spirit-like essence that stimulates the body to heal itself.

Finally, a homeopathic physician generally prescribes only a single remedy to cover all symptoms—mental as well as physical—the patient is experiencing. However, the use of multi-ingredient remedies is recognized as part of homeopathic practice.

106

FDA Regulation

In 1938, Sen. Royal Copeland of New York, the chief sponsor of the Food, Drug, and Cosmetic Act and a homeopathic physician, wrote into the law a recognition of any product listed in the Homeopathic Pharmacopeia of the United States. The Homeopathic Pharmacopeia includes a compilation of standards for source, composition and preparation of homeopathic drugs.

FDA regulates homeopathic drugs in several significantly different ways from other drugs.

Manufacturers of homeopathic drugs are deferred from submitting new drug applications to FDA. Their products are exempt from good manufacturing practice requirements related to expiration dating and from finished product testing for identity and strength. Homeopathic drugs in solid oral dosage form must have an imprint that identifies the manufacturer and indicates that the drug is homeopathic. The imprint on conventional products, unless specifically exempt, must identify the active ingredient and dosage strength as well as the manufacturer.

"The reasoning behind [the difference] is that homeopathic products contain little or no active ingredients," explains Edward Miracco, a consumer safety officer with FDA's Center for Drug Evaluation and Research. "From a toxicity, poison-control standpoint, [the active ingredient and strength] was deemed to be unnecessary."

Another difference involves alcohol. Conventional drugs for adults can contain no more than 10 percent alcohol, and the amount is even less for children's medications. But some homeopathic products contain much higher amounts because the agency has temporarily exempted these products from the alcohol limit rules.

"Alcohol is an integral part of many homeopathic products," says Miracco. For this reason, the agency has decided to delay its decision concerning alcohol in homeopathic products while it reviews the necessity of high levels of alcohol.

"Overall, the disparate treatment has been primarily based on the uniqueness of homeopathic products, the lack of any real concern over their safety because they have little or no pharmacologically active ingredients, and because of agency resources and priorities," explains Miracco.

However, homeopathic products are not exempt from all FDA regulations. If a homeopathic drug claims to treat a serious disease such as cancer it can be sold by prescription only. Only products sold for so-called self-limiting conditions—colds, headaches, and other minor

health problems that eventually go away on their own—can be sold without a prescription (over-the-counter).
Requirements for nonprescription labeling include:

• an ingredients list

• instructions for safe use

• at least one major indication

• dilution (for example 2X for one part per hundred, 3X for one part per thousand).

Over the past several years, the agency has issued about 12 warning letters to homeopathic marketers. The most common infraction was the sale of prescription homeopathic drugs over-the-counter. "It's illegal, it's in violation, and we're going to focus on it," says Miracco.
Other problems include:

• products promoted as homeopathic that contain nonhomeopathic active ingredients, such as vitamins or plants not listed in homeopathic references

• lack of tamper-resistant packaging

• lack of proper labeling

• vague indications for use that could encompass serious disease conditions. For example, a phrase like "treats gastrointestinal disorders" is too general, explains Miracco. "This phrase can encompass a wide variety of conditions, from stomachache or simple diarrhea to colon cancer," he says. "Claims need to be specific so the consumer knows what the product is intended to treat and the indication does not encompass serious disease conditions that would require prescription dispensing and labeling."

In addition to enforcement, the agency is also focusing on preventing problems by educating the homeopathic industry about FDA regulations. "Agency representatives continue to meet with homeopathic trade groups to tell them about problems we've had, difficulties we've seen, and trends we've noticed," says Miracco.
FDA is aware of a few reports of illness associated with the use of homeopathic products. However, agency review of those reported to FDA discounted the homeopathic product involved as the cause of the adverse reaction. In one instance, arsenic, which is a recognized homeopathic ingredient, was implicated. But, as would be expected, FDA

analysis revealed the concentration of arsenic was so minute there wasn't enough to cause concern, explains Miracco. "It's been diluted out."

Homeopathic Treatment

Homeopathy consists of highly individualized treatments based on a person's genetic history, personal health history, body type, and present status of all physical, emotional and mental symptoms.

Jennifer Jacobs, M.D., who has a family practice and is licensed to practice homeopathy in Washington state, spends at least an hour and a half with each new patient. "What I do is review the lifetime history of the patient's health," she explains. "Also I ask a lot of questions about certain general symptoms such as food preferences and sleep patterns that usually aren't seen as important in conventional medicine. In looking to make the match between the person and the remedy, I need to have all of this sort of information."

Why does someone trained in conventional medicine turn to homeopathy? "With chronic illnesses such as arthritis and allergies, conventional medicine has solutions that help control the symptoms but you don't really see the patients getting better," says Jacobs. "What I have seen in my homeopathic work is that it really does seem to help people get better. I'm not saying I can cure everyone but I do see where people's overall health is improved over the course of treatment."

Jacobs' hasn't abandoned conventional medicine completely. "My daughter is 17 and she's never taken antibiotics, but I would have no hesitation to use antibiotics if she had pneumonia, or meningitis, or a kidney infection," says Jacobs.

About a third of Jacobs' practice is children, and ear infections are one of the most common problems she treats. "Ear infections are something that seems to respond well to homeopathy," she says. "Of course, if a child is not better within two or three days, or if the child develops a high fever, or if I feel that there's a serious complication setting in, then of course I will use antibiotics. But I find that in the majority of cases, ear infections do resolve without antibiotics."

In addition to treating patients, Jacobs has conducted a clinical trial the results of which suggest that homeopathic treatment might be useful in the treatment of acute childhood diarrhea. The results were published in the May 1994 issue of *Pediatrics*. In the article, Jacobs concluded that further studies should be conducted to determine whether her findings were accurate. A subsequent article appearing in the November 1995 issue of *Pediatrics* indicated that Jacobs' study was flawed in several ways.

Although *Pediatrics* is published by the American Academy of Pediatrics, Jacobs' study and several others published in such journals as *The Lancet* and the *British Medical Journal* are considered "scanty at best" by the academy. "Given the plethora of studies that are published [on other topics] in scientific journals, I wouldn't say there are a lot of articles coming out," says Joe M. Sanders Jr., M.D., the executive director of the academy. "Just because an article appears in a scientific journal does not mean that it's absolute fact and should be immediately incorporated into therapeutic regimens. It just means that the study is [published] for critique and review and hopefully people will use that as a stepping stone for further research."

More studies are under way. For example, the Office of Alternative Medicine at the National Institutes of Health has awarded a grant for a clinical trial of the effects of homeopathic treatment on mild traumatic brain injury.

Even with the dearth of clinical research, homeopathy's popularity in the United States is growing. The 1995 retail sales of homeopathic medicines in the United States were estimated at $201 million and growing at a rate of 20 percent a year, according to the American Homeopathic Pharmaceutical Association. The number of homeopathic practitioners in the United States has increased from fewer than 200 in the 1970s to approximately 3,000 in 1996.

When looking for a homeopathic practitioner, it's important to find someone who is licensed, according to the National Center for Homeopathy. Each state has its own licensing requirements. "Whether that person is a medical doctor or a physician's assistant or a naturopathic physician, I feel that anyone who's treating people who are sick needs to have medical training," says Jacobs.

Real Medicine or Wishful Thinking?

Many who don't believe in homeopathy's effectiveness say any successful treatments are due to the placebo effect, or, in other words, positive thinking.

But homeopathy's supporters counter that their medicine works in groups like infants and even animals that can't be influenced by a pep talk. Jacobs adds that sometimes she mistakenly gives a patient the wrong remedy and he or she doesn't get better. "Then I give the right remedy, and the person does get better," she says. "So it's not like everybody gets better because it's all in their head. I think it's only because we don't understand the mechanism of action of homeopathy that so many people have trouble accepting it."

The American Medical Association does not accept homeopathy, but it doesn't reject it either. "The AMA encourages doctors to become aware of alternative therapies and use them when and where appropriate," says AMA spokesman Jim Fox.

Similarly, the American Academy of Pediatrics has no specific policy on homeopathy. If an adult asked the academy's Sanders about homeopathy, he would tell that person to "do your own investigation. I don't personally prescribe homeopathic remedies, but I would be open-minded." That open-mindedness applies only to adults, however. "I would have problems with somebody imposing other than conventional medicine onto a child who's incapable of making that decision," he says.

Even professionals who practice homeopathy warn that nothing in medicine—either conventional or alternative—is absolute. "I'm not saying we can cure everyone [with homeopathy]," says Jacobs.

Chapter 11

Native American Medicine

Defining Traditional Healing

The four elements of the person are the Spiritual, Emotional, Physical and Mental. The physical manifestations of a weakness are seen as disease or a bodily ailment. The disease is traditionally seen as a symptom of the weakness. The weakness may be derived within the spiritual, emotional, or psychological aspects of the person. When a person is inflicted with a disease, the traditional view is that it is an offering of a teaching to the individual. The teaching will ultimately be of oneself but the person may choose to deal only with the symptom of physical manifestation of the weakness and not address the root of the disease itself. If the person chooses to treat only the disease and ignores the teaching which it is offered, then the disease will return. Physical manifestations may continue to appear until the individual accepts the teaching.

The weaknesses are caused by being out of balance or off center. There are many reasons why an individual is out of balance. The reasons range from working too much in one area or over-working at a job, being too greedy, wanting too much, and not paying attention to the other parts of ones' self or ones' life and family. If we do not pay attention to all of our parts then we will become unbalanced and an

"Defining Traditional Healing" by Gloria Lee, from *Justice as Healing*, Volume 1, Number 4 (Winter 1996), the newsletter of The Native Law Centre of Canada, Saskatoon, Saskatchewan, Canada, © 1996 University of Saskatchewan; reprinted with permission.

illness may come forward to remind us of the fact that we have not paid attention to other parts of ourselves. Being out of balance may also be caused by not receiving the appropriate teachings from Elders because First Nations culture was hidden to protect it from total loss. There are traditional ways of dealing with illnesses. With the support of Elders and the assistance of Healers and Elder Apprentices we can find the right healing for the illness and an explanation for why the illness happened in the first place. If we ignore this explanation and continue with the same behavior or activity which is said to have caused the illness, the illness will return. Inevitably the illness is said to be caused because the person is out of balance. Being out of balance happens because one has not lived a "careful" life.

When speaking to a traditional healer, one will discover that much of what a healer does is sorting out the jumble of disorder found in and around the patient. The disorder has many causes but primarily is caused by not living life in a good way. The job of the Healer, simply put, is to help reorder the elements of the person and to explain why and how disorder was achieved. The Healer then explains how to ensure that the illness does not return.

Traditional healing by a Healer was utilized when a family determined that there was an "Indian" illness.

"When people discuss a particular case of illness, identifying the probable cause was often a central topic. Indeed, when the cause of a particular illness was not readily apparent, individuals would commonly note that the illness "just didn't occur for no reason." In conversations about serious or complex cases, several different explanations may be discussed."[2]

Understanding the cause of the illness or observable behavior was important in finding the appropriate treatment for the illness or behavior.

"Indian" illnesses are those which can be explained by reference to a potentially observable event. These include such things as colds, fevers, and respiratory infections, like bronchitis, attributed to exposure to excessive cold, or to being overheated and catching a chill; and stomach aches or diarrhea that come from overeating."[3]

These are physical manifestations of a problem. As part of the diagnosis, a Healer can determine if the physical manifestation is due to spiritual or emotional imbalance, this is part of the diagnosis.

Understanding begins with the Elders and what they have to teach. Their knowledge comes from the Creator. Because traditional healing is within each of us, we are all capable of healing ourselves, sometimes with the assistance or support of others such as Elders, Healers, and Helpers. Healing begins at one's own center, this is the ultimate responsibility for one's own well being.[4] This traditional approach to healing is found in discussions on the meaning of justice. For example, the meaning of 'justice' found in the *Report of the Aboriginal Justice Inquiry of Manitoba* states:

"The dominant society tries to control actions it considers potentially or actually harmful to society as a whole, to individuals or to the wrongdoers themselves by interdiction, enforcement or apprehension, The emphasis is on the punishment of the deviant as a means of making that person conform, or as a means of protecting other members of society.

"The purpose of a justice system in an Aboriginal society is to restore the peace and equilibrium within the community, and to reconcile the accused with his or her own conscience and with the individual or family who has been wronged. This is a primary difference. It is a difference that significantly challenges the appropriateness of the present legal system for Aboriginal people in the resolution of conflict, the reconciliation and the maintenance of community harmony and good orders."[5]

From the First Nations understanding, the Euro-Canadian concept of justice is too narrow and too confining for a complete appreciation of all the elements involved in a Wholistic perspective of justice. The Euro-Canadian justice model is focuses on delivering punishment for wrongdoing. In this model, justice is the maintenance or administration of what is righteous by determining awards or punishment; it is the quality of being just, impartial, or fair.

The First Nations' philosophy of justice is really an expanded understanding which, in the end, does not even mean 'justice' anymore. There is not an English word for the First Nations' Wholistic meaning. Aboriginal people have inherently a higher standard or a fuller concept of what is required to make things right. This understanding is guided by the spiritual realm and the teachings of the Creator. These teachings are sometimes referred to as Natural Laws. The following is an excerpt from the Federation of Saskatchewan Indian Nations' Justice Unit *Historical / Customary First Nations Law Practices—The Natural Law*, which is respectfully included:

"The teachings of our culture tell us that we as aboriginal people were placed here by our Creator, the same Creator who is responsible for all of creation. This of course includes all nations, regardless of race. Each nation was provided with a means of communication to the Creator, or as some would call it, a faith or religion for which to follow. These various religions are considered gifts to mankind and are to be treated with respect by all. Therefore, for one nation to denounce or show disrespect to another faith is in essence, committing an act of disrespect to the Creator even though it is done unintentionally. Once we, as a Nation of people, begin to acknowledge the existence of one Creator, a teaching of respect for mankind emerges.

"If one chooses to accept or acknowledge this concept, one can easily see that our culture, customs and traditions were also provided to us by the Creator. We are told that our culture in based on the natural law and that the natural law is connected to the natural universe."

Long ago our ancestors had a clear understanding of the natural law and they understood how all things were inter-connected. It was understood by our ancestors that when one walked with disrespect, their own spirit paid with retribution. Even by insulting the smallest child, one already insulted their own spirit. Such acts were considered an abuse or violations of the natural law and the individual was obligated to correct the wrong doing through service to mankind. We have been told that such teachings have not been a part of our people, as a nation, for several hundred years. This is not to suggest that natural law has diminished for the natural law is constant and does not change. Rather, our own understanding and practice of the natural law as a whole nation has diminished. This is not intended to discourage First Nations people as we are told that we as a nation, are entering a new cycle of life which will bring increased harmony and balance. As we learn more about our traditional past, we will be challenged to the degree that we will doubt our own ability to learn. We are to have faith in our Creator and the power of the Spirit and to continue no matter how it is perceived.

"The natural law as we know it, is connected to the natural universe which is comprised of positive and negative energy forces. Our white brothers and sisters understand this concept to a certain degree, however, they have chosen to acknowledge it in a different manner, namely in scientific terms. At times, they have chosen to direct these energies in a negative fashion, i.e.; splitting of the atom, thus allowing the creation of atomic weapons. We have, on the other hand, chosen to acknowledge and respect these energy forces in accordance with our traditions, for even the negative energy that is present in the universe can show us the beauty of love. The negative energy is used as a balance to maintain harmony within and by doing so, can provide a greater understanding of love. We are told that as humans, we have to maintain that balance."[6]

This brief introduction to natural law, while not a complete explanation does provides a sense that natural law encompasses the workings of the universe (physics) and emotions such as love which are all guided by the power of the Creator. The Euro Canadian understanding of justice does not consider neither physics nor love.

Cultural and Religious Contexts

The way in which an Individual chooses to relate to the Creator and to all of Creation will determine how justice is perceived and how restorative justice is viewed. This is attributed to fundamental beliefs and values which are inherently different and are in a state of ongoing conflict between Aboriginal and non-Aboriginal peoples' laws.

Hollow Water has discussed the meaning of justice and how different cultural perspectives define justice. The following is an extensive quote from the Hollow Water material which helps us understand that culture and values are important in determining what a society or community will accept and develop as justice. It is included because of its usefulness and clarity on the issue of cultural and spiritual contexts.

"In looking at the relationship between Community Holistic Circle Healing (CHCH) and the Manitoba justice system, it is useful to consider the cultural and religious contexts in which the respective views and systems of justice have been developed. This is not intended to be an in-depth analysis of the contexts, but rather an overview from which to understand the differences, and perhaps to understand the resulting tensions between the systems.

"A community's justice system reflects its culture and values, which are often entrenched in its religion. In comparing the Hollow Water notions of justice with those of the Euro-Canadian system, it is easy to perceive the religious roots.

"The over riding rational for the use of traditional teachings for CHCH is found in the importance of healing, which has an important spiritual significance due to the need to unite all aspects of a person's

117

being: the physical, the spiritual, the mental and the emotional elements. For CHCH the act of sexual abuse clearly indicates a lack of balance in all aspects of a person's being.

"Because the spiritual being is integrally interwoven into the relationship with the Creator, a lack of balance in the spiritual being has an impact on the relationship with the Creator.

"While it can perhaps be over-simplifying a very complex process, it can be said that justice for CHCH is restoring the balance.

"This implies, for the "justice process" of CHCH, not only a consideration of the imbalance that led to the wrongful act, but also the external forces that caused the imbalance, as well as the consequences of the act. One would be foolish to think, for example, that an act of sexual abuse would not affect the spiritual balance of the victim. Justice then would include righting that imbalance as well.

"One can easily see the role of Christianity in the concepts of the Canadian justice system. Christianity is a "top down" system with God at the top. In the Old Testament at least, God smote those who offended him. Christians pay for their sins with God doling out the punishment.

"In our justice system, the role of God is played by the judge. Christianity is founded on the notion of free will. People choose to sin and are held accountable for that choice. Sinners are punished.

"This context, translated into the Canadian system, makes justice focus on very simple issues. Free will is, in the justice system, translated into "mens rea" (guilty mind). It forms the most important concept in our justice system. It allows us to focus our attention on a single act."

"We never need to ask "Why?" because that answer is always supplied to us through the precepts. The presence of mens rea means the accused chose to commit the act, and that's all we need to know. The offender is then held blameworthy, ready to be punished.

"The result of the fact finding approach in a justice system which seeks to lay blame on an individual is to pit the offender and the victim against one another, thus further exacerbating the harm that has come between them.

"Having established guilt we then invoke the wisdom of experts, i.e. complete strangers to the protagonists, to advise us as to the implications of the wrong doing.

"The only time we look beyond the offender is in the punishment stage. But this is only to determine what caused the offender to go wrong. (We already know this because of our free will concept.)

"It arises in a concept called 'general deterrence'. Simply put, this amounts to punishing the offender for an offence someone else might commit in the future. No doubt the rationale for this can be traced back to the concept of 'original sin' which in essence makes us responsible for the sins of others.

"In Christianity the ultimate punishment is Hell. In our justice system it is jail, a place similar to Hell where we organized the gathering of wrongdoers to cohabit with one another. It is not a place designed to make the offender a better person, but simply to punish him for his wrongful acts, just like Hell.

"It is not far removed from the "eye for an eye" concept of justice, about which Ghandi once said, if we practice an eye for an eye as justice, soon we will all end up blind.

"Recent trends would not lead one to the conclusion that popular notions of justice are moving away from the notion that offenders deserve to have great amounts of suffering inflicted upon them in the name of justice.

"When one considers the two systems from this perspective, it is easier to understand the underlying causes of the tensions between them. If one accepts that the respective views of "justice," and the systems that have evolved around those views, are founded on the underlying belief structure of the culture, then it follows that each culture will have difficulty perceiving the merits of the other's approach to justice. It is difficult to accept as valid that which does not conform to one's fundamental beliefs. Even more problematic is the effort to inflict on one culture the justice system, and thus the underlying belief structure, of the other culture. Where the underlying belief structures are fundamentally inconsistent, the justice system of the one cannot work for the other, for in their eyes, what is being delivered is not justice."[7]

Notes

1. The information in this section was obtained through the oral tradition from Elders Mary Lee, Danny Musqua, Henry Ross and others, except where otherwise noted.

2. Linda C. Garro, "Ways of Talking About Illness in a Manitoba Anishinabe (Ojibway) Community" in *Circumpolar Health* 90, p. 226.

3. Ibid p. 226.

4. These concepts and others are discussed further by Edward A. Connors, Registered Mohawk Psychologist, in "How Well We

Can See The Whole Will Determine How Well We Are and How Well We Can Become" found in Sue Deranger, *Culturally Specific Helping with First Nations People*, 1996.

5. A.C. Hamilton & C.M. Sinclair, *Report of the Manitoba Justice Inquiry*, (Winnipeg, Manitoba: Queen's Printer, 1990) p. 22.

6. F.S.I.N. Justice Unit, *Historical/Customary Law, First Nations Law Practices: The Natural Law*, December 1995, pp. 3-4.

7. This section is respectfully included from the Hollow Water Community Holistic Circle Healing C.H.C.H. Discussion Paper.

Chapter 12

Naturopathic Medicine

The origin of naturopathy can be traced back to the ancient healing arts of a variety of cultures. Still, as a formal system of medicine and healing, it was developed in the United States nearly one hundred years ago by Benjamin Lust.

To heal in harmony with the natural functions of the body—without harm—is the underlying principle of the naturopathic system of medicine. The intent is to support the natural healing potential of the human body as validated by modern scientific research. It is this combination of the healing power of nature and scientific methods that makes naturopathic medicine an important system of medicine for today's health care.

Naturopathic medicine's basic principles are:

1. Utilize the healing power of nature

2. First, do no harm

3. Find the cause

4. Treat the whole person

5. Preventative medicine

The American Association of Naturopathic Physicians (AANP) more fully describes these tenets as:

Utilize the Healing Power of Nature: (Vis Medicatrix Naturae.) Nature acts powerfully through the healing mechanisms of the body and mind to maintain and restore health. Naturopathic physicians work to restore and support these inherent healing systems when they have broken down, by using methods, medicines, and techniques that are in harmony with natural processes.

First Do No Harm: (Prinum Non Nocere.) Naturopathic physicians prefer noninvasive treatments, which minimize the risks of harmful side effects. They are trained to know which patients they can treat safely, and which ones they need to refer to other health care practitioners.

Find the Cause: (Tolle Causam.) Every illness has an underlying cause, often an aspect of the lifestyle, diet, or habits of the individual. A naturopathic physician is trained to find and remove the underlying cause of a disease.

Treat the Whole Person: Health or disease results from a complex interaction of physical, emotional, dietary, genetic, environmental, lifestyle, and other factors. Naturopathic physicians treat the whole person, taking these factors into account.

Preventative Medicine: The naturopathic approach to health care can prevent minor illnesses from developing into more serious, chronic, or degenerative diseases. Patients are taught the principles with which to live a healthy life; by following these principles, they can prevent major illnesses.[12]

Above all, naturopathic physicians respect the natural healing power present in all systems of the human body and they attempt to focus and mobilize that power in their treatment process. N.D.'s have found that this natural healing power, if effectively mobilized, can destroy invading organisms, cast off toxins, as well as rebuild strength and vitality. Dr. Stephen Speidel, an N.D. practicing in Poulsbo, Washington, says, "A good example of how we in naturopathic medicine use the healing force in the body is what we do or don't do when a child has a fever. Often times a fever is a way that the body rids itself of a bacteria that only grows in certain temperatures.

"Most parents say, 'My child has a fever. We have to stop that fever. Give him aspirin or Tylenol.' I tell them, 'Imagine that your child has a helper, which is the immune system.' If you take the aspirin, it's like taking a sledge hammer to your child's immune system and saying, 'Be quiet and sit down!' And it will. You'll win. That helper will be quiet and sit down. But your child will stay sicker longer. There are a number of studies that show antihistamines prolong the course of a cold. But if the fever or cold is allowed to run its course, the body eliminates the problem and the child gets healthy."[13]

The role of a fever as healing process may seem strange to many health care consumers who are used to using medications to eliminate its presence. Yet, many systems of healing and medicine throughout the world since ancient times have recognized the healing wisdom of letting a fever run its course.

Clinical Nutrition

Clinical nutrition has been one of the main cornerstones of naturopathic medicine since its inception. Studies from around the world, in a variety of medical traditions, have validated the benefits of naturopathic's nutritional principles. A vast number of documented cases of physical problems, including heart disease and diabetes, have been helped by nutrition, without unpleasant side effects or complications.

Naturopathic theory suggests that most illnesses are caused by digestive disturbances, which have led to a toxic environment in the body. As the body is overwhelmed by toxins it cannot eliminate, the health or strength of the body breaks down and symptoms of various illnesses surface. Nutritional changes are a main component to changing the diseased situation because today's processed foods and poor eating habits are the source of many of the body's toxins.

To treat chronic illnesses, many times nutritional changes are the first step toward healing in naturopathic medicine. For example, simple vegetable soups are often recommended because, as they are easy to digest and assimilate, they provide the body with vitamin and mineral nutrients without adding toxins to the body.

Hydrotherapy

If nutritional therapy is the first cornerstone of naturopathic medicine, then hydrotherapy is the second. Hydrotherapy improves digestive function by bringing additional blood (and all of its healing components) to the inner organs. The most common form of hydrotherapy is called the "constitutional," where two towels dipped in hot water, then squeezed, are placed on the front of the patient for five minutes. The hot towels are replaced with one cold towel for ten minutes. The same procedure is done on the back of the patient. During the hot portion of the hydrotherapy, the upper blood vessels are dilated while the deeper ones constrict. The cold portion of the treatment constricts the outer blood vessels but dilates the internal ones. The combination drives more blood to both the inner and outer systems, allowing the body to bring more healing nutrients to its organs and to carry away toxins.

Homeopathy

Homeopathy is used by many naturopaths and is a primary treatment in their practices. Based on the "law of similars," it uses minuscule doses of naturally occurring substances to treat illness. Naturopaths have found that homeopathy fits well into their philosophical principles, since it stimulates the body's own immune system without producing unpleasant side effects. It is also documented to be effective for many illnesses, including migraines, headaches, rheumatoid arthritis, acute diarrhea, flu, and allergies.

The history of homeopathy's use spans two hundred years. Many countries embrace it as a viable healing treatment, including England, whose Royal family retains the services of a homeopath for their personal health care.

Herbs

Herbs are used by naturopathic physicians as medicine. As such, they can be extremely powerful and beneficial when used in the right dosage and in the correct combination with other herbs.

Though herbs are the main ingredient for some of the drugs used in conventional medicine, N.D.'s use herbs in a different manner than M.D.'s use them. Most drugs prescribed by M.D.'s are intended to impose an external order on the body. For example, a medicine prescribed to lower blood pressure forces the body to lower the pressure but doesn't correct the reason why the body has increased the pressure in the first place. Therefore, many patients taking blood pressure medicine as prescribed by a conventional medical doctor must continue to take blood pressure medication for the rest of their lives. Regrettably, the patient also endures the probable side effects: impotency, sexual dysfunction, and nervousness.

In contrast, an N.D.'s goal is not to impose an outside order but to correct the underlying problem. In the case of a weakened heart, an N.D. would accomplish this by using herbs that nourish and strengthen the heart, such as hawthorne berry, or herbs that disperse congestion or toxins in the body, such as dandelion root. When strengthening and detoxification occur, a patient's vitality becomes stronger, the root cause of the illness is addressed, and a permanent recovery becomes possible.

Chinese Medicine

The treatments and diagnostic techniques as well as the fundamentals of Chinese medicine are a part of all naturopathic physician's training at the accredited medical colleges. Some naturopaths do advanced training and become licensed practitioners of Chinese medicine, using Chinese herbs, acupuncture, and acupressure in their practice.

Natural Childbirth

Natural childbirth is offered by some naturopathic physicians in either a home or a clinic environment. N.D.'s are trained in natural prenatal and postnatal care involving noninvasive, nonpharmaceutical treatments. Through their treatments and techniques, N.D.'s continuously screen to make sure the mother and child are in a low-risk state. One important screening involves monitoring the mother's diet and supplements to ensure that the mother's inner nutrients are sufficient to create a healthy, normal baby. Naturopathic theory suggests that adequate nutrient levels in the mother minimize childbirth risks.

Naturopathic physicians believe counseling is an important component of their jobs as facilitators for childbirth care. Dr. Jared Zeff, a naturopathic physician and licensed practitioner of Chinese medicine, says that he requires the mother and partner to invite him and his assistant to dinner. "One factor that we found that can significantly disrupt a birth is the emotional state of the mother," he says. "If, during our dinner time with the mother/couple, we notice any significant stress, then we know that counseling will be needed to minimize the mother's emotional distress so that she can relax during labor and have a normal birth."[15]

N.D.'s use many different treatments during the various stages of gestation and birth, including some that most conventional doctors are unfamiliar with. For instance, some N.D.'s use homeopathy before labor begins to help a breach baby turn to the correct "head-down" position. In some cases, the homeopathic remedy Pulsatilla is used when the baby is not yet in the right position for delivery. Naturopathic physicians have seen that within twelve hours of giving a dose of Pulsatilla to the mother, the baby turns by itself. Another remedy used by naturopathic physicians is a preparation of the herb cottonroot. This herb, usually given to the mother in tincture form, helps bring the placenta down if she has not delivered it within a normal time.

Although N.D.'s are well trained in most birthing situations, they are also quick to refer mothers to the appropriate M.D. or hospital if a risk is present that disqualifies the mother and child from a natural childbirth experience.

Counseling and Stress Management

Naturopathic physicians believe the patient's emotional and psychological makeup can greatly influence the patient's ability to heal. Therefore, they are trained in many psychological techniques, including counseling, stress management, hypnotherapy, biofeedback, and nutritional balancing.

Minor Surgery

Most people would be surprised to know that minor surgery is a part of some naturopathic physicians' practices. In addition to natural treatments of illnesses, N.D.'s are also trained to mend surface wounds; to remove unwanted foreign masses, cysts, and other superficial bodies with local anesthesia; as well as to perform circumcisions, skin lesion removal, hemorrhoid surgery, and setting of fractures.

Ayurvedic Medicine

Ayurvedic medicine is an ancient system of holistic medicine and healing from India. Its focus is on treating the whole person with diet, nutrition, and lifestyle recommendations. One of the key components of this system of healing is an appreciation of the role that one's vital energy, called "prana," plays in the healing process. Bastyr University now offers a specialization in this ancient system of medicine. As a result, some N.D.'s have earned specialty degrees in ayurvedic medicine and have incorporated it into their practices.

Physical Medicine

Naturopathic physicians use a combination of manipulative therapies, which move soft tissue as well as skeletal bones. These are collectively called naturopathic manipulative therapy and in some ways are similar to the techniques used by osteopathic physicians, chiropractors, massage therapists, and body workers in that structure is realigned to support the innate healing process of the body.

Not all naturopathic doctors use this as a major component of their practice. However, when other treatments fail to bring the desired response, then manipulative therapies can be helpful. One gentleman who had tried a wide range of treatments to correct the weakness and pain he felt in his own right arm went to his N.D. for manipulative treatments. The N.D. found that the man had a combination of muscle spasm from stress and spinal misalignment. As a result, the nerve flow necessary for normal muscular activity was being blocked. The N.D. treated this man with manipulative therapy. The result: the gentleman felt better than he had in six months.

Misalignment of the spinal vertebrae as well as other skeletal structures can be the cause of pain or even illness in some cases. The return of vertebrae, bones, and joints to their optimal position can eliminate pain in as little as one treatment.

Health Condition that Respond Well to Naturopathic Medicine

Naturopathic medicine is beneficial for a wide range of physical illnesses and conditions. Naturopaths claim that their ability to determine the underlying cause of the illness and to stimulate the body's own healing ability is why their medicine can be so effective where other systems of medicine are not.

One area where modern naturopathic medicine has been very effective is in the natural treatment of women's health problems. One series of clinical research studies for women suffering from cervical dysplasia (abnormal Pap smears) produced results in which of the forty-three women in the study, thirty-eight returned to normal Pap smears and normal tissue biopsy by using naturopathic medical treatments. Naturopathic medical formulas are also effectively being used as a natural alternative to hormone replacement therapy for women.[16]

An excellent example of naturopathic medical principles in action is the recent success of Dean Ornish, M.D., director of the Preventive Medicine Research Institute in Sausalito, California, in his work with heart disease. Dr. Ornish found that his patients with chronic coronary heart disease could actually reverse their conditions without drugs or surgery, a concept that before his study was not only discounted, but unheard of by the conventional medical profession. This extraordinary feat was accomplished through an extremely low-fat diet, stress reduction through meditation and yoga practices, modest exercise, and weekly participation in an emotional support group.[17]

Dr. Ornish's success validated naturopathic medicine's basic tenets and treatment approaches. Not only that, healing through nutrition, exercise, and stress management has now been recognized by many insurance companies, who reimburse for Dr. Ornish's program as an alternative to expensive and risky heart bypass surgery.

Another area where naturopathic medicine has proven to be effective is in preventative medicine and health maintenance. "I think the best position for N.D.'s is in the family practice," Dr. Konrad Kail, a practicing naturopathic physician, says. "Naturopaths are the only physicians who have primary skills in health/risk analysis and disease prevention. We find that people do want more time with their physician, to be educated, to be given less toxic therapies. Most people are as yet unaware that naturopaths provide just those things." Kail says some of the benefits of using a naturopathic doctor are safer medicine, quicker recovery time, and, especially, prevention of future illness. "I tell my patients what they can do at home to keep themselves healthy," he says. "If we do our job right, then they don't have to see a [conventional] doctor as much. That saves money."[17]

Also, given that naturopaths are trained in natural childbirth, with their noninvasive and natural treatments, N.D.'s are able to avoid many of the complications associated with childbirth. The result is that births overseen by N.D.'s require far fewer cesarean sections than with conventional medical care.

Naturopathic medicine, although effective, does have its limitations. "The areas of expertise and efficacy of naturopathic medicine are not the same as conventional medicine," Dr. Zeff explains. "Conventional medicine excels in acute trauma care. We do not. If I were in an automobile accident, I'd want them to take me to a hospital where they can patch me up. The areas where I would not go to a naturopath are acute trauma, childbirth emergency, and orthopedic problems that require orthopedic surgery."[19]

Naturopathic medicine has been shown to be an effective approach for the treatment of ear inflammations, infections, and respiratory illnesses, as well as degenerative illnesses. Recently the National Institutes of Health took note of naturopathic medicine's success with terminal diseases and granted Bastyr University almost $1 million to research the effects of alternative therapies on HIV and AIDS patients. Leanna Standish, N.D., Ph.D., research director at Bastyr University of Natural Health Sciences and advisor to the Office of Alternative Medicine, states that initial research has found enhanced immune response and a decline in the progression of AIDS, when compared to the control study who only received conventional medical therapy.[20]

Whether patients need help in health maintenance or a reversal of a devastating disease, naturopathic medicine is a viable option worthy of consideration. If you decide to try the skills and expertise of a naturopathic physician, use the following questions to help you make your decision.

Get Good Referrals

The best referral source for licensed naturopathic physicians who have graduated from an accredited four-year naturopathic medical college is the American Association of Naturopathic Physicians (AANP). For a small fee, they will send you a list of qualified members who have satisfied their stringent requirements.

Screen the Candidates

Once you have a few naturopathic physicians to investigate, call their offices and ask to speak to someone on the staff. Asking well-targeted questions can assist you in determining if this is a good doctor for you. Here are a few suggestions:

What is the doctor's educational background?

If naturopathic medicine is new to you, it would be ideal if you could work with an N.D. who has completed all the hours of study and clinical residency to graduate from one of the three accredited naturopathic colleges: Bastyr University of Natural Sciences in Seattle, Washington; National College of Naturopathic Medicine in Portland, Oregon; the Canadian College of Naturopathic Medicine in Toronto, Ontario, Canada. A fourth college, Southwest College of Naturopathic Medicine and Health Sciences in Scottsdale, Arizona, is in the accreditation process.

However, since there are only about one thousand naturopathic physicians from these medical schools practicing across the nation, it is possible that a graduate of one of these institutions will not be available to you. In that case, you will need to determine if you want to work with a respected practicing naturopath in your area who received their education and training from other sources, such as competent apprenticeship programs and other viable training. Given that this particular group of naturopaths has not necessarily met the high standards required by the AANP, it is extremely important to use seven to ten years of full-time clinical experience as a guide when determining the competency of a naturopath who has not been formally trained at one of the accredited naturopathic medical schools.

Be very careful to thoroughly investigate N.D.'s who are not graduates of the three accredited naturopathic colleges. Not all "naturopaths" with the initials "N.D." after their name have competent training or the necessary expertise. For instance, some practitioners have been awarded Doctors of Naturopathy ("N.D.") after graduating from a mail order school. These graduates have had possibly no clinical residency and significantly fewer hours of education, than required of graduates of the accredited naturopathic medical colleges. Training from a mail order school is considered insufficient to legally gain licensure as an N.D. in the states that license naturopathic physicians as primary care providers.

Knowing your practitioner is a well trained, licensed N.D. assures a dependable level of competence. Someone who does not have that background can certainly be a risky choice and must be thoroughly investigated before beginning treatment.

Does the naturopath have experience with my condition?

Find out how many patients with your health care problem this doctor has successfully helped. The higher the number of successes by the naturopath, the better for you. Ask to talk to some of those patients. Make sure all your questions about their background, training, and expertise have been answered to your satisfaction before beginning treatment.

What is the doctor's specialty?

In most cases, in naturopathic medicine the answer to this question will be given in the types of treatment the N.D. specializes in rather than in specific physical conditions. Dr. Zeff explains, "We don't tend to specialize in systems like medical conventional doctors do, but we tend to create affinities for various therapeutic methods."[21] For instance, due to Dr. Kail's training in conventional medicine, he tends to prescribe antibiotics to avoid bacterial complications, while Dr.

Jared Zeff, who is also a licensed acupuncturist, tends to use more alternative treatments.

Does the doctor use health care techniques not taught in his or her formal training at medical school? If so, what are they, what training has the doctor had in them, and how long have they used them in practice?

Naturopathic medical education includes a wide variety of alternative health care modalities, but not all. Make sure your doctor is well trained in any technique that he or she may recommend for your recovery. Check for credit hours, board certifications, and certificates of completion.

Will my insurance cover naturopathic care?

There are about seventy health insurance companies that cover naturopathic medical fees at this time. Most naturopathic offices carry a list of insurance carriers that cover naturopathic medicine and should be able to verify whether your insurance company will reimburse you for their services.

Is this N.D. licensed?

At this writing, there are twelve states that license N.D.'s as primary-care providers: Alaska, Arizona, Connecticut, Florida, Hawaii, Maine, Montana, New Hampshire, Oregon, Utah, Vermont, and Washington. It is believed that by the year 2010, all fifty states will license naturopathic physicians.

If you live in a state where N.D.'s are not yet licensed, but you would still like to work with a naturopathic physician, there are four types of practitioners who call themselves "naturopaths" or "N.D.'s" that you will find in an "unlicensed" state.

The first type of practitioner:

• Has graduated from an accredited naturopathic medical school

• Is a recognized member of the American Association of Naturopathic Physicians

• Is licensed to practice in one of the "licensable" states

This practitioner is qualified to see you for almost any health condition.

The second type of practitioner:

- Has not graduated from one of the accredited naturopathic medical schools

- May have received a degree or certification from a correspondence school

- Has at least seven years of clinical experience through apprenticeship with a qualified naturopath coupled with full-time personal practice

This practitioner may be qualified enough to help you. However, it is essential that you investigate their exact education and training to make sure they are competent for your needs. Jim Massey, N.D., of Portland, Oregon, admits, "Not all effective healers have initials after their names."[22]

An example of an exceptional naturopathic practitioner who does not have the "N.D." initials after her name is Yvonne Sklar of Hermosa Beach, California. Yvonne is proficient at integrating holistic health alternatives and has provided service for thousands of people worldwide over the last twenty-five years. She earned her Master Herbalist Certification from John Christopher's School of Natural Healing in Utah, and received her certification in iridology from Bernard Jensen, D.C., and is a direct protégé of his. She has also received extensive training in fasting and tissue cleansing procedures. Yvonne is currently working alongside Dr. Hans Gruenn, M.D., at his practice in Marina Del Rey, California. Her main diagnostic and treatment tools are iridology, nutrition, and herbs.

Finding a naturopathic practitioner who is not an "N.D." and yet is also well trained and experienced like Yvonne is unusual, but not impossible. Again, if you are interested in trying naturopathic medicine but do not have an N.D. in your area, ask other respected alternative providers if they know of a good naturopath. Be sure to investigate the naturopath's training thoroughly.

The third type of practitioner:

- Has not graduated from one of the accredited naturopathic medical schools

- Received his or her degree from a correspondence school

- Has not gained enough training and experience to competently treat you in naturopathic medicine

We do not recommend that you work with practitioners in this category.

The fourth type of practitioner:

- Has no formal educational training

- Has voluntarily designated him or herself a "Naturopath" or an "N.D."

- Has little or no training to competently treat you

Working with someone in this category can be dangerous. We do not recommend practitioners in this category.

Take extra screening precautions before agreeing to treatment with any practitioners of naturopathic medicine who are not graduates of one of the three accredited naturopathic medical colleges.

Interview the Candidate

During an interview with a naturopathic physician, find out the personal philosophy of the naturopath. "I would need to know that I could trust the doctor and if they were well trained," Dr. Zeff suggests. "I would talk to them about what their ideas are about the nature of disease, the nature of my problem, and what approach they would take to improve it. I would ask how long I could expect improvement to take and what kinds of costs are involved. The most important thing is to get a sense of who this person is, what they have to offer, as well as their credentials. You are an individual. So choose someone who fits with you."[24]

If you're looking for an N.D. who is caring and capable, you may find your search fairly easy since naturopathic physicians value the healing power that can happen in the relationship between doctor and patient. Most take the time and effort to develop a good rapport with their patients.

What to Expect during a Naturopathic Medical Appointment

Naturopathic physicians use specific treatment(s) that can include homeopathy, Ayurveda, and Chinese medicine, or the traditional naturopathic approach of nutrition, herbology, and hydrotherapy in their practices. These "specialties," in addition to the specific health condition of the patient, make a session with each naturopath a unique experience. However, there are some standard procedures that all naturopathic physicians use.

Cost and Insurance

Cost

According to the American Association of Naturopathic Physicians [AANP], sessions with naturopathic physicians are about half the cost of visiting an M.D. Because naturopaths primarily rely on their own diagnostic skills, costs for extensive tests are usually minimal. This can substantially reduce the cost of naturopathic health care.

Also, naturopathic physicians are well trained in preventative medicine. Many insurance companies are realizing the long-term savings of keeping their plan members healthy. Naturopathic physicians excel at preventative medical techniques and can pass those long-term savings on to you.

Initial office visits are usually between $75 and $100 and follow-ups are in the range of $35-$50. The prescribed supplements are usually vitamin, mineral, herbal, and/or homeopathic. Each of these supplements are far less expensive than prescriptions filled at the pharmacy. However, in the states of Arizona, Oregon, and Washington, N.D.'s are licensed to prescribe antibiotics, thyroid medicine, progesterone, as well as other drugs that may end up costing you more.

Insurance

As mentioned above, a growing number of insurance companies have recognized the value of preventative health care, a specialty of naturopathic medicine. For this reason, naturopathic medicine is being covered by more and more insurance plans. If you are fortunate enough to live in the states of Connecticut or Washington, naturopathic medical coverage is mandatory by law from all health insurance companies.

For a list of insurance carriers that cover naturopathic medicine, call the AANP or your local naturopathic physician's office. Many N.D.'s carry a list of insurance providers who cover their services.

One insurance plan that has given special attention to naturopathic coverage is American Western Life Insurance Company of Foster City, California. Their "Wellness" medical director, Marcel Hernandez, is an N.D. American Western Life provides a twenty-four-hour hot line where you can talk directly to a licensed naturopathic physician at any time, day or night. In addition, they cover all naturopathic treatments, including homeopathy, nutritional counseling, Ayurveda, massage, and physical therapy.

Education, Training and Licensing

Education and Training

Naturopathic physicians are well educated in the basic clinical sciences as well as natural and alternative diagnostic and treatment methods. According to the American Association of Naturopathic Physicians, "Naturopathic physicians (N.D.'s) are general practitioners trained as specialists in natural medicine. They are educated in the conventional medical sciences, but they are not orthodox medical doctors (M.D.'s). Naturopathic physicians treat disease and restore health using therapies from the sciences of clinical nutrition, herbal medicine, homeopathy, physical medicine, exercise therapy, counseling, acupuncture, natural childbirth, and hydrotherapy. They tailor these approaches to the needs of an individual patient."[27]

Graduates of accredited four-year naturopathic medical schools are justifiably proud of their education. "Essentially, naturopathic medical training is similar to conventional medical training," Dr. Zeff explains. "The first two years are virtually the same as any medical school: anatomy, physiology, microbiology, biochemistry, etc. They are taught at the same level as any other medical school. If you look at the number of hours in our classroom situation, you'll find in most cases the number of hours we spend exceeds most medical schools." He adds, "We are required fifteen hundred hours of clinical education as a minimum to graduate from the school. This is under the supervision of naturopathic doctors."[28] Medical educators and legislators have been impressed with the high standard of education required of naturopathic physicians.

Licensing

There are currently twelve states in the U.S. and five provinces in Canada that license naturopathic doctors as primary care physicians: Alaska, Arizona, Connecticut, Florida, Hawaii, Maine, Montana, New Hampshire, Oregon, Utah, Vermont, Washington, Alberta, British Columbia, Manitoba, Ontario, and Saskatchewan. All other states in the U.S. have licensable, trained naturopaths practicing. In these states, many N.D.'s who graduated from an accredited four-year college opt to apply for licenses in other health care modalities, such as acupuncture or chiropractic, in order to stay protected by law. Others choose to practice without protection of the law. In most states, naturopathic medicine is "alegal" (neither "legal" nor "illegal"). In these states, naturopathic medicine is neither protected nor regulated. Regrettably, this can be somewhat confusing for the health care consumer.

Jim Massey, N.D., says, "When I was in North Carolina, there must have been thirty people practicing as N.D.'s. Only four of them had been to four-year medical schools. You could pay $25 and set up a tax I.D. number and start practicing immediately. You'd have to kill somebody before they'd come after you for practicing without a license. It isn't fair to the public to be duped by these people with the phony initials after their names."[29]

Again, to protect yourself and your health, call the American Association of Naturopathic Physicians. They represent the largest contingency of licensed naturopathic physicians who have graduated from an accredited school.

Licensed naturopathic physicians are filling an important need as primary health care providers who are experts in nontoxic, noninvasive treatments. As highly skilled and well educated about the human body as graduates of Stanford or Yale medical schools, they bring the best of ancient natural treatments and scientific research to their medicine. Naturopathic medicine could serve you as well as the growing number of Americans who are calling their naturopathic physician first for their health care needs.

Notes

1. Senator Claiborne Pell. Personal letter to Mrs. Hillary Rodham Clinton, March 31, 1993.

2. Burton Goldberg. *Alternative Medicine: The Definitive Guide* (Future Medicine Publishing, 1993), 360.

3. Bastyr University press release, October 4, 1994.

4. "Naturopathic and Major Medical Schools, Comparative Curricula." Document from the American Association of Naturopathic Physicians.

5. "Twenty Questions About Naturopathic Medicine." Document from the American Association of Naturopathic Medicine.

6. "Naturopathic and Major Medical Schools: Comparative Curricula." Document from the American Association of Naturopathic Physicians.

7. William Collinge. *The American Holistic Health Association Complete Guide to Alternative Medicine* (Warner Books, 1996), 125.

8. NIH. *Alternative Medicine: Expanding Medical Horizons* (U.S. Government Printing Office, 1993), 88.

9. American Association of Naturopathic Physicians brochure.

10. Ibid.

11. Bastyr University press release, February 27, 1995.

12. American Association of Naturopathic Physicians brochure.

13. Stephen Speidel, N.D. Personal interview, Summer 1990.

14. Jared Zeff, N.D., L.Ac., Personal interview, June 1996.

16. NIH. *Alternative Medicine: Expanding Medical Horizons* (U.S. Government Printing Office, 1993), 89.

17. Dean Ornish, M.D. *Dr. Dean Ornish's Program for Reversing Heart Disease* (Ivy Books, 1996).

18. Konrad Kail, N.D. Personal interview, Fall 1990.

19. Jared Zeff, N.D., L.Ac. Personal interview, June 1996.

20. "NIH Exploratory Study Coordination Centers for Alternative Medical Research." NIH Office of Alternative Medicine press release, June 1995.

21. Jared Zeff, N.D., L.Ac. Personal interview, June 1996.

22. Jim Massey, N.D. Personal interview, August 1990.

23. Yvonne Sklar. Personal correspondence, July 1996.

24. Jared Zeff, N.D., L.Ac. Personal interview, June 1996.

25. Konrad Kail, N.D. Personal interview, Fall 1990.

26. Ibid.

27. American Association of Naturopathic Physicians brochure.

28. Jared Zeff, N.D., L.Ac. Personal interview, June 1996.

29. Jim Massey, N.D. Personal interview, Summer 1990.

Chapter 13

Yoga

All people wish to be happy. This seemingly simple desire appears to elude the best-intentioned efforts of even the most intelligent among us. Yet almost everyone has had glimpses of deep peacefulness when they have felt connected both to themselves, to others, and to nature.

Curiously, the state of feeling good and whole does not seem to be something we can order up on demand but rather appears to happen spontaneously. In such moments we experience a sense of translucence such that that which we see, feel, sense, hear, or touch no longer feels separate from us but is experienced as a part of our own totality. When our hand resting over the heart of the beloved merges and becomes one with his or her body, when we become the same midnight sky that fills us with awe, we remember, however briefly, our place in the scheme of things. These brief flickers of remembrance imbue our vision with freshness and innocence so that we can see things as they truly are. Because these moments of lucidity are so blissful, we wish that they may become the base state of our lives rather than the brief and oftentimes tenuous experience to which such happiness is usually assigned. These moments of clarity have nothing to do with the caricatures of happiness presented to us through the media or popular culture. These moments have always been there. The beloved's heartbeat and the sky have always been there. These moments are simply awaiting our arrival.

"What Is Yoga?" © 2000 Donna Farhi, excerpted from *Yoga Mind, Body, and Spirit: A Return to Wholeness*, (Henry Holt and Co., April 2000); reprinted with permission.

Yoga is a technology for arriving in this present moment. It is a means of waking up from our spiritual amnesia, so that we can remember all that we already know. It is a way of remembering our true nature, which is essentially joyful and peaceful. Developed as a pragmatic science by ancient seers centuries ago, yoga is a practice that any person, regardless of age, sex, race, or religious belief, can use to realize her full potential. It is a means of staying in intimate communication with the formative core matrix of yourself and those forces that serve to bind all living beings together. As you establish and sustain this intimate connection, this state of equanimity becomes the core of your experience rather than the rare exception.

Through observing nature and through intense self-observation and inquiry, the ancient yogis were able to codify the conditions that must be present for realizing our intrinsic wholeness. Although such realization can occur spontaneously, more often than not it is the result of a sustained commitment to practice over a lifetime. This is not to imply that yoga is a goal which we strive toward, or that there is some kind of chronological progression toward "self-improvement." Rather, it is the recognition that each individual can achieve understanding only through his own exploration and discovery, and that all of life is a continual process of refinement which allows us to see more clearly. When we clean the windshield of our car, we suddenly see the road ahead as bright and defined. The road, the image before us, is exactly as it was before we cleaned the window. The trees are the same green, the sky the same vivid blue, and the markers just as defined, only now we see what is there. We start to be able to see the potholes in the road ahead and to avoid them. We start to remember such dangerous roads and steer our way clear to safer routes in the future. In the same way, yoga is not about self-improvement or making ourselves better. It is a process of deconstructing all the barriers we may have erected that prevent us from having an authentic connection with ourselves and with the world. This tenet is an extremely important one because the effort to change and improve ourselves is fraught with the risk of subtle self-aggression that only produces more unhappiness. We cannot strive toward something that we already are.

Nonetheless, there is work to be done. And this work is not about following a formula, or strictly adhering to rules, because yoga is not a paint-by-numbers affair. Nor does yoga require blind faith in an outside authority or dogma. Nor is it a religion, although the practice of its central precepts inevitably draws each individual to the direct experience of those truths on which religion rests. Rather, yoga is a way of living and being that makes real happiness possible. Yoga is also a science that incorporates a broad range of practices and techniques that can be tailored and adapted, to best suit your personal constitution and personality. We are not asked to believe anything until we have experimented, tested, and found our direct experience to be sound. The great paradox of this "work" is that there is no reward to strive toward, because the practice is the reward. In the very moment you focus your attention by coming back into your body, your breath, and your immediate sensate reality, you will experience a deep sense of vibrant stillness. This feeling is so pleasurable, so joyful and revitalizing that you will be drawn toward lifestyle choices that nourish your well being. This work is not about forcing yourself to give up anything, because that which is no longer nourishing to you will gradually drop away effortlessly. There is no waiting and no delayed gratification because yoga is both the means and the result, and the seed of all that is possible is present at the very beginning. This experience of stillness is possible in the first ten minutes of your first yoga class. It is possible in this very breath. Sadly, if we approach and practice yoga with the same cultural dictum of striving and effort, force and self-coercion that we may have applied to other aspects of our lives, we may practice diligently for decades while never allowing our self to appreciate the simple truth of its own wholeness.

Although there are many branches to the tree of yoga, from devotional methods to more intellectual approaches, from schools that emphasize service toward others to those that focus on physical purification, Patanja Sutras, clearly defines an eight-limbed path (ashtanga) that forms the structural framework for whatever emphasis upon which an individual wishes to concentrate. The Yoga Sutras, or "threads," consist of four books produced sometime in the third century before Christ. Such was the clarity of Patanjali's vision of wholeness that he consolidated the entirety of yoga philosophy in a series of 196 lucid aphorisms. Each thread of the Yoga Sutras is revealed as a part of a woven fabric, with each aphorism merely a mark or color within the whole pattern. The threads, however, begin to make sense only through a direct experience of their meaning. This is not a linear process but rather an organic one in which colors and markings gradually become more clear until a pattern forms. And this pattern that Patanjali weaves for us is a description of the process of unbinding our limited ideas about ourselves and becoming free.

The eight limbs of yoga are traditionally presented as a hierarchical progression, but this linear progression toward an idealized goal tends only to reinforce the dualistic idea that yoga is something to "get." It may be more helpful to imagine the eight limbs as the arms and legs of a body—connected to one another through the central body of yoga just as a child's limbs grow in proportion to one another, whatever limb of practice we focus upon inevitably causes the other limbs to grow as well. People who begin yoga through the limb of meditation are often later drawn to practice more physical postures. Those who are drawn to vigorous physical practice later find themselves being drawn into the quieter, more meditative practices just as each limb is essential for the optimal functioning of your body, every limb of yoga practice is important. Growth in practice happens naturally when a person is sincere in her wish to grow.

The eight limbs emanating from a central core consist of the following:

- *Yamas and Niyamas:* Ten ethical precepts that allow us to be at peace with ourselves, our family, and our community.

- *Asanas:* Dynarmic internal dances in the form of postures. These help to keep the body strong, flexible, and relaxed. Their practice strengthens the nervous system and refines our process of inner perception.

- *Pranayama:* Roughly defined as breathing practices, and more specifically defined as practices that help us to develop constancy in the movement of prana, or life force.

- *Pratyahara:* The drawing of one's attention toward silence rather than toward things.

- *Dharana:* Focusing attention and cultivating inner perceptual awareness.

- *Dhyana:* Sustaining awareness under all conditions.

- *Samadhi:* The return of the mind into original silence.

The greater part of this chapter will focus on the most down-to-earth practices—the asanas and the practices of breathing and meditation. These form an embodied approach to spiritual practice, where we use the body and all our sensual capacities in the service of regeneration and transformation. This is contrasted to many approaches in which the body is seen as an obstacle that must be transcended. Let us first look at the core principles for living, the yamas and niyamas that form the central vein from which all other yoga practices spring.

The Ten Living Principles

The first limb, or the yamas, consists of characteristics observed and codified by wise people since the beginning of time as being central to any life lived in freedom. They are mostly concerned with how we use our energy in relationship to others and in a subtler sense, our relationship to ourselves. The sages recognized that stealing from your neighbor was likely to promote discord, lying to your wife would cause suffering, and violence begets more violence; the results are hardly conducive to living a peaceful life. The second limb, the niyamas, constitutes a code for living in a way that fosters the soulfulness of the individual and has to do with the choices we make. The yamas and niyamas are emphatic descriptions of what we are when we are connected to our source. Rather than a list of dos and don'ts, they tell us that our fundamental nature is compassionate, generous, honest, and, peaceful.

In the West we are taught from an early age that what we do and what we own sole components for measuring whether we are "successful." We measure our success and that of others through this limited vantage point, judging and dismissing anything that falls outside these narrow parameters. What yoga teaches us is that who we are and how we are constitute the ultimate proof of a life lived in freedom. If you do not truly believe this, it is likely that you will measure success in your yoga practice through the achievement of external forms. This tendency has produced a whole subculture of yoga in the West that is nothing more than sophisticated calisthenics, with those who can bend the farthest or do the most extraordinary yoga postures being deemed masters.

Because it's easy to measure physical prowess, we may compare ourselves to others who are more flexible, or more "advanced" in their yoga postures, getting trapped in the belief that the forms of the practice are the goal. These outward feats do not necessarily constitute any evidence of a balanced practice or a balanced life. What these first central precepts the yamas and niyamas ask us to remember is that the techniques and forms are not goals in themselves but vehicles for getting to the essence of who we are.

One of our greatest challenges as Westerners practicing yoga is to learn to perceive progress through "invisible" signs, signs that are quite often unacknowledged by the culture at large. Are we moving toward greater kindness, patience, or tolerance toward others? Are we able to remain calm and centered even when others around us become agitated and angry? How we speak, how we treat others, and how we live are more subjective qualities and attributes we need to learn to recognize in ourselves as a testament to our own progress and as gauges of authenticity in our potential teachers. When we remain committed to our most deeply held values we can begin to discern the difference between the appearance of achievement and the true experience of transformation, and thereby free ourselves to pursue those things of real value.

As you read through the precepts that follow, take the time to dwell upon their relevance to your life and to consider your own personal experiences both past and present in reference to them. You can take almost any situation that arises in your life and consider it from the vantage point of one or more of these precepts. It can also be valuable consciously to choose a precept that you'd like to explore in depth for a month or even a year at a time investigating how the precept works in all aspects of your life. And last, the way in which you approach the practices that follow in this book, and your underlying intentions, will ultimately determine whether your practice bears fruit. As you progress in your yoga practice, take the time to pause frequently and ask "Who am I becoming through this practice? Am I becoming the kind of person I would like to have as a friend?"

Yamas—Wise Characteristics

Ahimsa—Compassion for All Living Things

Ahimsa is usually translated as nonviolence, but this precept goes far and beyond the limited penal sense of not killing others. First and foremost we have to learn how to be nonviolent toward ourselves. If we were able to play back the often unkind, unhelpful, and destructive comments and judgments silently made toward our self in any given day, this may give us some idea of the enormity of the challenge of self-acceptance. If we were to speak these thoughts out loud to another person, we would realize how truly devastating violence to the self can be. In truth, few of us would dare to be as unkind to others as we are to ourselves. This can be as subtle as the criticism of our body when we look in the mirror in the morning, or when we denigrate our best efforts. Any thought, word, or action that prevents us (or someone else) from growing and living freely is one that is harmful.

Extending this compassion to all living creatures is dependent on our recognition of the underlying unity of all sentient beings. When we begin to recognize that the streams and rivers of the earth are no different from the blood coursing through our arteries, it becomes difficult to remain indifferent to the plight of the world. We naturally find ourselves wanting to protect all living things. It becomes difficult to toss a can into a stream or carve our names in the bark of a tree, for each act would be an act of violence toward ourselves as well. Cultivating an attitude and mode of behavior of harmlessness does not mean that we no longer feel strong emotions such as anger, jealously, or hatred. Learning to see everything through the eyes of compassion demands that we look at even these aspects of our self with acceptance. Paradoxically, when we welcome our feelings of anger, jealousy, or rage rather than see them as signs of our spiritual failure, we can begin to understand the root causes of these feelings and move beyond them. By getting close enough to our own violent tendencies we can begin to understand the root causes of them and learn to contain these energies for our own well being and for the protection of others. Underneath these feelings we discover a much stronger desire that we all share—to be loved. It is impossible to come to this deeper understanding if we bypass the tough work of facing our inner demons.

In considering ahimsa it's helpful to ask; Are my thoughts, actions, and deeds fostering the growth and well being of all beings?

Satya—Commitment to the Truth

This precept is based on the understanding that honest communication and action form the bedrock of any healthy relationship, community, or government, and that deliberate deception, exaggerations, and mistruths harm others. One of the best ways we can develop this capacity is to practice right speech. This means that when we say something, we are sure of its truth. If we were to follow this precept with commitment, many of us would have a great deal less to say each day! A large part of our everyday comments and conversations are not based upon what we know to be true but are based on our imagination, suppositions, erroneous conclusions, and sometimes out-and-out exaggerations. Gossip is probably the worst form of this miscommunication.

Commitment to the truth isn't always easy, but with practice, it's a great deal less complicated and ultimately less painful than avoidance and self-deception. Proper communication allows us to deal with immediate concerns taking care of little matters before they become big ones.

Probably the hardest form of this practice is being true to our own heart and inner destiny. Confusion and mistrust of our inner values can make it difficult to know the nature of our heart's desire, but even when we become clear enough to recognize what truth means for us, we may lack the courage and conviction to live our truth. Following what we know to be essential for our growth may mean leaving unhealthy relationships or jobs and taking risks that jeopardize our own comfortable position. It may mean making choices that are not supported by consensual reality or ratified by the outer culture. The truth is rarely convenient. One way we can know we are living the truth is that while our choices may not be easy, at the end of the day we feel at peace with ourselves.

Asteya—Not Stealing

Asteya arises out of the understanding that all misappropriation is an expression of a feeling of lack. And this feeling of lack usually comes from a belief that our happiness is contingent on external circumstances and material possessions. Within Western industrialized countries satisfaction can be contingent upon so many improbable conditions and terms that it is not uncommon to spend all of one's time hoping for some better life, and imagining that others (who possess what we do not) have that better life. In constantly looking outside of ourselves for satisfaction, we are less able to appreciate the abundance that already exists. That is what really matters—our health and the riches of our inner life and the joy and love we are able to give and receive from others. It becomes difficult to appreciate that we have hot running water when all we can think about is whether our towels are color-coordinated. How can we appreciate our good fortune in having enough food to eat when we wish we could afford to eat out more often?

The practice of asteya asks us to be careful not to take anything that has not been freely given. This can be as subtle as inquiring whether someone is free to speak with us on the phone before we launch into a tirade about our problems. Or reserving our questions after a class for another time, rather than hoarding a teacher's attention long after the official class time has ended. In taking someone's time that may not have been freely given, we are, in effect, stealing. The paradox of practicing asteya is that when we relate to others from the vantage point of abundance rather than neediness, we find that others are more generous with us and that life's real treasures begin to flow our way.

This may seem unlikely, so let me share an example. Paul was a medical student and past acquaintance who seemed always to be helping others and sharing his seemingly limited resources. One evening when it became too late for a commute home, I offered Paul my guest room for the night. On awakening in the morning I discovered he had cleaned my refrigerator ("It looked like you'd been busy"). Paul had few financial resources but always seemed to be having wonderful dinner feasts to share with his friends. Later, I found out that he worked late at a local health-food restaurant, and, thankful for the extra hours Paul spent helping out, the owner gave him many of the leftover vegetables, breads, and prepared dishes to take home. When a number of friends joined Paul at a holiday home for a week, Paul initiated a special "clean up and dust" party that lasted all day ("Just think how great it will be for the owner when he comes back after his trip overseas . . !").

Paul rarely asked for anything but was always surprising his friends with his new acquisitions. People gave things to Paul all the time—even large items like cars and washing machines—not because they felt sorry for him but because his own sense of intrinsic abundance and his own generosity tended to make you feel that, like him, you had a lot to give.

Not stealing demands that we cultivate a certain level of self-sufficiency so that we do not demand more of others, our family, or our community than we need. It means that we don't take any more than we need, because that would be taking from others. A helpful way of practicing asteya when you find yourself dwelling on the "not enoughs" of your life is to ask: "How is this attitude preventing me from enjoying the things I already have?" Another way of fostering this sense of abundance is to take a moment before going to sleep to dwell on at least one gift in your life. This can be as simple as the gift of having a loving partner or loyal pet, the grace of having good health, or the pleasure of having a garden.

Brahmacharya—Merging with the One

Of all the precepts, the call to brahmacharya is the least understood and the most feared by Westerners. Commonly translated as celibacy, this precept wreaks havoc in the minds and lives of those who interpret brahmacharya as a necessary act of sexual suppression or sublimation. All spiritual traditions and religions have wrestled with the dilemma of how to use sexual energy wisely. Practicing brahmacharya means that we use our sexual energy to regenerate our connection to our spiritual self. It also means that we don't use this energy in any way that might harm another.

147

It doesn't take a genius to recognize that manipulating and using others sexually creates a host of bad feelings, with the top contenders being pain, jealousy, attachment, resentment, and blinding hatred. This is one realm of human experience that is guaranteed to bring out the best and worst in people, so the ancient Yogis went to great lengths to observe and experiment with this particular form of energy. It may be easier to understand brahmacharya if we remove the sexual designation and look at it purely as energy. Brahmacharya means merging one's energy with God. While the communion we may experience through making love with another gives us one of the clearest experiences of this meshing of energies, this experience is meant to be extended beyond discrete events into a way of life—a kind of omnidimensional celebration of Eros in all its forms. Whether we achieve this through feeling our breath as it caresses our lungs, through orgasm, or through celibacy is not important.

Given the pragmatism of the ancient yogis, it is hard to believe that Patanjali would have put forth a precept that would be so undeniably unsuccessful as selfwined denial. The fall from grace of countless gurus who, while admonishing their devotees to practice celibacy, have wantonly misused their own sexual power gives cause to consider more deeply the appropriateness of such an interpretation. When any energy is sublimated or suppressed, it has the tendency to backfire, expressing itself in life-negating ways. This is not to say that celibacy in and of itself is an unsound practice. When embraced joyfully the containment of sexual energy can be enormously self-nourishing and vitalizing and, at the very least, can provide an opportunity to learn how to use this energy wisely. When celibacy is practiced in this way, there is no sense of stopping oneself from doing or having what one really wants. Ultimately it is not a matter of whether we use our sexual energy but how we use it.

In looking at your own relationship to sexual energy, consider whether the ways you express that energy bring you closer to or farther away from your spiritual self.

Aparigraha—Not Grasping

Holding on to things and being free are two mutually exclusive states. The ordinary mind is constantly manipulating reality to get ground underneath it, building more and more concretized images of how things are and how others are, as a way of generating confidence and security. We build self-images and construct concepts and paradigms that feed our sense of certainty, and we then defend this edifice by bending every situation to reinforce our certainty. This would be fine if life were indeed a homogeneous event in which nothing ever changed; but life does change, and it demands that we adapt and change with it. The resistance to change, and tenaciously holding on to things, causes great suffering and prevents us from growing and living life in a more vital and pleasurable way. What yoga philosophy and all the great Buddhist teachings tells us is that solidity is a creation of the ordinary mind and that there never was anything permanent to begin with that we could hold on to. Life would be much easier and substantially less painful if we lived with the knowledge of impermanence as the only constant. As we all have discovered at some time in our lives, whenever we have tried to hold on too tightly to anything, whether it be possessiveness of our partner or our youthful identity, this has only led to the destruction of those very things we most value. Our best security lies in taking down our fences and barricades and allowing ourselves to grow, and through that growth becoming stronger and yet more resilient.

The practice of aparigraha also requires that we look at the way we use things to reinforce our sense of identity. The executive ego loves to believe in its own power but unfortunately requires a retinue of foot soldiers in the way of external objects such as the right clothes, car, house, job, or image to maintain this illusion. Because this executive ego is but an illusion created by our sense of separateness, it requires ever greater and more elaborate strategies to keep it clothed. Although the practice of not grasping may first begin as consciously withdrawing our hand from reaching for external things, eventually the need to reach outward at all diminishes until there is a recognition that that which is essential to us is already at hand.

Niyamas—Codes for Living Soulfully

Shaucha—Purity

Shaucha, or living purely, involves maintaining a cleanliness in body, mind, and environment so that we can experience ourselves at a higher resolution. The word pure comes from the Latin purus, which means clean and unadulterated. When we take in healthy food, untainted by pesticides and unnatural additives, the body starts to function more smoothly. When we read books that elevate our consciousness, see movies that inspire, and associate with gentle people, we are feeding the mind in a way that nourishes our own peacefulness. Creating a home environment that is elegant, simple, and uncluttered generates an atmosphere where we are not constantly distracted by the paraphernalia of yesterday's projects and last year's knickknacks. Shaucha is a testament to the positive power of association.

Practicing shaucha, meaning "that and nothing else," involves making choices about what you want and don't want in your life. Far from self-deprivation or dry piety, the practice of shaucha allows you to experience life more vividly. A clean plate enjoys the sweetness of an apple and the taste of pure water; a clear mind can appreciate the beauty of poetry and the wisdom imparted in a story; a polished table reveals the deep grain of the wood. This practice both generates beauty and allows us to appreciate it in all its many forms.

Santosha—Contentment

Santosha, or the practice of contentment, is the ability to feel satisfied within the container of one's immediate experience. Contentment shouldn't be confused with happiness, for we can be in difficult, even painful circumstances and still find some semblance of contentment if we are able to see things as they are without the conflictual pull of our expectations. Contentment also should not be confused with complacency, in which we allow ourselves to stagnate in our growth. Rather it is a sign that we are at peace with whatever stage of growth we are in and the circumstances we find ourselves in. This doesn't mean that we accept or tolerate unhealthy relationships or working conditions. But it may mean that we practice patience and attempt to live as best we can within our situation until we are able to better our conditions.

Contentment not only implies acceptance of the present but tends to generate the capacity for hopefulness. This may seem contradictory but is not. When you are equanimous within any situation, this strengthens your faith that there is the possibility of living even more fully. This possibility is not held out as something to look forward to, nor does it have the negative effect of making you feel dissatisfied until those hopes are gratified. Rather, the ability to sustain one's spirits even in dire situations, is proof that a central sense of balance is rarely contingent on circumstances. And, sustaining hopefulness, even when there are few signs that things win improve, is one very good way of fostering contentment.

Tapas—Burning Enthusiasm

Literally translated as "fire" or "heat," tapas is the disciplined use of our energy. Because the word discipline has the negative connotation of self-coercion, I take the liberty here of translating this central precept as "burning enthusiasm." When we can generate an attitude of burning ardor, the strength of our convictions generates a momentum that carries us forward. We all know how even a seemingly boring or unpleasant task like cleaning the house can be transformed when we work with vigor and impulsion. Suddenly cleaning the toilet becomes fun, hauling heavy loads invigorating, and dusting the furniture absorbing. Tapas is a way of directing our energy. Like a focused beam of light cutting through the dark, tapas keeps us on track so that we don't waste our time and energy on superfluous or trivial matters. When this energy is strong, so also are the processes of transmutation and metamorphism.

We are not all equally possessed of the disciplined energy of tapas. Some people need to work more earnestly to kindle the flames of tapas, and it is at these times that it is helpful to have a kind of parental consciousness coupled with a good sense of humor. Our actions are then guided by a part of the self that knows what's good for it, which is aided by the ability to laugh in the face of one's neuroses, lethargy, or addictions. Even the laser minds among us have days when it takes a sheer act of will to get out of bed, turn to our studies, or withdraw the hand that reaches for a second slice of cake. If you have little enthusiasm yourself, it can be enormously helpful to seek the company of those who have this quality in abundance. Attending a class with an inspiring teacher or practicing yoga with a friend who has already established a strong practice can help to stimulate tapas within yourself. Once activated, however, the embers of tapas tend to generate more and more heat and momentum, which makes each subsequent effort less difficult. The analogy of a fire is fitting for this precept. Once a fire has completely died out it can take a great deal of effort to start it up again. When you do get a fire to light, the tentative embers must be fed at regular intervals or the fire dies out again. But once the fire is roaring, it is easy to sustain.

For what greater purpose do we need tapas, or discipline? Pema Chödrön, the Abbot of Gampo Abbey in Cape Breton, Nova Scotia, and the author of many books on Tibetan Buddhism, tells us that "what we discipline is not our 'badness' or our 'wrongness.' What we discipline is any form of potential escape from reality." When we're not living in this disciplined awareness, our willing tactics of avoidance create an endless cycle of more suffering for ourselves. These avoidance tactics may temporarily placate our senses, but they create a deep form of unhappiness. On some level we know we're not being true to ourselves or our potential. Discipline is having enough respect for yourself to make choices that truly nourish your well being and provide opportunities for expansive growth. Far from being a kind of medicinal punishment, tapas allows us to direct our energy toward a fulfilled life of meaning and one that is exciting and pleasurable.

Swadhyaya—Self-Study

Any activity that cultivates self-reflective consciousness can be considered swadhyaya. The soul tends to be lured by those activities that will best illuminate it. Because people are so different in their proclivities, one person may be drawn to write, while another will discover herself through painting or athletics. Another person may come to know himself through mastering an instrument, or through service at a hospice. Still another may learn hidden aspects of herself through the practice of meditation. The form that this self-study takes is inconsequential. Whatever the practice, as long as there is an intention to know yourself through it, and the commitment to see the process through, almost any activity can become an opportunity for learning about yourself. Swadhyaya means staying with our process through thick and thin because it's usually when the going gets rough that we have the greatest opportunity to learn about ourselves.

While self-study uncovers our strengths, authentic swadhyaya also ruthlessly uncovers our weakness, foibles, addictions, habit patterns, and negative tendencies. This isn't always the most cheering news. The worst thing we can do at these times is give ourselves the double whammy of both uncovering a soft spot and beating ourselves up for what we perceive as a fatal flaw. At these times, it's important actually to welcome and accept our limitations. When we welcome a limitation, we can get close enough to ourselves to see the roots of our anger, impatience, or self-loathing. We can have a little compassion, for the forces and conditions that molded our behaviors and beliefs, and in so doing develop more skill in handling, containing, and redirecting previously self-destructive tendencies. The degree to which we can do this for ourselves is the degree to which we will be tolerant of other people's weaknesses and flaws. Self-study is a big task.

Self-study also can become psychically incestuous when the same self that may be confused and fragmented attempts to see itself. This is why it can be so helpful (not to mention expedient) to secure the help of a mentor, teacher, or close friend to support your self-study. If you've ever said that someone "just doesn't see himself" and watched him enact the same self-destructive behaviors again and again, just consider how likely it is that you too are blind to your own faults. A skillful mentor, and that can be anyone from a wise aunt to a therapist to a bona fide guru, can find loving ways to help you see yourself as you really are.

Ishvarapranidhana—Celebration of the Spiritual

Life is not inherently meaningful. We make meaning happen through the attention and care we express through our actions. We make meaning happen when we set a table with care, when we light a candle before practicing, or when we remove our shoes before entering a temple. Yoga tells us that the spiritual suffuses everything it is simply that we are too busy, too distracted, or too insensitive to notice the extraordinary omnipresence that dwells in all things. So one of the first ways that we can practice ishvarapranidhana is by putting aside some time each day, even a few minutes, to avail ourselves of an intelligence larger than our own. This might take the form of communing with your garden at dawn, taking a few moments on the bus to breathe slowly and clear your mind, or engaging in a more formal practice such as a daily reading, prayer, ritual, or meditation. This practice requires that we have recognized that there is some omnipresent force larger than ourselves that is guiding and directing the course of our lives. We all have had the experience of looking back at some event in our life that at the time may have seemed painful, confusing and disruptive, but later, in retrospect, made perfect sense in the context of our personal destiny. We recognize that the change that occurred during that time was necessary for our growth, and that we are happier for it. The catch is that it's hard to see the bigger picture when you think you are the great controller of your life. When you are the great controller, you fail to recognize that supposed coincidences, accidents and chance meetings all have some greater significance in the larger scheme of your destiny. When you are the master of your universe, it's hard to trust anything but your own self-made plans. When we don't have this recognition that there's a bigger story going on, we get caught up in our personal drama and a frustrating cycle of resistance to change. Ishvarapranidhana asks us to go quietly, even when it's not possible to see exactly where things are headed. At first this can be frightening, like being suspended in the air between one trapeze bar and another, but, over time, this not knowing exactly how life is going to unfold and the giving up of our frantic attempts to manipulate and control makes each day an adventure. It makes our life a horse race right up until the very finish!

Ultimately, ishvarapranidhana means surrendering our personal will to this intelligence so we can fulfill our destiny. The first step in this practice is attuning ourselves to perceive a larger perspective. By setting aside enough time to get quiet and clear, we can begin to differentiate between the cluttered thoughts of our ordinary mind and the resonant intelligence that comes through as intuition. Rather than trying to unravel the mystery, we start to embody the mystery of life. When we embody the mystery, we begin to experience meaning. Where before we experienced numbness. When we drink a glass of water, we taste it; when a cool breeze brushes our bare skin, we feel it; and when a stranger speaks to us, we listen. Everything and anything can become a sign of this intelligence. Eventually we are spontaneously drawn to look at the purpose of our life with a new eye. One starts to ask, How can my life be useful to others? Living the insurance nor a guarantee but it is neither spiritual rain against living a meaningless life, a life that at its end we regret.

What Are Yoga Asanas and Why Practice Them?

Given the central importance of the yamas and niyamas, one might wonder why it would be necessary to practice the other limbs of yoga. Would it not be enough to be compassionate, truthful, and content? Why would it be important to take the time to stretch our backs or to listen to our breath? If not for the tremendous importance of grounding spirituality in the body, it's unlikely that the great sages would have listed asana practice as the second limb. This is why I have chosen to focus in such detail on this dimension of practice. What is asana practice all about?

The word asana is usually translated as "pose" or "posture," but its more literal meaning is "comfortable seat." Through their observations of nature, the yogis discovered a vast repertoire of energetic expressions, strong physical effect on the body but also a concomitant psychological effect. Each movement demands that we hone some aspect of our consciousness and use ourselves in a new way. The vast diversity of asanas is no accident, for through exploring both familiar and unfamiliar postures we are also expanding our consciousness, so that regardless of the situation or form we find ourselves in, we can remain "comfortably seated" in our center. Intrinsic to this practice is the uncompromising belief that every aspect of the body is pervaded by consciousness. Asana practice is a way to develop this interior awareness.

While a dancer's or athlete's internal impulses result in movement that takes him into space, in asana practice our internal impulses are contained inside the dynamic form of the posture. When you witness a yoga practitioner skilled in this dynamic internal dance, you have the sense that the body is in continuous subtle motion. What distinguishes an asana from a stretch or calisthenic exercise is that in asana practice we focus our mind's attention completely in the body so that we can move as a unified whole and so we can perceive what the body has to tell us. We don't do something to the body, we become the body. In the West we rarely do this. We watch TV while we stretch; we read a book while we climb the StairMaster; we think about our problems while we take a walk, all the time living a short distance from the body. So asana practice is a reunion between the usually separated body-mind.

Apart from the vibrant health, flexibility, and stamina this unified body-mind brings us, living in the body is also an integral aspect of spiritual practice. The most tangible way that we can know what it means to be compassionate or not grasping is directly through the cellular experience of the body. The most direct way that we can learn what it means to let go is through the body. When we have a self-destructive addiction—the impulse to overeat or to take drugs—this happens through the entrenchment of neurological and physiological patterns in our bodies. And on a more basic level, it's hard to feel focused and purposeful when our bodies are full of aches and pains or burdened with illness and disease.

While I have given the practice of asanas great emphasis in this book, it is not because the perfection of the body or of yoga postures is the goal of yoga practice. This down-to-earth, flesh-and-bones practice is simply one of the most direct and expedient ways to meet yourself. It is a good place to begin. Whether you meet yourself through standing on your feet or standing on your head is irrelevant. It's important, therefore, not to make the mistake of thinking that the perfection of the yoga asanas is the goal, or that you'll be good at yoga only once you've mastered the more difficult postures. The asanas are useful maps to explore yourself, but they are not the territory. The goal of asana practice is to live in your body and to learn to perceive clearly through it. If you can master the Four Noble Acts, as I like to call them, of sitting, standing, walking, and lying down with ease, you will have mastered the basics of living an embodied spiritual life.

The emphasis on asana practice is also specific to the age we live in, for we live in a time of extreme dissociation from bodily experience. When we are not in our bodies we are dissociated from our instincts, intuitions, feelings and insights, and it becomes possible to dissociate ourselves from other people's feelings, and other people's suffering. The insidious ways in which we become numb to our bodily experience and the feelings and perceptions that arise from them leave us powerless to know who we are, what we believe in, and what kind of world we wish to create. If we do not know when we are breathing in and when we are breathing out, when we are unable to perceive gross levels of tension, how then can we possibly know how to create a balanced world?

Every violent impulse begins in a body filled with tension; every failure to reach out to someone in need begins in a body that has forgotten how to feel. There has never been a back problem or a mental problem that didn't have a body attached to it. This limb of yoga practice reattaches us to our body. In reattaching ourselves to our bodies we reattach ourselves to the responsibility of living a life guided by the undeniable wisdom of our body.

Practicing with Joyfulness

When we begin practice, we may feel far from happy within ourselves. In fact, even the semblance of happiness may seem as remote to us as winning the lottery. We may feel utterly confused, buried in self-destructive habits, and encumbered by difficulties, whether emotional, physical, or material, that appear insurmountable. Our bodies may feel as stiff and knotted as an old tree, and our minds a jumble of worries and neuroses. Platitudes about the peace and happiness available to us right now sound empty in the face of our very real pain. Most of us begin like this, and even those who feel some sense of inner balance often find that underneath the thin veneer of appearances, there is much work to be done.

How do we go about doing this work without becoming discouraged by the enormity of the task? Unless we can find a way to practice with joyfulness, working with our difficulties rather than against, them, practice will be an experience of frustration and disappointment. Unless we can find a way to enjoy what we are doing right now, yoga practice will become a negative time, and ultimately we'll develop a strong resistance even to stepping onto the mat.

A story may help you to understand what I mean. Many years ago I moved into a derelict house. The back door was nailed shut and had not been opened for fifteen years; once pried open it revealed a six-foot wall of seemingly impenetrable blackberry bushes, vines, and crabgrass. I wanted a garden. For many months I looked in despair through the window of the back door. The task seemed too large and. too difficult. Then I decided upon a strategy that my mind could grasp.

I decided that I would divide the project into four-foot increments. Every week I would clear a four-foot patch of garden. The backyard was sixty-five feet long! As I would begin to dig and root, cutting and pulling my tiny patch, I resolved that I would focus my attention only on the four-foot patch. I would not even look at the other sixty-one feet of garden left to clear. Within minutes of beginning I would become completely absorbed in the insects, the tiny plants uncovered, and the pleasure of digging my hands into the brown earth. Each four-foot patch took about three hours because the crabgrass had to be dug out completely and the earth was rock hard. But three hours a week was an easily manageable commitment. When I was finished with the patch, I would step back and admire my good work, never allowing myself to consider the chaotic mess left remaining. How wonderful it looked! Each four-foot patch was a unique wonder. Pathways buried two feet under emerged. A lawn mower, enveloped by grass (proof of the law of karma), was discovered. Not only was the task challenging, it became an adventure, and I eagerly anticipated what I might find each week. Within a year I had a beautiful lawn, an herb garden, and a patch of flowers to enjoy. But, more important, I enjoyed the process of transforming an inhospitable patch of ground into an urban paradise.

When you begin to practice, you may feel very bound in your body and mind, not unlike the densely woven crabgrass of my garden. You can choose to fight with yourself, pulling and tugging on yourself as a way to force your own metamorphosis. If you've ever encountered a weed with deep roots, you know the futility of pulling at the stem knowing full well some digging is in order! There's a moment when you can cheerfully accept the task and set to it with full vigor, or turn sour and miserable in the face of such work. There's a moment when you can resign yourself to the patient work ahead or give in to the impulse to pull on the stem before the ground has been dug deep enough. The first step is accepting that some deep work needs to be done and then deciding to make this a positive, uplifting experience.

In yoga practice you can do this by dividing your experience into incremental breaths and taking care of only that which arises in one breath cycle and no more. In this way almost any difficulty becomes manageable. Rather than focusing on how much further you wish you could go, or comparing your meager efforts with those of someone who is more adept, you can choose to focus on what you are accomplishing in each breath. Maybe today you open your hip five millimeters farther, or you manage to sit comfortably in meditation for the first time. As you investigate the tightness around your hip you discover ways to release it; as you sit for five more minutes you discover that those "urgent" matters were really not so urgent. It is only through these tiny, slow, and progressive openings that deep, profound change occurs. It is your choice to take pleasure in these small awakenings or to disregard your efforts as insignificant in the face of how much further you have to go. You can choose to have a sense of humor about your dilemma or fester in negativity. Whom would you like to garden with?

When we make practice a joyful time, it is also much more likely that we are growing more deeply within our spiritual life. When we get hooked into striving toward where we think we should be and how far we ought to be able to go, in truth we are somewhere else all the time. We are in our fantasy, our ideas, our concepts, and our judgments. There's not much room in there to perceive and appreciate what's actually happening. Even when we feel pain, even when we face great difficulty, we can take refuge in our practice. There will inevitably be times when progress is slow, when injury or illness or life circumstances limit our ability to do the outward forms. But this doesn't limit our ability to plumb the depths of our inner life.

Each day as you step onto your mat, make a decision to enjoy just where you are right now. Take a few moments, too, to contemplate how fortunate you are to be practicing this wonderful art. A casual glance at the morning paper is proof enough of the vast suffering, poverty, violence, and homelessness that is the lot of so many human beings. If you are standing on a yoga mat and have the time to practice even fifteen minutes, you are a fortunate person. If you have a yoga teacher, you have an invaluable gift and life tool available to very few people. In the spirit of this gratefulness, let your practice begin.

Part Three

Mind-Body Interventions

Chapter 14

Biofeedback

Biofeedback is a treatment technique in which people are trained to improve their health by using signals from their own bodies. Physical therapists use biofeedback to help stroke victims regain movement in paralyzed muscles. Psychologists use it to help tense and anxious clients learn to relax. Specialists in many different fields use biofeedback to help their patients cope with pain.

Chances are you have used biofeedback yourself. You've used it if you have ever taken your temperature or stepped on a scale. The thermometer tells you whether you're running a fever, the scale whether you've gained weight. Both devices "feedback" information about your body's condition. Armed with this information, you can take steps you've learned to improve the condition. When you're running a fever, you go to bed and drink plenty of fluids. When you've gained weight, you resolve to eat less and sometimes you do.

Clinicians reply on complicated biofeedback machines in somewhat the same way that you rely on your scale or thermometer. Their machines can detect a person's internal bodily functions with far greater sensitivity and precision than a person can alone. This information may be valuable. Both patients and therapists use it to gauge and direct the progress of treatment.

"What Is Biofeedback?" by Bette Runck, and undated fact sheet produced by the Department of Health and Human Services (DHHS), DHHS Publication No. (ADM) 83-1273, cited December 2001. Despite the original date of this publication, people interested in understanding the basic principles of biofeedback will still find this information useful.

For patients, the biofeedback machine acts as a kind of sixth sense which allows them to "see" or "hear" activity inside their bodies. One commonly used type of machine, for example, picks up electrical signals in the muscles. It translates these signals into a form that patients can detect. It triggers a flashing light bulb, perhaps, or activates a beeper every time muscles grow more tense. If patients want to relax tense muscles, they try to slow down the flashing or beeping.

Like a pitcher learning to throw a ball across a home plate, the biofeedback trainee, in an attempt to improve a skill, monitors the performance. When a pitch is off the mark, the ballplayer adjusts the delivery so that he performs better the next time he tries. When the light flashes or the beeper beeps too often, the biofeedback trainee makes internal adjustments which alter the signals. The biofeedback therapist acts as a coach, standing at the sidelines setting goals and limits on what to expect and giving hints on how to improve performance.

The Beginnings of Biofeedback

The word "biofeedback" was coined in the late 1960s to describe laboratory procedures then being used to train experimental research subjects to alter brain activity, blood pressure, heart rate, and other bodily functions that normally are not controlled voluntarily.

At the time, many scientists looked forward to the day when biofeedback would give us a major degree of control over our bodies. They thought, for instance, that we might be able to "will" ourselves to be more creative by changing the patterns of our brainwaves. Some believed that biofeedback would one day make it possible to do away with drug treatments that often cause uncomfortable side effects in patients with high blood pressure and other serious conditions.

Today, most scientists agree that such high hopes were not realistic. Research has demonstrated that biofeedback can help in the treatment of many diseases and painful conditions. It has shown that we have more control over so-called involuntary bodily function than we once though possible. But it has also shown that nature limits the extent of such control. Scientists are now trying to determine just how much voluntary control we can exert.

How Is Biofeedback Used Today?

Clinical biofeedback techniques that grew out of the early laboratory procedures are now widely used to treat an ever-lengthening list of conditions. These include:

162

- Migraine headaches, tension headaches, and many other types of pain
- Disorders of the digestive system
- High blood pressure and its opposite, low blood pressure
- Cardiac arrhythmias (abnormalities, sometimes dangerous, in the rhythm of the heartbeat)
- Raynaud's disease (a circulatory disorder that causes uncomfortably cold hands)
- Epilepsy
- Paralysis and other movement disorders

Specialists who provide biofeedback training range from psychiatrists and psychologists to dentists, internists, nurses, and physical therapists. Most rely on many other techniques in addition to biofeedback. Patients usually are taught some form of relaxation exercise. Some learn to identify the circumstances that trigger their symptoms. They may also be taught how to avoid or cope with these stressful events. Most are encouraged to change their habits, and some are trained in special techniques for gaining such self-control. Biofeedback is not magic. It cannot cure disease or by itself make a person healthy. It is a tool, one of many available to health care professionals. It reminds physicians that behavior, thoughts, and feelings profoundly influence physical health. And it helps both patients and doctors understand that they must work together as a team.

Patients' Responsibilities

Biofeedback places unusual demands on patients. They must examine their day-to-day lives to learn if they may be contributing to their own distress. They must recognize that they can, by their own efforts, remedy some physical ailments. They must commit themselves to practicing biofeedback or relaxation exercises every day. They must change bad habits, even ease up on some good ones. Most important, they must accept much of the responsibility for maintaining their own health.

How Does Biofeedback Work?

Scientists cannot yet explain how biofeedback works. Most patients who benefit from biofeedback are trained to relax and modify their behavior. Most scientists believe that relaxation is a key component in biofeedback treatment of many disorders, particularly those brought on or made worse by stress.

Their reasoning is based on what is known about the effects of stress on the body. In brief, the argument goes like this: Stressful events produce strong emotions, which arouse certain physical responses. Many of these responses are controlled by the sympathetic nervous system, the network of nerve tissues that helps prepare the body to meet emergencies by "flight or fight."

The typical pattern of response to emergencies probably emerged during the time when all humans faced mostly physical threats. Although the "threats" we now live with are seldom physical, the body reacts as if they were: The pupils dilate to let in more light. Sweat pours out, reducing the chance of skin cuts. Blood vessels near the skin contract to reduce bleeding, while those in the brain and muscles dilate to increase the oxygen supply. The gastrointestinal tract, including the stomach and intestines, slows down to reduce the energy expensed in digestion. The heart beats faster, and blood pressure rises.

Normally, people calm down when a stressful event is over especially if they have done something to cope with it. For instance, imagine your own reactions if you're walking down a dark street and hear someone running toward you. You get scared. Your body prepared you to ward off an attacker or run fast enough to get away. When you do escape, you gradually relax.

If you get angry at your boss, it's a different matter. Your body may prepare to fight. But since you want to keep your job, you try to ignore the angry feelings. Similarly, if on the way home you get stalled in traffic, there's nothing you can do to get away. These situations can literally may you sick. Your body has prepared for action, but you cannot act.

Individuals differ in the way they respond to stress. In some, one function, such as blood pressure, becomes more active while others remain normal. Many experts believe that these individual physical responses to stress can become habitual. When the body is repeatedly aroused, one or more functions may become permanently overactive. Actual damage to bodily tissues may eventually result.

Biofeedback is often aimed at changing habitual reactions to stress that can cause pain or disease. Many clinicians believe that some of their patients and clients have forgotten how to relax. Feedback of physical responses such as skin temperature and muscle tension provides information to help patients recognize a relaxed state. The feedback signal may also act as a kind of reward for reducing tension. It's like a piano teacher whose frown turns to a smile when a young musician finally plays a tune properly.

The value of a feedback signal as information and reward may be even greater in the treatment of patients with paralyzed or spastic muscles. With these patients, biofeedback seems to be primarily a form of skill training like learning to pitch a ball. Instead of watching the ball, the patient watches the machine, which monitors activity in the affected muscle. Stroke victims with paralyzed arms and legs, for example, see that some part of their affected limbs remains active. The signal from the biofeedback machine proves it.

This signal can guide the exercises that help patients regain use of their limbs. Perhaps just as important, the feedback convinces patients that the limbs are still alive. This reassurance often encourages them to continue their efforts.

Should You Try Biofeedback?

If you think you might benefit from biofeedback training, you should discuss it with your physician or other health care professional, who may wish to conduct tests to make certain that your condition does not require conventional medical treatment first. Responsible biofeedback therapists will not treat you for headaches, hypertension, or most disorders until you have had a thorough physical examination. Some require neurological tests as well.

How do you find a biofeedback therapist? First, ask your doctor or dentist, or contact the nearest community health center, medical society, or State biofeedback society for a referral. The psychology or psychiatry departments at nearby universities may also be able to help you. Most experts recommend that you consult only a health care professional, a physician, psychologist, psychiatrist, nurse, social worker, dentist, physical therapist, for example who has been trained to use biofeedback.

Professional Associations

The Association for Applied Psychophysiology and Biofeedback
10200 W. 44th Avenue
Suite 304
Wheat Ridge, CO 80033-2840
Toll Free: 800-477-8892
Tel: 303-422-8436

The Association for Applied Psychophysiology and Biofeedback (continued)

Fax: 303-422-8894
Website: http://www.aapg.org
E-Mail: AAPB@resourcenter.com

AAPB is the national membership association for professionals using biofeedback. AAPB holds a national meeting, offers CE programs, produces a journal and newsmagazine and other biofeedback related publications.

The Biofeedback Certification Institute of America

10200 W. 44th Avenue
Suite 304
Wheat Ridge, CO 80033-2840
Website: http://www.bcia.org

The BCIA was established as an independent agency to provide national certification for biofeedback providers.

Chapter 15

Guided Imagery

Imagery is a flow of thoughts you can see, hear, feel, smell, or taste. An image is an inner representation of your experience or your fantasies—a way your mind codes, stores, and expresses information. Imagery is the currency of dreams and daydreams; memories and reminiscence; plans, projections, and possibilities. It is the language of the arts, the emotions, and most important, of the deeper self.

Imagery is a window on your inner world; a way of viewing your own ideas, feelings, and interpretations. But it is more than a mere window—it is a means of transformation and liberation from distortions in this realm that may unconsciously direct your life and shape your health.

Imagination, in this sense, is not sufficiently valued in our culture. The imaginary is equated with the fanciful, the unreal, and the impractical. In school we are taught the three R's while creativity, uniqueness, and interpersonal skills are either barely tolerated or frankly discouraged. As adults, we are usually paid to perform tasks, not to think creatively. The premium is on the practical, the useful, the real, as it should be—but imagination nurtures human reality as a river brings life to a desert.

Without imagination, humanity would be long extinct. It took imagination—the ability to conceive of new possibilities—to make fire,

"What Is Imagery, and How Does it Work?" from the book *Guided Imagery for Self-Healing,* © 2000 Martin L. Rossman, M.D. Reprinted with permission of HJ Kramer/New World Library, Novato, CA. 800-972-6657 ext. 52 or http://www.newworldlibrary.com.

create weapons, and cultivate crops; to construct buildings, invent cars, airplanes, space shuttles, television, and computers.

Paradoxically, our collective imagination, which has allowed us to overcome so many natural threats, has been instrumental in creating the major survival problems we face on earth today—pollution, exhaustion of natural resources, and the threat of nuclear annihilation. Yet imagination, teamed with will, remains our best hope for overcoming these same problems.

Imagery and Physiologic Change

Imagery in healing is probably best known for its direct effects on physiology. Through imagery, you can stimulate changes in many body functions usually considered inaccessible to conscious influence.

A simple example: Touch your finger to your nose. How did you do that? You may be surprised to learn that nobody knows.

A neuroanatomist can tell us the area of the brain where the first nerve impulses fire to begin that movement. We can also trace the chain of nerves that conduct impulses from the brain to the appropriate muscles. But no one knows how you go from thinking about touching your nose to firing the first cell in that chain. You just decide to do it and you do it, without having to worry about the details.

Now make yourself salivate.

You probably didn't find that as easy, and may not have been able to do it at all. That's because salivation is not usually under our conscious control. It is controlled by a different part of the nervous system than the one that governs movement. While the central nervous system governs voluntary movement, the autonomic nervous system regulates salivation and other physiologic functions that normally operate without conscious control. The autonomic nervous system doesn't readily respond to ordinary thoughts like "salivate." But it does respond to imagery.

Relax for a moment and imagine you are holding a juicy yellow lemon. Feel its coolness, its texture, and weight in your hand. Imagine cutting it in half and squeezing the juice of one half into a glass. Perhaps some pulp and a seed or two drop into the glass. Imagine raising the glass to your lips and taking a good mouthful of the tart juice. Swish it around in your mouth, taste its sourness, and swallow.

Now did you salivate? Did you pucker your lips or make a sour face when you imagined that? If you did, that's because your autonomic nervous system responded to your imaginary lemon juice. You probably don't spend much time thinking about drinking lemon juice, but what you do habitually think about may have important effects on your body through a similar mechanism. If your mind is full of thoughts of danger, your nervous system will prepare you to meet that danger by initiating the stress response, a high level of arousal and tension. If you imagine peaceful, relaxing scenes instead, it sends out an "all-clear" signal, and your body relaxes.

Research in biofeedback, hypnosis, and meditative states has demonstrated a remarkable range of human self-regulatory capacities. Focused imagery in a relaxed state of mind seems to be the common factor among these approaches.

Imagery of various types has been shown to affect heart rate, blood pressure, respiratory patterns, oxygen consumption, carbon dioxide elimination, brain wave rhythms and patterns, electrical characteristics of the skin, local blood flow and temperature, gastrointestinal motility and secretions, sexual arousal, levels of various hormones and neurotransmitters in the blood, and immune system function.[1] But the healing potentials of imagery go far beyond simple effects on physiology.

Imagery in the Larger Context of Healing

Recovering from a serious or chronic illness may well demand more from you than simple imagery techniques. It may also require changes in your lifestyle, your attitudes, your relationships, or your emotional state. Imagery can be an effective tool for helping you see what changes need to be made, and how you can go about making them.

Imagery is the interface language between body and mind. It can help you understand the needs that may be represented by an illness and can help you develop healthy ways to meet those needs. Let me give you another example from my practice. Jeffrey was a successful middle manager in his thirties who had recurrent peptic ulcers for many years. In our work together he learned to relax and use simple visualization to give himself temporary relief from his stomach pain. He pictured the pain as a fire in his stomach and would then imagine an ice-cold mountain stream extinguishing the fire and cooling the scorched area beneath it. He was surprised and pleased to find that relaxing and imagining this process for a few minutes would relieve his pain for several hours to a day at a time, and he used it successfully for about two weeks. Then it stopped working. His pain grew worse in spite of his visualizations, and he began to despair. In our next session I suggested he focus once more on the pain and allow an image to arise that might help him understand why the pain had returned. He soon became aware of an image of a hand pinching the inside of his stomach.

At my suggestion, he mentally asked the hand if it would tell him why it was pinching him, and it changed into an arm shaking a clenched fist. He asked the arm why it was angry, and it replied, "Because there's a part of you locked away where no one can see it, and it's getting badly hurt." I asked him to form an image of the part that was locked away, and he saw a transparent sack that contained a "chaotic whirling of things inside nothing is clear, everything is zooming around, bumping into everything else." All he could make out were colors and shapes and a sense of discomfort. After observing them for a while, he quietly said, "My heart is in there, and it's getting bumped and bruised by all these things."

I asked Jeffrey to imagine opening the bag, but as he began he became afraid and said there was too much pain there to let out all at once. I asked him to let just one thing out of the bag and let an image form for it. He imagined his father's face and recalled a number of painful childhood interactions with his father, who was quite emotionally abusive. Over a series of sessions, he began to come to terms with the feelings he had locked away about this and started to feel much better emotionally and physically. In this way, he not only obtained relief from his ulcer pain, he learned a method to better express and respond to his own emotional needs.

Using imagery in this way can allow illness to become a teacher of wellness. Symptoms and illnesses indicate that something is out of balance, something needs to be adjusted, adapted to, or changed. Imagery can allow you to understand more about your illness and respond to its message in the healthiest imaginable way.

How Does Imagery Work?

The ultimate mechanisms of imagery are still a mystery. in the last twenty years, however, we have learned that imagery is a natural language of a major part of our nervous system. Critical to this understanding is the Nobel-prize-winning work of Dr. Roger Sperry and his collaborators at the University of Chicago and later at the California Institute of Technology. They have shown that the two sides of the human brain think in very different ways and are simultaneously capable of independent thought. In a real sense, we each have two brains. One thinks as we are accustomed to thinking, with words and logic. The other, however, thinks in terms of images and feelings.

170

In most people, the left brain is primarily responsible for speaking, writing, and understanding language; it thinks logically and analytically, and identifies itself by the name of the person to whom it belongs. The right brain, in contrast, thinks in pictures, sounds, spatial relationships, and feelings. It is relatively silent, though highly intelligent. The left brain analyzes, taking things apart, while the right brain synthesizes, putting pieces together. The left is a better logical thinker, the right is more attuned to emotions. The left is most concerned with the outer world of culture, agreements, business, and time, while the right is more concerned with the inner world of perception, physiology, form, and emotion.

The essential difference between the two brains is in the way each processes information. The left brain processes information sequentially, while the right brain processes it simultaneously. Imagine a train coming around a curve in the track. An observer is positioned on the ground, on the outside of the curve, and he observes the train to be a succession of separate though connected cars passing him one at a time. He can see just a little bit of the cars ahead of and behind the one he is watching. This observer has a "left-brain" view of the train.

The "right-brain" observer would be in a balloon several hundred feet above the tracks. From here he could not only see the whole train, but also the track on which it was traveling, the countryside through which it was passing, the town it had just left, and the town to which it was headed.

This ability of the right hemisphere to grasp the larger context of events is one of the specialized functions that make it invaluable to us in healing. The imagery it produces often lets you see the "big picture" and experience the way an illness is related to events and feelings you might not have considered important. You can see not only the single piece, but the way it's connected to the whole. This change of perspective may allow you to put ideas together in new ways to produce new solutions to old problems. A right-brain point of view may reveal the opportunity hidden in what seems to be a problem.

The right brain has a special relationship not only to imagery but to emotions. This is another of the major strengths it brings to the healing adventure. Many studies have shown that the right brain is specialized to recognize emotion in facial expressions, body language, speech, and even music. This is critical to healing because emotions are not only psychological but physical states that are at the root of a great deal of illness and disease. Rudolph Virchow, a nineteenth century physician and founding father of the science of pathology, remarked that "Much illness is unhappiness sailing under a physiologic flag." Studies in England and the United States have found that from 50 to 75 percent of all problems presenting to a primary care clinic are emotional, social, or familial in origin, though they are being expressed by pain or illness.[2]

Emotions themselves are, of course, not unhealthy. On the contrary, they are a normal response to certain life events. Failure to acknowledge and express important emotions, however, is an important factor in illness, and one that is widespread in our society. In many ways we are emotional illiterates, lacking clear guidelines and traditions for expressing emotions in healthy ways. It is difficult to know what to do with distressing emotions such as grief, fear, and anger, so we cope as best we can. We may unconsciously build layer upon layer of inner defenses to protect us from feeling unpleasant feelings. But strong emotion has a way of finding routes of expression. If not recognized and dealt with for what it is, it may manifest as pain or illness.

Social and family relationships to some extent depend on our ability to process emotions internally. We don't need to express every emotion we feel. But strong, persistent emotions need to be expressed or resolved, as their chronic denial may lead to physiologic imbalance and disease.

Most of us understand and use left-brain language and logic every day. We are relatively familiar with our conscious needs and desires. Imagery gives the silent right brain a chance to bring its needs to light and to contribute its special qualities to the healing process.

Frankly, calling verbal or logical thinking "left-brained," and symbolic, imaginal thinking "right-brained" is an oversimplification, but it is a useful model for thinking about some uses of imagery. Imagery allows you to communicate with your own silent mind in its native tongue. Imagery is a rich, symbolic, and highly personal language, and the more time you spend observing and interacting with your own image-making brain, the more quickly and effectively you will use it to improve your health.

If you are ill, you have undoubtedly thought long and hard about why you fell ill and what you need to do to get better. If your illness is chronic, or severe, you have probably consulted many doctors, whose highly educated, logical analyses may have led to a diagnosis. Yet the diagnosis may not have led to a cure, or even relief.

What Kinds of Illnesses Can Be Treated with Imagery?

While preliminary studies have demonstrated that imagery can be an effective part of treatment in a wide variety of illnesses, I am

172

reluctant to offer a list of "diseases that can be treated with imagery." Imagery can be helpful in so many ways that it is more accurate to think of it as a way of treating people than a way of treating illnesses.

Imagery can help you whether you have simple tension headaches or a life-threatening disease. Through imagery, you can learn to relax and be more comfortable in any situation, whether you are ill or well. You may be able to reduce, modify, or eliminate pain. You can use imagery to help you see if your lifestyle habits have contributed to your illness and to see what changes you can make to support your recovery. Imagery can help you tap inner strengths and find hope, courage, patience, perseverance, love, and other qualities that can help you cope with, transcend, or recover from almost any illness.

There are, of course, certain symptoms and illnesses that seem to be more readily responsive to imagery than others. Conditions that are caused by or aggravated by stress often respond very well to imagery techniques. These include such common problems as headaches, neck pain, back pain, "nervous stomach," spastic colon, allergies, palpitations, dizziness, fatigue, and anxiety. Other major health problems including heart disease, cancer, arthritis, and neurological illnesses are often complicated by or themselves cause stress, anxiety, and depression. The emotional aspects of any illness can often be helped through imagery, and relieving the emotional distress may in turn encourage physical healing.

I must repeat that good medical care for the serious problems mentioned above is essential and perfectly compatible with imagery. If you choose to have therapeutic treatments of any kind, acknowledge them as your allies in healing and include them in your imagery. If you are taking an antibiotic or chemotherapy, imagine the medicines coursing through your tissues, finding and eliminating the bacteria or tumor cells you are fighting. If you have surgery, imagine the operation going smoothly and successfully, and your recovery being rapid and complete. There is good evidence that this type of preoperative preparation reduces recovery time and complications from surgery.[3]

Notes

1. A very good review of this literature is found in "Imagery, physiology, and psychosomatic illness," Sheikh, A., and Kunzendorf, R. G. (1984). In *International Review of Mental Imagery*, Vol. 1, ed. Sheikh, A. New York: Human Sciences Press.

2. Rosen, G., Kleinman, A., and Katon, W. (1982), "Somatization in family practice: a biopsychosocial approach." *Journal of Family Practice*, 14:3, 493-502. Stoeckle,J. D., Zola, I. K., and Davidson, G. E. (1964), "The quantity and significance of psychological distress in medical patients." *Journal of Chronic Disease*, 17:959.

3. An excellent review of psychological factors in surgical outcome is found in "Behavioral Anesthesia," by Henry L. Bennett, Ph.D., in *Aduances*, 2:4, Fall, 1985. Pickett, C., and Clum, G. A. (1982), "Comparative treatment strategies and their interaction with locus of control in the reduction of post-surgical pain and anxiety." *Journal of Consulting and Clinical Psychology*, 50:3, 439-441.

Chapter 16

Hypnosis

Hypnosis is a state of inner absorption, concentration and focused attention. It is like using a magnifying glass to focus the rays of the sun and make them more powerful. Similarly, when our minds are concentrated and focused, we are able to use our minds more powerfully. Because hypnosis allows people to use more of their potential, learning self-hypnosis is the ultimate act of self-control.

Everyone has experienced a trance many times, but we don't usually call it hypnosis. All of us have been so absorbed in thought—while reading a book, or riding the bus to work—that we fail to notice what is happening around us. While we were zoned out, another level of consciousness, which we refer to as our unconscious mind, took over. These are very focused states of attention similar to hypnosis.

Clinical hypnotists do essentially three things with hypnosis. They encourage the use of imagination. Mental imagery is very powerful, especially in a focused state of attention. The mind seems capable of using imagery, even if it is only symbolic, to assist us in bringing about the things we are imagining. For example, a patient with ulcerative colitis may be asked to imagine what her distressed colon looks like. If she imagines it as being like a tunnel, with very red, inflamed walls that are rough in texture, the patient may be encouraged in hypnosis (and in self-hypnosis) to imagine this image changing to a healthy one.

"How to Find a Hypnotherapist," an undated fact sheet, © American Society of Clinical Hypnosis, cited January 2002; reprinted with permission. For further information, contact the American Society of Clinical Hypnosis, 140 North Bloomingdale Road, Bloomingdale, IL 60108, Telephone: 630-980-4740, Website: http://www.asch.net, E-Mail info@asch.net.

Another basic hypnotic method is to present ideas or suggestions to the patient. In a state of concentrated attention, ideas and suggestions that are compatible with what the patient wants seem to have a more powerful impact on the mind.

Finally, hypnosis may be used for unconscious exploration, to better understand underlying motivations or identify whether past events or experiences are associated with causing a problem. Hypnosis avoids the critical censor of the conscious mind, which often defeats what we know to be in our best interests.

Myths about Hypnosis

People often fear that being hypnotized will make them lose control, surrender their will, and result in their being dominated, but a hypnotic state is not the same thing as gullibility or weakness. Many people base their assumptions about hypnotism on stage acts but fail to take into account that stage hypnotists screen their volunteers to select those who are cooperative, with possible exhibitionist tendencies, as well as responsive to hypnosis. Stage acts help create a myth about hypnosis which discourages people from seeking legitimate hypnotherapy.

Another myth about hypnosis is that people lose consciousness and have amnesia. A small percentage of subjects, who go into very deep levels of trance will fit this stereotype and have spontaneous amnesia. The majority of people remember everything that occurs in hypnosis. This is beneficial, because the most of what we want to accomplish in hypnosis may be done in a medium depth trance, where people tend to remember everything.

In hypnosis, the patient is not under the control of the hypnotist. Hypnosis is not something imposed on people, but something they do for themselves. A hypnotist simply serves as a facilitator to guide them.

When Will Hypnosis Be Beneficial?

We believe that hypnosis will be optimally effective when the patient is highly motivated to overcome a problem and when the hypnotherapist is well trained in both hypnosis and in general considerations relating to the treatment of the particular problem. Some individuals seem to have higher native hypnotic talent and capacity that may allow them to benefit more readily from hypnosis.

It is important to keep in mind that hypnosis is like any other therapeutic modality: it is of major benefit to some patients with some problems, and it is helpful with many other patients, but it can fail, just like any other clinical method. For this reason, we emphasize that we are not "hypnotists," but health care professionals who use hypnosis along with other tools of our professions.

Selecting a Qualified Hypnotherapist

As in choosing any health care professional, care should be exercised in selecting a hypnotherapist. Hypnosis and the use of hypnotic therapies are not regulated in most states, and hypnotherapists are, in most cases, not state licensed in hypnosis. Lay hypnotists are people who are trained in hypnosis but lack medical, psychological, dental or other professional health care training. A lay hypnotist may be certified and claim to have received 200 or more hours of training, but licensed health care professionals typically have seven to nine years of university coursework, plus additional supervised training in internship and residency programs. Their hypnosis training is in addition to their medical, psychological, dental or social work training. Careful questioning can help you avoid a lay hypnotist who may engage in fraudulent or unethical practices.

Ask if the person is licensed (not certified) in their field by the state. If they are not legitimately licensed, they probably lack the education required for licensure. Find out what their degree is in. If it is in hypnosis or hypnotherapy, rather than a state-recognized health care profession, the person is a lay hypnotist. Check for membership in the American Society of Clinical Hypnosis or the Society for Clinical and Experimental Hypnosis (which are the only nationally recognized organizations for licensed health care professionals using hypnosis) as well as membership in the American Medical Association, the American Dental Association, the American Psychological Association, etc. Contact a state or local component section of the American Society of Clinical Hypnosis to see if the person is a reputable member. If you have doubts about their qualifications, keep looking.

Uses of Hypnosis in Medicine and Psychotherapy

- Gastrointestinal Disorders (Ulcers, Irritable Bowel Syndrome, Colitis, Crohn's Disease)

- Dermatologic Disorders (Eczema, Herpes, Neurodermatitis, Pruritus [itching], Psoriasis, Warts)

- Surgery/Anesthesiology (In unusual circumstances, hypnosis has been used as the sole anesthetic for surgery, including the removal of the gall bladder, amputation, cesarean section, and hysterectomy. Reasons for using hypnosis as the sole anesthetic may include: situations where chemical anesthesia is contraindicated because of allergies or hyper-sensitivities; when organic problems increase the risk of using chemoanesthesia; and in some conditions where it is ideal for the patient to be able to respond to questions or directives from the surgeon)

- Pain (back pain, cancer pain, dental anesthesia, headaches and migraines, arthritis or rheumatism)

- Burns: Hypnosis is not only effective for the pain, but when hypnotic anesthesia and feelings of coolness are created in the first few hours after a significant burn, it appears that it also reduces inflammation and promotes healing. We believe that a second degree burn can often be kept from going third degree if hypnosis is used soon after the injury.

- Nausea and Vomiting associated with chemotherapy and pregnancy (hyperemisis gravidarum)

- Childbirth: Based upon our members' anecdotal evidence, approximately two thirds of women have been found capable of using hypnosis as the sole analgesic for labor. This eliminates the risks that medications can pose to both the mother and child.

- Hemophilia: Hemophilia patients can often be taught to use self-hypnosis to control vascular flow and keep from requiring a blood transfusion.

- Victims of Abuse (incest, rape, physical abuse, cult abuse)

Other areas of application include: Allergies; anxiety and stress management; asthma; bed-wetting; depression; sports and athletic performance; smoking cessation; obesity and weight control; sleep disorders; Raynaud's disease; high blood pressure; sexual dysfunctions; concentration, test anxiety and learning disorders.

Chapter 17

Meditation and Relaxation

For thousands of years, religions the world over have extolled the benefits of meditation and quiet contemplation. In Islam and Catholicism, Judaism and Buddhism, Hinduism and Taoism, and in religious practice from the Americas to Africa to Asia, the value of sitting quietly, using various techniques to cultivate stillness or focused attention of the mind, has been well recognized.

The goals of religious meditation extend far beyond its potential physical health benefits and also extend beyond the scope of this book. Higher human function of body, mind, and spirit is explored in sacred literature throughout the world. An excellent summary of ancient and contemporary information on the subject can be found in Michael Murphy's landmark book *The Future of the Body: Explorations Into the Further Evolution of Human Nature.*

In the closing years of the Twentieth Century, the intimate connection between body and mind is widely acknowledged. Once the domain of speculation by mystics and philosophers, this realm has in recent decades been visited and revisited by scientists, who have produced an impressive array of documentation. Most of this research appeared after 1970, and there currently exists a state of informational jet lag, in which the available documentation has not yet fully percolated through the scientific community. Thus, meditation remains a tool drastically underutilized within the medical fields.

"Meditation and Relaxation," by Daniel Redwood, D.C., © Daniel Redwood, D.C., an undated document, cited January 2002; reprinted with permission.

179

The data pool is now so substantial that it can be stated, without fear of contradiction, that meditation and related relaxation techniques have been scientifically shown to be highly beneficial to health. Over a thousand research studies, most of them published in well-respected scientific journals, attest to a wide range of measurable improvements in human function as a result of meditative practices.

Herbert Benson, M.D., and the Relaxation Response

Herbert Benson's research at Harvard in the early 1970s led the way. Benson's impeccable credentials and university affiliation, along with the world-class quality of his work, led to publication of breakthrough articles on meditation in the *Scientific American* and the *American Journal of Physiology*. His book, *The Relaxation Response* topped the bestseller lists in the mid-1970s, and is still widely read.

In *The Relaxation Response*, Benson concluded, based on his research, that meditation acted as an antidote to stress. The body's physical response under stress is well known; when a real or imagined threat is present, the human nervous system activates the "fight-or-flight" mechanism. The activity of the sympathetic portion of the nervous system increases, causing an increased heartbeat, increased respiratory rate, elevation of blood pressure, and increase in oxygen consumption.

This fight-or-flight response has a purpose. If you need to run quickly to escape an attack by a wild animal or need increased strength to battle an invader, you will be better equipped to do so if the fight-or-flight mechanism is turned up to maximum intensity. But this mechanism functions best when used occasionally, for brief periods only. If activated repeatedly, the effects are harmful and potentially disastrous. It is not uncommon for people in modern societies to maintain high stress levels most of the time. The current epidemic of hypertension and heart disease in the Western world is in part a direct result.

The effects of meditation, Benson demonstrated, are essentially the opposite of the fight-or-flight response. Benson's research showed that meditation:

- Decreases the heart rate

- Decreases the respiratory rate

- Decreases blood pressure in people who have normal or mildly elevated blood pressure

- Decreases oxygen consumption

These basic findings have been replicated by so many subsequent studies that they are not in dispute. They also established once and for all that meditation is physiologically distinct from sleep. In sleep, oxygen consumption drops about 8 percent below the waking rate, and this decrease occurs slowly over a period of five or six hours. In meditation, it drops 10 to 20 percent in minutes. Moreover, alpha waves, which indicate a state of relaxed alertness, are abundant during meditation, and rarely noted in the sleep state.[1]

Meditation's Effects on Muscle Tension and Pain

Numerous studies have shown a decrease in muscle tension during meditation. As Michael Murphy points out, this "contributes to the body's lowered need for energy, the slowing of respiration, and the lowering of stress-related hormones in the blood." In some studies, the decrease in muscle tension as a result of meditation even exceeded the impressive effects of biofeedback training. One interesting study measured the electrical patterns in muscles, and demonstrated that the lotus position (seated with legs fully crossed), a traditional posture for meditation, is the only position in which the body's muscles are as relaxed as they are when lying down.[2]

Meditation has also been shown to aid in the alleviation of pain. Extensive studies on chronic pain patients have been conducted by John Kabat-Zinn, Ph.D., the founder and Director of the Stress Reduction Clinic at the University of Massachusetts Medical Center, and Associate Professor of Medicine in the Division of Preventative and Behavioral Medicine at the University of Massachusetts Medical School. Kabat-Zinn and his program were featured on the American public television (PBS) series *Healing and the Mind*, with Bill Moyers.

Dr. Kabat-Zinn's studies have demonstrated decreases in many kinds of pain in people who had been unresponsive to standard medical treatment. A large majority of the patients in Kabat-Zinn's studies who were taught to meditate improved, while control groups of similar patients showed no significant improvement. Various related studies have shown improvement in pain from muscle tension, headaches, dysmenorrhea, and other conditions.[3]

Changes in Brainwaves and Enhanced Perception

It should come as no surprise that among the well-documented effects of meditation is the alteration of brain-wave patterns. Dozens of studies have shown an increase in alpha rhythms, which are correlated with a state of relaxed alertness. In addition, numerous studies have shown enhanced synchronization of alpha rhythms among four regions of the brain—right, left, front, and back. This may be an indication of increased coherence of brain-wave activity.[4]

Some researchers have demonstrated positive effects of meditation on mind-body coordination, exploring this area by measuring such parameters as visual sensitivity to light flashes,[5] response to auditory stimuli,[6] and ability to remember and discriminate musical tones.[7] There are also indications that during meditation the function of the right hemisphere of the brain (generally correlated with creativity and imagination) is enhanced, while that of the left hemisphere (generally correlated with linear, intellectual thought) is inhibited.[8]

Despite the encouraging trend of increased research attention to the subject in recent years, scientific evaluation of meditation is still in its early stages. While certain benefits have been proven, much remains untested. Furthermore, the technology may not yet exist to validate many of the most profound effects of meditation. It is likely that research in the coming decades will take us far beyond our current knowledge, just as today's level of understanding far exceeds that which existed prior to 1970.

Meditation Methods

Now that the value of meditation has been established, one might reasonably ask next: What exactly is meditation, and how do I meditate? Ironically, these questions are not easy to answer, because there are so many different approaches.

Most widely used meditation methods evolved as part of religious traditions and, as such, each of them may be controversial for people who do not identify with the tradition in which the particular method developed. Since this chapter is on health rather than religion, I want to tread lightly when discussing religious meditation. I personally have found value in meditative techniques of religious origin, whether it has been the Vedic roots of Transcendental Meditation, the Judeo-Christian orientation of Edgar Cayce's method, or the Buddhist origin of various Tibetan, Chinese or Japanese practices.

I have personally practiced several of these techniques and feel that I have benefited from each. But out of respect for all who have qualms about mixing their health care with religion, when I speak to patients about meditation I always encourage use of a method consistent with their own beliefs. I usually say something like, "I'm not selling a particular brand." I also emphasize to my patients, and wish to reiterate here, that the physical health benefits of meditation can be attained through the practice of any of the methods in this chapter, and through other methods as well.

The Relaxation Response

Aside from generating groundbreaking research, it may be that Herbert Benson's most lasting contribution is the development and popularization of a meditative technique with no religious overlay. This approach allows those who are not religious, or whose beliefs may appear to conflict with the teachings connected to a particular meditation system, to nonetheless participate fully in this worthwhile, health-giving activity.

According to Benson, the relaxation response technique produces the same physiological changes as does Transcendental Meditation, the method which has been most fully researched in scientific settings.

Here are Benson's directions for evoking the relaxation response.

1. Sit quietly in a comfortable position.

2. Close your eyes.

3. Deeply relax all your muscles, beginning at your feet and progressing up to your face. Keep them relaxed.

4. Breathe through your nose. Become aware of your breathing. As you breathe out, say the word "ONE," silently to yourself. For one example, breathe IN. . . OUT, "ONE"; IN. . . OUT, "ONE,": etc. Breathe easily and naturally.

5. Continue for 10 to 20 minutes. You may open your eyes to check the time, but do not use an alarm. When you finish, sit quietly for several minutes, at first with your eyes closed and later with your eyes opened. Do not stand up for a few minutes.

6. Do not worry about whether you are successful in achieving a deep level of relaxation.

Maintain a passive attitude and permit relaxation to occur at its own pace. When distracting thoughts occur, try to ignore them by not dwelling upon them and return to repeating "ONE." With practice, the response should come with little effort. Practice the technique once or twice daily, but not within two hours after any meal, since the digestive processes seem to interfere with the elicitation of the relaxation response.[9]

Transcendental Meditation (TM) and the Use of Mantras

TM was brought to the Western world in the mid-twentieth century by Maharishi Mahesh Yogi, an Indian spiritual teacher. The Maharishi's method has been taught to hundreds of thousands of people, and is widely credited with being the first form of Eastern meditation to be practiced on a mass scale in the West.

Herbert Benson's original research subjects were TM practitioners (they were the ones who approached him with the idea of doing research on meditation), and it is TM that Benson used as the basis for formulating his relaxation response method. The relaxation response incorporates many of the principles of TM, but with the Indian tradition removed. TM organizations assert that something significant is lost when the traditional methods are not followed in full.

I cannot provide a step-by-step series of instructions for TM as I did for the relaxation response, because those who receive instruction in TM agree not to reveal the details of what they have learned. I feel it is appropriate to share certain general principles of the TM teachings, however, since they may well be applicable elsewhere. TM is presented as a method that involves neither concentration nor contemplation. That is, unlike some meditative practices, you do not attempt one-pointed focus on an idea or a visual image nor do you pursue trains of thought, however interesting, worthwhile, or inspired they may seem.

Instead, you use a mantra (a seed-syllable or primordial sound) given to you by a TM teacher. The sounds used for mantras, which are derived from Sanskrit, do not have a verbal meaning, and thus are not intended to engage the cognitive mind. The mantra is a sound you say silently to yourself, which functions something like the ringing of a bell. Just as Benson used the word "ONE" in the sample directions given for the relaxation response, TM practitioners use their mantras to help still the mind when distracting thoughts intrude.

The internal chatter created by these thoughts is a normal occurrence. (What shall I wear this morning? How will I ever solve that problem at work?) But meditation time is not for working on problem solving. When the thought arises, you should acknowledge it, and then let it pass, silently repeating the mantra to yourself.

Eknath Easwaran, an Indian-born meditation teacher, philosopher and author, speaks of the purpose of the mantra in his book *Meditation*. He says, "Our aim, remember, is to drive the mantra to the deepest levels of consciousness, where it operates not as words but as healing power."[10]

For those who do not practice TM, some possible mantras from various traditions are:

- Peace
- Love
- Om Mani Padme Hum
- Om Nima Shivaya
- So Hum
- Hari Om
- Tat twam asi
- Thank You
- The Lord is My Shepherd
- Thy Will Be Done

It is common for beginners at meditation (of all types) to experience a great deal of mental chatter and clutter. If this happens to you, it does not mean that you are doing anything wrong. Just notice each thought as it comes, and then let it pass on by, using the mantra to, as it were, break the spell. As a rule, people who are patient enough to continue the practice of meditation for months or years note gradual changes in the ratio between silence and internal chatter. Step by step, there is more silence and less chatter. Even experienced meditators, however, are likely to have periodic increases in the amount of internal chatter, especially in times of stress.

Deepak Chopra on Meditation and Health

Deepak Chopra, M.D., is a physician and author who practices TM. Trained as an endocrinologist, he now practices traditional Indian Ayurvedic medicine (which emphasizes the use of herbs and meditation) in Massachusetts, and has authored several best-selling, highly influential books on holism, the best-known of which is *Quantum Healing*. Dr. Chopra also serves on a review panel for the National Institutes of Health Office of Alternative Medicine.

In his book *Unconditional Life: Discovering the Power to Fulfill Your Dreams*, he provides a set of questions with which to evaluate meditative practices.

"There are any number of important issues to consider when evaluating a form of meditation-above all: Did my mind actually

185

find the silence I was seeking? Was I psychologically comfortable during and after meditation? Did my old self begin to change as a result of having meditated? Is there more truth in my self?"[11]

For Dr. Chopra, TM provided what he sought. Similarly, I know people who have practiced TM for years, enjoy it greatly, and find it to be supportive of their physical well being and personal growth.

I interviewed Dr. Chopra, and asked how he views the relationship between meditation and healing. His answer draws on some of the concepts explored in depth in *Quantum Healing*:

"Our bodies ultimately are fields of information, intelligence and energy. Quantum healing involves a shift in the fields of energy information, so as to bring about a correction in an idea that has gone wrong. So quantum healing involves healing one mode of consciousness, mind, to bring about changes in another mode of consciousness, body.

"Meditation is a very important aspect of all the approaches that one can use in quantum healing, because it allows you to experience your own source. When you experience your own source, you realize that you are not the patterns and eddies of desire and memory that flow and swirl in your consciousness. Although these patterns of desire and memory are the field of your manifestation, you are in fact not these swirling fluctuations of thought.

"You are the thinker behind the thought, the observer behind the observation, the flow of attention, the flow of awareness, the unbounded ocean of consciousness. When you have that on the experiential level, you spontaneously realize that you have choices, and that you can exercise these choices, not through some sheer will power, but spontaneously."[12]

I asked Chopra whether he felt that TM was superior to other forms of meditation, and his answer reflected a broadminded respect for other approaches:

"I feel that all forms of traditional meditation which are time-tested are worthwhile. My experience is with TM, therefore I am best qualified to speak about TM . . . My experience is that it is effortless, easy, spontaneous. It allows the mind to simply transcend to its source. This does not mean I think Zen is not a good form of meditation, or that Vipassana is not. They are all authentic forms of meditation. That is why they have survived over thousands of years."[13]

The quest for profound inner silence and stillness is the essence of meditation. Chopra illumines this beautifully in the following passage from Unconditional Life, as he converses with a patient who has had anxiety attacks since childhood. The man is concerned that he never actually experiences periods of silence in meditation. " . . . But intellectually," I [Chopra] said, "you realize that the mind can be silent?" "Not mine," he said. "Why not?" "It's too quick." "But even a quick mind has gaps between thoughts," I pointed out. "Each gap is like a tiny window onto silence, and through that window one actually contacts the source of the mind. As we're talking here now, there are gaps between our words, aren't there? When you meditate, you take a vertical dive into that gap."

"Sure, I can see that," he rejoined, "but I don't think I experience it in meditation." I asked him what he did experience. He said, "The only thing that makes meditation different from just sitting in a chair is that when I open my eyes after twenty minutes, I often feel that only two or three minutes have passed—I am intrigued by that."

"I said, 'But you see, this is the very best clue that you have gone beyond thought. When you don't have thoughts, there is silence. Silence does not occupy time, and in order to contact the Self, one has to go into the field of the timeless. Your mind might not be able to register this experience at first, because it is so accustomed to thinking. You may feel that time has simply flown by, or that it was lost somewhere. But the 'lost' time was actually spent immersed in the Self.'"[14]

Meditation as Taught by Edgar Cayce

The Cayce method was my first introduction to meditation, and is one to which I have returned in recent years. I am particularly attracted to its underlying intention—the integration of body, mind, and spirit. The goal of meditation, say the Cayce readings, goes beyond attunement within the individual; it includes service to humankind and a heightened relationship to God, or the Creative Forces.

"What is meditation? . . . it is the attuning of the mental body and the physical body to its spiritual source . . . it is the attuning of . . . physical and mental attributes seeking to know the relationships to the Maker. That is true meditation."[15]

187

Cayce said that we must learn to meditate, just as we once learned to walk. It is very important not to mistake beginnings for failures. We each must begin at the beginning, and should understand that we may falter in some of our early steps. The place to start, Cayce asserted, is not with technique but with an examination of our purpose. Find your ideal, he urged, so that your practice of meditation will be grounded in a positive purpose. This ideal might be "love," "compassion," "serving others," or any of a host of other worthwhile guiding principles. What matters most is that it truly be an ideal that embodies service, and that it be something you have a sincere commitment to live up to.

In her book, *Healing Through Meditation and Prayer*, Meredith Puryear offers a clear and concise introduction to Edgar Cayce's approach to meditation. Before laying out a specific set of directions, Puryear asks us to remember why we are meditating, and offers suggestions on how to enhance the effects of meditation. "When we ask how to meditate, the real question we are asking is: How do we learn to commune with God? The answer lies not in some technique, though every activity will have some form to it, but with the desire of the heart to know our oneness with Him. To awaken this desire we must feed our soul and mind a more spiritual diet. We must begin to take time to listen to beautiful, uplifting music, to read inspirational poetry and prose and the great scriptures of the ages: the Bible, the Koran, the Talmud, the Bhagavad-Gita.

"Even five minutes a day with some uplifting word will change the direction of our lives. We must also make some real choices about the kind of reading, TV, and movie diet we choose . . . These choices involve voluntary use of time, energy, and money; they also entail involuntary glandular involvement, because the glandular centers and secretions play a part in every activity of our lives. With every activity in which we engage, we are building toward something either constructive or destructive. The choices themselves may at first be a matter of discipline; but as we continue to do with persistence what we know to do, we will find it becoming easier and easier, because the process of meditation or communion changes our desires, and we begin to want different things and activities than we had heretofore."[16]

The following set of directions for meditation is adapted from Puryear's book, which in turn is based on the Cayce readings.[17]

1. Set the ideal.

2. Set a time—be regular, persistent and patient.

188

3. Prepare—physically, mentally, spiritually.

    Immediate Preparation:

    *   A. Posture: spine straight (feet on floor, or lying on back, or sitting cross-legged)
    *   B. Head-and-neck exercise
    *   C. Breathing exercise

4. Invite protection

    Surround yourself with the consciousness of the presence of the Christ Spirit (alternatives might include surrounding yourself with the love of God, a pure white light, or any other healing and uplifting image or thought)

5. Use an affirmation

    Cayce recommended beginning with the Lord's Prayer. This may be followed by a specific affirmation, such as "Make me an instrument of Thy peace." (You may, as always, substitute an phrase which has deep meaning for you).

6. Silence!

    Return to the affirmation (or a shortened version of it) as distracting thoughts arise. Continue for 10-30 minutes, or whatever period of time feels intuitively appropriate to you.

7. Pray for others

    What is called the "affirmation" in these directions is the structural equivalent of the mantra in TM, and the word "One" in Dr. Benson's relaxation response method. It is the meditator's all-purpose tool, the one used for prying ourselves out of all the dead-end nooks and crannies the mind invents to distract us from the depths of silence, and the heights of revelation.

Edgar Cayce said that "meditation is listening to the Divine within."[18] May we all become good listeners.

Notes

1. Dietnstfrey, Harris. *Where Mind Meets Body*, p. 31.

2. Murphy and Donovan, *The Physical and Psychological Effects of Meditation*, p. 27.

3. Ibid., p. 30.

4. Ibid., p. 15-18.

5. Brown, D.P., Engler, J. "The Stages of Mindfulness Meditation: A Validation Study." *Journal of Transpersonal Psychology*, 1980, 12 (2), 143-192.

6. McEvoy, T.M., Frumkin, L.R., Harkins, S.W. "Effects of Meditation on Brainstem Auditory Evoked Potentials." *International Journal of Neuroscience*, 1980, 10, 165-170.

7. Pagano, R.R., Frumkin, L.R. "The Effect of Transcendental Meditation on Right Hemisphere Functioning, Biofeedback and Self-Regulation," 1977, 2 (4) 407-415.

8. Pagano and Frumkin, Ibid.

9. Benson, *The Relaxation Response*, p. 162-163.

10. Easwaran, Eknath. *Meditation*. p. 71.

11. Chopra, Deepak. *Unconditional Life*, p. 161.

12. Redwood, Daniel, "The Pathways Interview: Deepak Chopra," *Pathways*, December 1991. pp. 5-7.

13. Ibid. p.7.

14. Chopra, op. cit.. p. 190.

15. Edgar Cayce Reading 281-41.

16. Puryear, *Healing through Meditation and Prayer*, p. 4-5.

17. Ibid. p. 6.

18. ECR 1861-19.

Chapter 18

Prayer

You can't go through years of education here in the U.S. without being exposed to the idea that everything is physical. If you have a metaphysical, cosmic experience, well, that's just a chemical reaction. If you have a born-again experience, lithium will take care of it! We come out of our schools with no appreciation of the mind or even the presence of consciousness.

In reality, you can't find anything in the body that defines consciousness. It's hard to find anything that you can pinpoint as "the mind." It's time we admitted that nothing in chemistry or physics has even a remote bearing on consciousness. As David Chalmers, a philosopher at the University of California at Santa Cruz said in a recent article in *Scientific American*, it's time to bite the bullet and admit that consciousness is another force altogether, on a par with matter and energy.

When we talk of prayer we are talking about distant manifestations of consciousness. To talk in this way is to break some kind of taboo. We can accept the power of the mind in affecting bodily processes, but to talk interpersonally—that my consciousness can have an effect on other persons and events—is a major paradigm shift.

The first major shift in our thinking about health came in the mid 1800s when we began to view the body scientifically and mechanically.

"Prayer as a Healing Force," ©1996, updated 2001. Larry Dossey, M.D. Larry Dossey is Executive Editor of the peer-reviewed journal *Alternative Therapies in Health and Medicine* and the author of nine books that examine the role of consciousness and spirituality in health, most recently *Healing Beyond the Body* (Boston: Shambhala, 2001). Reprinted with permission.

You identify what's not working right and fix it. The second era brought in the connection between mind and body. We began to talk about psychosomatic illness. The third era introduces the idea of non-local medicine.

Local medicine believes that my mind is localized in my brain. Non-local medicine says that my mind may not be localized to my brain and body or even to the present moment. One way to define intercessory prayer is as a "positive, distant, non-local manifestation of conciousness." This includes born-again Christians' prayers as well as the Buddhists'. It can include rejoicing, talking, silence, be addressed to God or to the universe. How you pray is up to you.

People get upset with this kind of broad definition. Most people in this culture define prayer as talking aloud to oneself or to some white, male parent figure, usually in the English language. But there are many cultures and religions with prayer practices. Unless you want to disenfranchize lots of people, we need a broader definition. And interestingly, the studies on prayer show no correlation between religious affiliation and the effects of prayer in the laboratory. The factors that seems to work are love, compassion, empathy and deep caring.

The most famous prayer study was conducted by Dr. Randolph Byrd, a cardiologist at the University of California at San Francisco Medical Center. He took 393 people who had been admitted to the hospital with a heart attack. All of the subjects received the same high-tech, state-of-the-art coronary care, but half were also prayed for by name by prayer groups around the country. No one knew who was being prayed for—the patients, the doctors, the nurses. The prayed-for group had fewer deaths, less need for CPR, less intubations, and used fewer potent medications.

If the subject of this study had been a new medication instead of prayer, this would have been considered a medical break through. Up until then, most medical people had considered prayer a nice thing. It didn't hurt much, but they certainly didn't consider it a matter of life and death.

One of the complaints about Byrd's and others' studies is that they are not rigorously done. In writing my books I looked at all of the studies, some 160 of them. While it is true that some have problems, many are fanatically precise and admirably designed. Two-thirds show that the impact of distant prayer is statistically significant.

Some scientists have talked of the "problem of extraneous prayer." How do we know that those cardiac patients in the control group weren't being prayed for by friends and family? People often pray in a crisis. Now, I for one am glad that this problem of extraneous prayer exists. If I have a heart attack, I want to have a lot of this problem! But for research purposes, scientists have gotten around this by doing studies of the growth of bacteria in test tubes. That way you guarantee the purity of the control group. This kind of study might seem outrageous but this is where precise science can be done.

Some people have told me, "You can't afford to talk about prayer stuff like this. You'll make people feel guilty. What if someone is on this wonderful spiritual path but the pathology report comes back positive? They may feel shame and blame and guilt. They may feel they haven't prayed hard enough or been spiritual enough. So don't bring it up and make them feel uncomfortable."

I think we who believe in the connection between body, mind and spirit have to take this problem very seriously. In some circles there is the belief that if you stay on a spiritual path everything will turn out all right. There's even a book that says that you'll never die if you achieve spiritual perfection. So if you get sick, that means you had some more spiritual work to do.

We need to say emphatically that there is not a one-to-one correlation. One's well-being is not just as simple as being happy and being aware or praying properly. Any model we create about the relationship between spiritual achievement and good health has to account for two groups of people. I call them the Healthy Reprobates and the Unhealthy Saints. One of the oldest men on earth lives in Iraq; he's at least 120 years old and drinks and smokes all the time. And history is full of very spiritual people who were sick all the time. In the Bible, Job was described as perfect, and look what happened to him. The Buddha died of food poisoning.

We should understand that prayer does have an impact, but it can't save us from death or guarantee we won't get sick. There's no historical or clinical evidence that this is true. I would say to you though, don't wait for the results of more double-blind studies to pray. We can stand to have more extraneous prayer in this world of ours.

Part Four

Dietary Interventions

Chapter 19

Special Dietary Therapy

Have you noticed how sometimes chance provides you with little hints of life's irony? As I was researching, I ventured into a major bookstore to seek out more of the information available to the general public on nutrition therapies. After wandering through racks and racks of books and magazines, I finally came upon the nutrition section. Right next to the "Science Fiction and Fantasy" section!

Fitting, isn't it? After all, nutrition is a science, but most of what is written about it is fiction. My goal in this chapter is to tell you about that science, and let you make an informed decision about what you want—or don't want—to do. Let's leave fiction out of the equation.

More and more people are turning to nutritional and herbal supplements as an alternative to conventional medicine. It is estimated that 90% of HIV positive people try some form of non-traditional approach to HIV therapy. Seventy percent take at least one unproven supplement from their local health food stores. Do you? If so, read on.

Before deciding what is appropriate and what is not, one must differentiate between vitamin supplements (A, B, C, E) and mineral supplements (selenium, iron, zinc, calcium to name a few) and herbal supplements (echinacea, ginseng, ginger and others).

"Nutrition: The Science behind the Fiction," by Marianne Friedman, from *Being Alive,* June 1998; © 1998 Being Alive (www.beingalivela.org); reprinted with permission.

An Integral Part of Therapy

Scientific studies indicate that supplementation with vitamins and minerals can be an integral part of therapy, along with anti-retroviral drugs, and can actually help maintain the immune system, which is placed under exceedingly high demand both by the infection and by the medications themselves. These vitamins and minerals do not act on the enemy (the virus) but they help maintain the defending army (the immune system), keeping it in shape for the continuous battle.

Supplementation with selenium (200–600 micrograms/day), beta-carotene (23 x RDA), vitamins C (500 mg2 g/day) and E (400–800 IU/day) has been shown to have beneficial effects in protecting the immune system against natural damage by our environment (air pollution, sun, and the like). These vitamins are called anti-oxidants because they protect against damage called oxidation (one example of oxidation is rust.) Some recent reports suggest that alpha lipoic acid or ALA (600–1000 mg/day) as well as N-acetyl-cysteine (12 g/day) may also play a role in protecting the immune system against oxidation.

Omega-3 fatty acids (in capsules labeled DHA and EPA, also referred to as fish fatty acids), are also increasingly recommended to support immune function, because of their role in preventing the inflammation that accompanies chronic infections.

But besides those well-recognized (and well-studied) vitamins and minerals, several new herbal compounds have appeared on the market as "food supplements." Some of them may be useful while others may actually be harmful.

Not Subject to FDA Regulations

Unlike medications, herbal or nutritional supplements are not subject to FDA regulations. This means that no warning about toxicity is required on the label, and any claim about beneficial effects can be made without supporting evidence. This also means that no quality control exists as to the composition or purity of a supplement. Thus extreme caution has to be exercised when choosing herb-based supplements so that they do not do more harm than good.

Keep in mind that no matter how efficient an herbal remedy may be at possibly maintaining your immune system, it is nowhere near as efficient as medical anti-retroviral therapy at decreasing your viral load. If you choose to use any type of alternative therapy in addition to conventional medicine, make sure you let your physician know about it, since some of these herbs may interact with your medications and place you at risk for serious side effects.

Echinacea

One of the most publicized herbal remedies today is echinacea (*Echinacea angustifolia*). Acclaimed as the "universal remedy," its uses range from treatment of the common cold to chronic infections. Studies still differ in their conclusions about its efficacy, but supplementation in people with a weakened immune system has so far been contraindicated until more is known about its effects.

However, one preliminary study done in test tubes and on 14 HIV positive people suggests that at doses of up to 1 gram three times a day, echinacea may be helpful at controlling the viral load by stimulating natural killer cells (an essential component of your defense system) with little toxicity and at little cost. More research is needed to confirm these findings. What is known is that the prolonged use of echinacea may actually depress the immune system, maybe by overstimulating it.

Therefore it should be taken in on-and-off alternating periods of two to three months, with breaks of three to four weeks to allow for the immune cells to renew themselves.

Ginseng

Ginseng is another herbal remedy that has been used for centuries in traditional Chinese medicine. Of the three types available on the market (Siberian, American or Korean), only the Korean or Asian type (*Panax ginseng*) appears to have beneficial effects on the immune system, at doses from 100 to 300 mg of ginseng extract per day.

Several adverse reactions to ginseng have occurred, but they may have been related to other components, since the compositions of the products vary widely, and labeling is not always accurate. People using insulin, anticoagulants or anti-depressants should avoid ginseng because of possible drug interactions.

Garlic

Garlic has been used since the Middle Ages as a protection against infection. It has been shown to have some anti-oxidant activity along with anti-bacterial and possibly immuno-stimulating effects. Other beneficial effects include a lowering of blood cholesterol levels and a decrease in blood pressure. No toxicity but what a breath!!! Unless you choose to use odorless garlic pills, two cloves a day of raw garlic is the recommended dose.

DHEA

DHEA is one of the latest "food supplements" to be closely looked at for its promising effects in stimulating the natural killer cells of the immune system and controlling the viral load in HIV positive people.

Recommended doses for men range from 50 to 200 mg/day in men and from 25 to 50 mg/day in women (overdosing in women may cause the appearance of male characteristics, including hair growth and voice changes.) However, DHEA may be associated with increased risks of breast or prostate cancer and should not be used if you have any risk factors for either (previous occurrence or family history.)

Glutamine and Lecithin

Glutamine, from 1 teaspoon/day to 1 tablespoon/day, helps maintain both the immune system and intestinal function and may be used regularly at the lower dose, with increases to the higher dose during bouts of diarrhea (along with acidophilus and bifidus-enriched products.)

Lecithin granules (not in tablet form which is not absorbed as well) mixed with lemon juice and olive oil have been reported to boost the immune system by increasing natural killer cell activity, without any toxicity. The cocktail is made of 2 teaspoons of lemon juice, 2 tablespoons of olive oil and 2 tablespoons of lecithin granules. (You could add the two cloves of garlic I previously talked about.)

Astragalus and "Cat's Claw"

Astragalus (or Huang ch'i) has been used for centuries in Chinese medicine to stimulate the immune system, and may help fight infections, but caution must be exercised, since overdose may actually cause the opposite effect and suppress the immune system. Too much may actually may be worse than none at all. Beware!

"Cat's Claw" (Uncaria tomentosa or una de gato) is one herb product, which, in one study, was found to be extremely powerful at killing in the test tube all cells including natural killer cells (an essential part of your immune system). Thus this compound could actually further weaken the body's natural defenses and may be very dangerous for HIV infected people.

Bittermelon enemas, Compound Q (sea cucumber extract), and Essiac tea (a mixture of sheepshead sorrel, Indian rhubarb, burdock and slippery elm) have not been shown to have any effect on the viral load or the immune system. Keep in mind that enemas are always dangerous because of the increased risks of damaging or irritating the colon, leading to diarrhea or intestinal infections.

Kombucha Mushrooms

Kombucha mushroom tea (the mushroom is actually a sac formed by the growth of various yeasts and bacteria) may actually be associated with increased risks of fungal infections (because of the fermentation process of the yeast and bacteria with sugar), without any demonstrated positive effect on the immune system. Home-brewed preparations are prone to microbial contamination and may increase risks of parasitic infections.

I hope that I have shed some light on the science behind the fiction. This is meant to help you, but in no way constitutes a recommendation. Let me once again remind you to let your physician know about any supplements or herbal preparations you are taking. Although sold over the counter, herbal remedies are chemicals and therefore could have severe side effects or interactions with medications you are currently taking.

And remember that if you are already taking a lot of pills, priority must be given to your medications over any supplement. Do not forget to take your medications under any circumstance. Forgeting to take your vitamins will not be harmful. Forgeting to take your medications could be.

Chapter 20

Dietary Supplements

Quick Definition

The Dietary Supplement Health and Education Act defines dietary supplements as a:

- product (other than tobacco) intended to supplement the diet that bears or contains one or more of the following dietary ingredients: a vitamin, mineral, amino acid, herb or other botanical;

OR

- a dietary substance for use to supplement the diet by increasing the total dietary intake;

OR

- a concentrate, metabolite, constituent, extract, or combination of any ingredient described above;

AND

- intended for ingestion in the form of a capsule, powder, softgel, or gelcap, and not represented as a conventional food or as a sole item of a meal or the diet.

"What are Dietary Supplements?" and undated document from the National Institutes of Health (NIH), Office of Dietary Supplements (ODS), cited December 2001.

Full Definition and Explanation

Dietary supplements are available widely through many commercial sources including health food stores, grocery stores, pharmacies, and by mail. Dietary supplements are provided in many forms including tablets, capsules, powders, geltabs, extracts, liquids, etc. Historically in the United States, the most prevalent type of dietary supplement was a multivitamin/mineral tablet or capsule that was available in pharmacies by prescription or "over the counter." Supplements containing strictly herbal preparations were less widely available. Currently in the United States, a wide array of supplement products are available and they include vitamin, mineral, other nutrients, and botanical supplements as well as ingredients and extracts of animal and plant origin.

The term "dietary supplement" for the United States Government offices such as the Office of Dietary Supplements (ODS) at the National Institutes of Health (NIH) was more formally defined in 1994 with the passage by the United States Congress of the Dietary Supplement Health and Education Act (DSHEA, Public Law 103-417, October 25, 1994). DSHEA is an amendment to the Federal Food, Drug, and Cosmetic Act "to establish standards with respect to dietary supplements..." One provision of DSHEA provides the following definitions for dietary supplements:

Section 3. Definitions

The term "dietary supplement means a product (other than tobacco) intended to supplement the diet that bears or contains one or more of the following dietary ingredients:

(A) a vitamin;

(B) a mineral;

(C) an herb or other botanical;

(D) an amino acid;

(E) a dietary substance for use by man to supplement the diet by increasing the total dietary intake; or

(F) a concentrate, metabolite, constituent, extract, or combination of any ingredient described in (A), (B), (C), (D), or (E);

It means a product that:

(A) is intended for ingestion in a form described above.

(B) is not represented for use as a conventional food or as a sole item of a meal or the diet; and

(C) is labeled as a dietary supplement.

Chapter 21

Folate

Folate: What Is It?

Folate and folic acid are forms of a water-soluble B vitamin. Folate occurs naturally in food. Folic acid is the synthetic form of this vitamin that is found in supplements and fortified foods. Folate gets its name from the Latin word "folium" for leaf. A key observation of researcher Lucy Wills nearly 70 years ago led to the identification of folate as the nutrient needed to prevent the anemia of pregnancy. Dr. Wills demonstrated that the anemia could be corrected by a yeast extract. Folate was identified as the corrective substance in yeast extract in the late 1930s and was extracted from spinach leaves in 1941. Folate is necessary for the production and maintenance of new cells. This is especially important during periods of rapid cell division and growth such as infancy and pregnancy. Folate is needed to make DNA and RNA, the building blocks of cells. It also helps prevent changes to DNA that may lead to cancer. Both adults and children need folate to make normal red blood cells and prevent anemia.

What Foods Provide Folate?

Leafy greens such as spinach and turnip greens, dry beans and peas, fortified cereals and grain products, and some fruits and vegetables

This text was developed by the Clinical Nutrition Service, Warren Grant Magnuson Clinical Center, in conjunction with the Office of Dietary Supplements (ODS), National Institutes of Health (NIH), January 2001.

are rich food sources of folate. Some breakfast cereals (ready-to-eat and others) are fortified with 25 percent or 100 percent of the Daily Value (DV) for folic acid. Table 21.2 suggests dietary sources of this vitamin. In 1996, the Food and Drug Administration (FDA) published regulations requiring the addition of folic acid to enriched breads, cereals, flours, corn meals, pastas, rice, and other grain products. This ruling took effect January 1, 1998, and was specifically targeted to reduce the risk of neural tube birth defects in newborns. Since the folic acid fortification program took effect, fortified foods have become a major source of folic acid in the American diet. Synthetic folic acid that is added to fortified foods and dietary supplements has a simpler chemical structure than the natural form of folate, and is absorbed more easily by the body. After digestion and absorption however, the two forms are identical and function in exactly the same manner.

What Is the Recommended Dietary Allowance for Folate for Adults?

The Recommended Dietary Allowance (RDA) is the average daily dietary intake level that is sufficient to meet the nutrient requirements of nearly all (97 to 98 percent) healthy individuals in each life-stage and gender group. The 1998 RDAs for folate are expressed in a term called the Dietary Folate Equivalent. The Dietary Folate Equivalent (DFE) was developed to help account for the differences in absorption of naturally occurring dietary folate and the more bioavailable synthetic folic acid. The 1998 RDAs for folate expressed in micrograms (mcg) of DFE for adults are shown in Table 21.1.

The National Health and Nutrition Examination Survey (NHANES III 1988-91) and the Continuing Survey of Food Intakes by Individuals (1994-96 CSFII) indicated that most adults did not consume adequate

Table 21.1. RDAs for Folate

Life Stage	Men	Women	Pregnancy	Lactation
Ages 19+	400 mcg	400 mcg		
All ages			600 mcg	500 mcg

1 mcg of food folate = 0.6 mcg folic acid from supplements and fortified foods

folate. However, the folic acid fortification program has increased folic acid content of commonly eaten foods such as cereals and grains, and as a result diets of most adults now provide recommended amounts of folate equivalents.

When Can Folate Deficiency Occur?

A deficiency of folate can occur when your need for folate is increased, when dietary intake of folate is inadequate, and when your body excretes (or loses) more folate than usual. Medications that interfere with your body's ability to use folate may also increase the need for this vitamin. Some situations that increase the need for folate include:

- pregnancy and lactation (breastfeeding)
- alcohol abuse
- malabsorption
- kidney dialysis
- liver disease
- certain anemias

Medications can interfere with folate utilization, including:

- anti-convulsant medications (such as dilantin, phenytoin, and primidone)
- Metformin (sometimes prescribed to control blood sugar in type 2 diabetes)
- Sulfasalazine (used to control inflammation associated with Crohn's disease and ulcerative colitis)
- Triamterene (a diuretic)
- Methotrexate

Signs of Folate Deficiency

Signs of folic acid deficiency are often subtle. Diarrhea, loss of appetite, and weight loss can occur. Additional signs are weakness, sore tongue, headaches, heart palpitations, irritability, and behavioral disorders. Women with folate deficiency who become pregnant are more likely to give birth to low birth weight and premature infants, and infants with neural tube defects. In adults, anemia is a sign of advanced folate deficiency. In infants and children, folate deficiency can slow growth rate. Some of these symptoms can also result from a variety of medical conditions other than folate deficiency. It is important to have a physician evaluate these symptoms so that appropriate medical care can be given.

Who May Need Extra Folic Acid to Prevent a Deficiency?

Women of childbearing age, people who abuse alcohol, anyone taking anti-convulsants or other medications that interfere with the action of folate, individuals diagnosed with anemia from folate deficiency, and individuals with malabsorption, liver disease, or who are receiving kidney dialysis treatment may benefit from a folic acid supplement.

Folic acid is very important for all women who may become pregnant. Adequate folate intake during the periconceptual period, the time just before and just after a woman becomes pregnant, protects against a number of congenital malformations including neural tube defects. Neural tube defects result in malformations of the spine (spina bifida), skull, and brain (anencephaly). The risk of neural tube defects is significantly reduced when supplemental folic acid is consumed in addition to a healthful diet prior to and during the first month following conception. Women who could become pregnant are advised to eat foods fortified with folic acid or take supplements in addition to eating folate-rich foods to reduce the risk of some serious birth defects. Taking 400 micrograms of synthetic folic acid daily from fortified foods and/or supplements has been suggested. The Recommended Dietary Allowance (RDA) for folate equivalents for pregnant women is 600 micrograms.

Folate deficiency has been observed in alcoholics. A 1997 review of the nutritional status of chronic alcoholics found low folate status in more than 50 percent of those surveyed. Alcohol interferes with the absorption of folate and increases excretion of folate by the kidney. In addition, many alcohol abusers have poor quality diets that do not provide the recommended intake of folate. Increasing folate intake through diet, or folic acid intake through fortified foods or supplements, may be beneficial to the health of alcoholics.

Anti-convulsant medications such as dilantin increase the need for folate. Anyone taking anti-convulsants and other medications that interfere with the body's ability to use folate should consult with a medical doctor about the need to take a folic acid supplement.

Anemia is a condition that occurs when red blood cells cannot carry enough oxygen. It can result from a wide variety of medical problems, including folate deficiency. Folate deficiency can result in the formation of large red blood cells that do not contain adequate hemoglobin, the substance in red blood cells that carries oxygen to your body's cells. Your physician can determine whether an anemia is associated with folate deficiency and whether supplemental folic acid is indicated.

Several medical conditions increase the risk of folic acid deficiency. Liver disease and kidney dialysis increase excretion (loss) of folic acid. Malabsorption can prevent your body from using folate in food. Medical doctors treating individuals with these disorders will evaluate the need for a folic acid supplement.

Caution about Folic Acid Supplements

Beware of the interaction between vitamin B12 and folic acid. Folic acid supplements can correct the anemia associated with vitamin B12 deficiency. Unfortunately, folic acid will not correct changes in the nervous system that result from vitamin B12 deficiency. Permanent nerve damage can occur if vitamin B12 deficiency is not treated. Intake of supplemental folic acid should not exceed 1,000 micrograms (mcg) per day to prevent folic acid from masking symptoms of vitamin B12 deficiency.

It is very important for older adults to be aware of the relationship between folic acid and vitamin B12 because they are at greater risk of having a vitamin B12 deficiency. If you are 50 years of age or older, ask your physician to check your B12 status before you take a supplement that contains folic acid.

What Are Some Current Issues and Controversies about Folate?

Folic Acid and Heart Disease

A deficiency of folate, vitamin B12, or vitamin B6 may increase your level of homocysteine, an amino acid normally found in your blood. There is evidence that an elevated homocysteine level is an independent risk factor for heart disease and stroke. The evidence suggests that high levels of homocysteine may damage coronary arteries or make it easier for blood clotting cells called platelets to clump together and form a clot. However, there is currently no evidence available to suggest that lowering homocysteine with vitamins will reduce your risk of heart disease. Clinical intervention trials are needed to determine whether supplementation with folic acid, vitamin B12 or vitamin B6 can lower your risk of developing coronary heart disease.

Folic Acid and Cancer

Some evidence associates low blood levels of folate with a greater risk of cancer. Folate is involved in the synthesis, repair, and functioning of DNA, our genetic map, and a deficiency of folate may result in damage to DNA that may lead to cancer. Several studies have

Table 21.2. Table of Food Sources of Folate (continued on next page)

Food	Dietary Folate Equivalents in Micrograms	%DV*
Ready to eat cereal, fortified with 100% of the DV, 3/4 c	400	100
Beef liver, cooked, braised, 3 oz	185	45
Cowpeas (blackeyes), immature, cooked, boiled, 1/2 c	105	25
Breakfast cereals, fortified with 25% of the DV, 3/4 c	100	25
Spinach, frozen, cooked, boiled, 1/2 c	100	25
Great Northern beans, boiled, 1/2 c	90	20
Asparagus, boiled, 4 spears	85	20
Wheat germ, toasted, 1/4 c	80	20
Orange juice, chilled, includes concentrate, 3/4 c	70	20
Turnip Greens, frozen, cooked, boiled, 1/2 c	65	15
Vegetarian baked beans, canned, 1 c	60	15
Spinach, raw, 1 c	60	15
Green peas, boiled, 1/2 c	50	15
Broccoli, chopped, frozen, cooked, 1/2 c	50	15
Egg noodles, cooked, enriched, 1/2 c	50	15
Rice, white, long-grain, parboiled, cooked, enriched, 1/2 c	45	10
Avocado, raw, all varieties, sliced, 1/2 c sliced	45	10
Peanuts, all types, dry roasted, 1 oz	40	10

associated diets low in folate with increased risk of breast, pancreatic, and colon cancer. Findings from a study of over 121,000 nurses suggested that long-term folic acid supplementation (for 15 years) was associated with a decreased risk of colon cancer in women aged 55 to 69 years of age. However, associations between diet and disease do not indicate a direct cause. Researchers are continuing to investigate whether enhanced folate intake from foods or folic acid supplements may reduce the risk of cancer. Until results from such clinical trials are available, folic acid supplements should not be recommended to reduce the risk of cancer.

Table 21.2. Table of Food Sources of Folate (continued from previous page)

Food	Dietary Folate Equivalents in Micrograms	%DV*
Lettuce, Romaine, shredded, 1/2 c	40	10
Tomato Juice, canned, 6 oz	35	10
Orange, all commercial varieties, fresh, 1 small	30	8
Bread, white, enriched, 1 slice	25	6
Egg, whole, raw, fresh, 1 large	25	6
Cantaloupe, raw, 1/4 medium	25	6
Papaya, raw, 1/2 c cubes	25	6
Banana, raw, 1 medium	20	6
Broccoli, raw, 1 spear (about 5 inches long)	20	6
Lettuce, iceberg, shredded, 1/2 c	15	4
Bread, whole wheat, 1 slice	15	4

* DV = Daily Value. DVs are reference numbers based on the Recommended Dietary Allowance (RDA). They were developed to help consumers determine if a food contains a lot or a little of a specific nutrient. The DV for folic acid is 400 micrograms (mcg). The percent DV (%DV) listed on the nutrition facts panel of food labels tells adults what percentage of the DV is provided by one serving. Percent DVs are based on a 2,000 calorie diet. Your Daily Values may be higher or lower depending on your calorie needs. Foods that provide lower percentages of the DV also contribute to a healthful diet.

Folic Acid and Methotrexate for Cancer

Folate is important for cells and tissues that rapidly divide. Cancer cells divide rapidly, and drugs that interfere with folate metabolism are used to treat cancer. Methotrexate is a drug often used to treat cancer because it limits the activity of enzymes that need folate. Unfortunately, methotrexate can be toxic, producing side effects such as inflammation in the digestive tract that make it difficult to eat normally. Leucovorin is a form of folate that can help "rescue" or reverse the toxic effects of methotrexate. It is not known whether folic acid supplements can help control the side effects of methotrexate without decreasing its effectiveness in chemotherapy. It is important for anyone receiving methotrexate to follow a medical doctor's advice on the use of folic acid supplements.

Folic Acid and Methotrexate for Non-Cancerous Diseases

Low dose methotrexate is used to treat a wide variety of non-cancerous diseases such as rheumatoid arthritis, lupus, psoriasis, asthma, sarcoidoisis, primary biliary cirrhosis, and inflammatory bowel disease. Low doses of methotrexate can deplete folate stores and cause side effects that are similar to folate deficiency. Both high folate diets and supplemental folic acid may help reduce the toxic side effects of low dose methotrexate without decreasing its effectiveness. Anyone taking low dose methotrexate for the health problems listed above should consult with a physician about the need for a folic acid supplement.

What Is the Health Risk of Too Much Folic Acid?

The risk of toxicity from folic acid is low. The Institute of Medicine has established a tolerable upper intake level (UL) for folate of 1,000 mcg for adult men and women, and a UL of 800 mcg for pregnant and lactating (breast-feeding) women less than 18 years of age. Supplemental folic acid should not exceed the UL to prevent folic acid from masking symptoms of vitamin B12 deficiency.

Selected Food Sources of Folate and Folic Acid

As the *2000 Dietary Guidelines for Americans* states, "Different foods contain different nutrients and other healthful substances. No single food can supply all the nutrients in the amounts you need."

Table 21.2 suggests dietary sources of folate. As the table indicates, green leafy vegetables, dry beans and peas, and many other types of vegetables and fruits are good sources of folate. In addition, fortified foods are a major source of folic acid. It is not unusual to find foods such as cereals fortified with 100 percent of the RDA for folate. The variety of fortified foods available has made it easier for women of childbearing age to consume the recommended 400 mcg of folic acid per day from fortified foods and/or supplements. The large numbers of fortified foods on the market, however, also raise concern that intake may exceed the UL. This is especially important for anyone at risk of vitamin B12 deficiency, which can be masked by too much folic acid. It is important for anyone who is considering taking a folic acid supplement to first consider whether their needs are being met by adequate sources of dietary folate and folic acid from fortified foods.

Chapter 22

Magnesium

Magnesium: What Is It?

Magnesium is a mineral needed by every cell of your body. About half of your body's magnesium stores are found inside cells of body tissues and organs, and half are combined with calcium and phosphorus in bone. Only 1 percent of the magnesium in your body is found in blood. Your body works very hard to keep blood levels of magnesium constant.

Magnesium is needed for more than 300 biochemical reactions in the body. It helps maintain normal muscle and nerve function, keeps heart rhythm steady, and bones strong. It is also involved in energy metabolism and protein synthesis.

What Foods Provide Magnesium?

Green vegetables such as spinach provide magnesium because the center of the chlorophyll molecule contains magnesium. Nuts, seeds, and some whole grains are also good sources of magnesium.

Although magnesium is present in many foods, it usually occurs in small amounts. As with most nutrients, daily needs for magnesium cannot be met from a single food. Eating a wide variety of foods, including five servings of fruits and vegetables daily and plenty of whole grains, helps to ensure an adequate intake of magnesium.

This text was developed by the Clinical Nutrition Service, Warren Grant Magnuson Clinical Center, in conjunction with the Office of Dietary Supplements (ODS), National Institutes of Health (NIH), January 2001.

The magnesium content of refined foods is usually low. Whole-wheat bread, for example, has twice as much magnesium as white bread because the magnesium-rich germ and bran are removed when white flour is processed. The table of food sources of magnesium suggests many dietary sources of magnesium.

Water can provide magnesium, but the amount varies according to the water supply. "Hard" water contains more magnesium than "soft" water. Dietary surveys do not estimate magnesium intake from water, which may lead to underestimating total magnesium intake and its variability.

What Is the Recommended Dietary Allowance for Magnesium?

The Recommended Dietary Allowance (RDA) is the average daily dietary intake level that is sufficient to meet the nutrient requirements of nearly all (97-98 percent) individuals in each life-stage and gender group. The 1999 RDAs for magnesium for adults, in milligrams (mg), are presented in Table 22.1.

Table 22.1. RDAs for Magnesium for Adults

Life-Stage	Men	Women	Pregnancy	Lactation
Ages 14-18	410 mg	360 mg	400 mg	360 mg
Ages 19-30	400 mg	310 mg	350 mg	310 mg
Ages 31 +	420 mg	320 mg	360 mg	320 mg

Results of two national surveys, the National Health and Nutrition Examination Survey (NHANES III-1988-91) and the Continuing Survey of Food Intakes of Individuals (1994 CSFII), indicated that the diets of most adult men and women do not provide the recommended amounts of magnesium. The surveys also suggested that adults age 70 and over eat less magnesium than younger adults, and that non-Hispanic black subjects consumed less magnesium than either non-Hispanic white or Hispanic subjects.

When Can Magnesium Deficiency Occur?

Even though dietary surveys suggest that many Americans do not consume magnesium in recommended amounts, magnesium deficiency is rarely seen in the United States in adults. When magnesium deficiency does occur, it is usually due to excessive loss of magnesium in urine, gastrointestinal system disorders that cause a loss of magnesium or limit magnesium absorption, or a chronically low intake of magnesium.

Treatment with diuretics (water pills), some antibiotics, and some medicine used to treat cancer, such as Cisplatin, can increase the loss of magnesium in urine. Poorly controlled diabetes increases loss of magnesium in urine, causing a depletion of magnesium stores. Alcohol also increases excretion of magnesium in urine, and a high alcohol intake has been associated with magnesium deficiency.

Gastrointestinal problems, such as malabsorption disorders, can cause magnesium depletion by preventing the body from using the magnesium in food. Chronic or excessive vomiting and diarrhea may also result in magnesium depletion.

Signs of magnesium deficiency include confusion, disorientation, loss of appetite, depression, muscle contractions and cramps, tingling, numbness, abnormal heart rhythms, coronary spasm, and seizures.

Who May Need Extra Magnesium?

Healthy adults who eat a varied diet do not generally need to take a magnesium supplement. Magnesium supplementation is usually indicated when a specific health problem or condition causes an excessive loss of magnesium or limits magnesium absorption.

Extra magnesium may be required by individuals with conditions that cause excessive urinary loss of magnesium, chronic malabsorption, severe diarrhea and steatorrhea, and chronic or severe vomiting.

Loop and thiazide diuretics, such as Lasix, Bumex, Edecrin, and Hydrochlorothiazide, can increase loss of magnesium in urine. Medicines such as Cisplatin, which is widely used to treat cancer, and the antibiotics Gentamicin, Amphotericin, and Cyclosporin also cause the kidneys to excrete (lose) more magnesium in urine. Doctors routinely monitor magnesium levels of individuals who take these medicines and prescribe magnesium supplements if indicated.

Poorly controlled diabetes increases loss of magnesium in urine and may increase an individual's need for magnesium. A medical doctor would determine the need for extra magnesium in this situation. Routine supplementation with magnesium is not indicated for individuals with well-controlled diabetes.

People who abuse alcohol are at high risk for magnesium deficiency because alcohol increases urinary excretion of magnesium. Low blood levels of magnesium occur in 30 percent to 60 percent of alcoholics, and in nearly 90 percent of patients experiencing alcohol withdrawal. In addition, alcoholics who substitute alcohol for food will usually have lower magnesium intakes. Medical doctors routinely evaluate the need for extra magnesium in this population.

The loss of magnesium through diarrhea and fat malabsorption usually occurs after intestinal surgery or infection, but it can occur with chronic malabsorptive problems such as Crohn's disease, gluten sensitive enteropathy, and regional enteritis. Individuals with these conditions may need extra magnesium. The most common symptom of fat malabsorption, or steatorrhea, is passing greasy, offensive-smelling stools.

Occasional vomiting should not cause an excessive loss of magnesium, but conditions that cause frequent or severe vomiting may result in a loss of magnesium large enough to require supplementation. In these situations, your medical doctor would determine the need for a magnesium supplement.

Individuals with chronically low blood levels of potassium and calcium may have an underlying problem with magnesium deficiency. Adding magnesium supplements to their diets may make potassium and calcium supplementation more effective for them. Doctors routinely evaluate magnesium status when potassium and calcium levels are abnormal, and prescribe a magnesium supplement when indicated.

What Is the Best Way to Get Extra Magnesium?

Doctors will measure blood levels of magnesium whenever a magnesium deficiency is suspected. When levels are mildly depleted, increasing dietary intake of magnesium can help restore blood levels to normal. Eating at least five servings of fruits and vegetables daily, and choosing dark-green leafy vegetables often, as recommended by the Dietary Guidelines for Americans, the Food Guide Pyramid, and the Five-a-Day program, will help adults at-risk of having a magnesium deficiency consume recommended amounts of magnesium. When blood levels of magnesium are very low, an intravenous drip (IV drip) may be needed to return levels to normal. Magnesium tablets also may be prescribed, but some forms, in particular magnesium salts, can cause diarrhea. Your medical doctor or qualified health-care provider can recommend the best way to get extra magnesium when it is needed.

What are Some Current Issues and Controversies about Magnesium?

Magnesium and Blood Pressure

Evidence suggests that magnesium may play an important role in regulating blood pressure. Diets that provide plenty of fruits and vegetables, which are good sources of potassium and magnesium, are consistently associated with lower blood pressure. The DASH study (Dietary Approaches to Stop Hypertension) suggested that high blood pressure could be significantly lowered by a diet high in magnesium, potassium, and calcium, and low in sodium and fat. In another study, the effect of various nutritional factors on incidence of high blood pressure was examined in over 30,000 U.S. male health professionals. After four years of follow-up, it was found that a greater magnesium intake was significantly associated with a lower risk of hypertension. The evidence is strong enough that the Joint National Committee on Prevention, Detection, Evaluation, and Treatment of High Blood Pressure recommends maintaining an adequate magnesium intake as a positive lifestyle modification for preventing and managing high blood pressure.

Magnesium and Heart Disease

Magnesium deficiency can cause metabolic changes that may contribute to heart attacks and strokes. There is also evidence that low body stores of magnesium increase the risk of abnormal heart rhythms, which may increase the risk of complications associated with a heart attack.

Population surveys have associated higher blood levels of magnesium with lower risk of coronary heart disease. In addition, dietary surveys have suggested that a higher magnesium intake is associated with a lower risk of stroke. Further studies are needed to understand the complex relationships between dietary magnesium intake, indicators of magnesium status, and heart disease.

Magnesium and Osteoporosis

Magnesium deficiency may be a risk factor for postmenopausal osteoporosis. This may be due to the fact that magnesium deficiency alters calcium metabolism and the hormone that regulates calcium. Several studies have suggested that magnesium supplementation may improve bone mineral density, but researchers believe that further investigation on the role of magnesium in bone metabolism and osteoporosis is needed.

Magnesium and Diabetes

Magnesium is important to carbohydrate metabolism. It may influence the release and activity of insulin, the hormone that helps control blood glucose levels. Elevated blood glucose levels increase the loss of magnesium in the urine, which in turn lowers blood levels of magnesium. This explains why low blood levels of magnesium

Table 22.2. Table of Food Sources of Magnesium (continued on next page)

Food	Milligrams	%DV*
100 percent Bran, 2 Tbs	44	11
Avocado, Florida, 1/2 med	103	26
Wheat germ, toasted, 1 oz	90	22
Almonds, dry roasted, 1 oz	86	21
Cereal, shredded wheat, 2 rectangular biscuits	80	20
Seeds, pumpkin, 1/2 oz	75	19
Cashews, dry roasted, 1 oz	73	18
Nuts, mixed, dry roasted, 1 oz	66	17
Spinach, cooked, 1/2 c	65	16
Bran flakes, 1/2 c	60	15
Cereal, oats, instant/fortified, cooked w/ water, 1 c	56	14
Potato, baked w/ skin, 1 med	55	14
Soybeans, cooked, 1/2 c	54	14
Peanuts, dry roasted, 1 oz	50	13
Peanut butter, 2 Tbs.	50	13
Chocolate bar, 1.45 oz	45	11
Vegetarian baked beans, 1/2 c	40	10
Potato, baked w/out skin, 1 med	40	10

(hypomagnesemia) are seen in poorly controlled type 1 and type 2 diabetes.

In 1992, the American Diabetes Association issued a consensus statement that concluded: "Adequate dietary magnesium intake can generally be achieved by a nutritionally balanced meal plan as recommended by the American Diabetes Association." It recommended that "... only diabetic patients at high risk of hypomagnesemia should have total serum (blood) magnesium assessed, and such levels should be repleted (replaced) only if hypomagnesemia can be demonstrated."

Table 22.2. Table of Food Sources of Magnesium (continued from previous page)

Food	Milligrams	%DV*
Avocado, California, 1/2 med	35	9
Lentils, cooked, 1/2 c	35	9
Banana, raw, 1 medium	34	9
Shrimp, mixed species, raw, 3 oz (12 large)	29	7
Tahini, 2 Tbs	28	7
Raisins, golden seedless, 1/2 c packed	28	7
Cocoa powder, unsweetened, 1 Tbs	27	7
Bread, whole wheat, 1 slice	24	6
Spinach, raw, 1 c	24	6
Kiwi fruit, raw, 1 med	23	6
Hummus, 2 Tbs	20	5
Broccoli, chopped, boiled, 1/2 c	19	5

*DV = Daily Value. DVs are reference numbers based on the Recommended Dietary Allowance (RDA). They were developed to help consumers determine if a food contains very much of a specific nutrient. The DV for magnesium is 400 milligrams (mg). The percent DV (%DV) listed on the nutrition facts panel of food labels tells adults what percentage of the DV is provided by one serving. Even foods that provide lower percentages of the DV will contribute to a healthful diet.

What Is the Health Risk of Too Much Magnesium?

Dietary magnesium does not pose a health risk, however very high doses of magnesium supplements, which may be added to laxatives, can promote adverse effects such as diarrhea. Magnesium toxicity is more often associated with kidney failure, when the kidney loses the ability to remove excess magnesium. Very large doses of laxatives also have been associated with magnesium toxicity, even with normal kidney function. The elderly are at risk of magnesium toxicity because kidney function declines with age and they are more likely to take magnesium-containing laxatives and antacids.

Signs of excess magnesium can be similar to magnesium deficiency and include mental status changes, nausea, diarrhea, appetite loss, muscle weakness, difficulty breathing, extremely low blood pressure, and irregular heartbeat.

The Institute of Medicine of the National Academy of Sciences has established a tolerable upper intake level (UL) for supplementary magnesium for adolescents and adults at 350 mg daily. As intake increases above the UL, the risk of adverse effects increases.

Chapter 23

Selenium

Selenium: What Is It?

Selenium is an essential trace mineral in the human body. This nutrient is an important part of antioxidant enzymes that protect cells against the effects of free radicals that are produced during normal oxygen metabolism. The body has developed defenses such as antioxidants to control levels of free radicals because they can damage cells and contribute to the development of some chronic diseases. Selenium is also essential for normal functioning of the immune system and thyroid gland.

What Foods Provide Selenium?

Plant foods are the major dietary sources of selenium in most countries throughout the world. The amount of selenium in soil, which varies by region, determines the amount of selenium in the plant foods that are grown in that soil. Researchers know that soils in the high plains of northern Nebraska and the Dakotas have very high levels of selenium. People living in those regions generally have the highest selenium intakes in the United States. Soils in some parts of China and Russia have very low amounts of selenium and dietary selenium deficiency is often reported in those regions.

This text was developed by the Clinical Nutrition Service, Warren Grant Magnuson Clinical Center, in conjunction with the Office of Dietary Supplements (ODS), National Institutes of Health (NIH), January 2001.

Table 23.1. Food Sources of Selenium

The selenium content of foods varies according to the growing area. The following table lists the mean selenium content of foods identified in the Total Diet Study and in the USDA data bank.

Food	Micrograms	% DV*
Brazil nuts, dried, unblanched, 1 oz	840	1200
Tuna, canned in oil, drained, 3 1/2 oz	78	111
Beef / calf liver, 3 oz	48	69
Cod, cooked, dry heat, 3 oz	40	57
Noodles, enriched, boiled, 1 c	35	50
Macaroni and cheese (box mix), 1 c	32	46
Turkey, breast, oven roasted, 3 1/2 oz	31	44
Macaroni, elbow, enriched, boiled, 1 c	30	43
Spaghetti w/ meat sauce, 1 c	25	36
Chicken, meat only, 1/2 breast	24	34
Beef chuck roast, lean only, oven roasted, 3 oz	23	33
Bread, enriched, whole wheat, 2 slices	20	29
Oatmeal, 1 c cooked	16	23
Egg, raw, whole, 1 large	15	21
Bread, enriched, white, 2 slices	14	20
Rice, enriched, long grain, cooked, 1 c	14	20
Cottage cheese, lowfat 2%, 1/2 c	11	16
Walnuts, black, dried, 1 oz	5	7
Cheddar cheese, 1 oz	4	6

*DV = Daily Value. DVs are reference numbers based on the Recommended Dietary Allowance (RDA). They were developed to help consumers determine if a food contains very much of a specific nutrient. The DV for selenium is 70 micrograms (mcg). The percent DV (%DV) listed on the nutrition facts panel of food labels tells adults what percentage of the DV is provided by one serving. Even foods that provide lower percentages of the DV will contribute to a healthful diet.

Selenium also can be found in some meats and seafood. Animals that eat grains or plants that were grown in selenium-rich soil have higher levels of selenium in their muscle. In the United States, meats and bread are common sources of dietary selenium. Some nuts, in particular Brazil nuts and walnuts, are also very good sources of selenium. Table 23.1 suggests many dietary sources of selenium.

What Is the Recommended Dietary Allowance for Selenium for Adults?

The Recommended Dietary Allowance (RDA) is the average daily dietary intake level that is sufficient to meet the nutrient requirements of nearly all (97-98%) individuals in each life-stage and gender group. Table 23.2 shows the 2000 RDAs for selenium for adults (9), in micrograms (mcg).

Table 23.2. 2000 RDAs for Selenium for Adults

Life-Stage	Men	Women	Pregnancy	Lactation
Ages 19 +	55 mcg	55 mcg		
All ages			60 mcg	70 mcg

Results of the Total Diet Study, a national survey conducted by the U.S. Food and Drug Administration (1982-86), indicated that the diets of most adult men and women provide recommended amounts of selenium.

When Can Selenium Deficiency Occur?

Selenium deficiency is most commonly seen in parts of China where the selenium content in the soil, and therefore selenium intake, is very low. Selenium deficiency is linked to Keshan Disease. The most common signs of selenium deficiency seen in Keshan Disease are an enlarged heart and poor heart function. Keshan disease has been observed in low-selenium areas of China, where dietary intake is less than 19 mcg per day for men and less than 13 mcg per day for women. This intake is significantly lower than the current RDA for selenium.

Selenium deficiency also may affect thyroid function because selenium is essential for the synthesis of active thyroid hormone. Researchers

227

also believe selenium deficiency may worsen the effects of iodine deficiency on thyroid function, and that adequate selenium nutritional status may help protect against some of the neurologic effects of iodine deficiency.

Selenium deficiency has been seen in people who rely on total parenteral nutrition (TPN) as their sole source of nutrition. TPN is a method of feeding nutrients through an intravenous (IV) line to people whose digestive systems do not function. Forms of nutrients that do not require digestion are dissolved in liquid and infused through the IV line. It is important for TPN solutions to provide selenium in order to prevent a deficiency. Physicians can monitor the selenium status of individuals receiving TPN to make sure they are receiving adequate amounts.

Severe gastrointestinal disorders may decrease the absorption of selenium, resulting in selenium depletion or deficiency. Gastrointestinal problems that impair selenium absorption usually affect absorption of other nutrients as well, and require routine monitoring of nutritional status so that physicians can recommend appropriate treatment.

Who May Need Extra Selenium?

Selenium supplementation is essential for anyone relying on TPN as the sole source of nutrition, and selenium supplementation has become routine during TPN administration since the relationship between selenium deficiency and TPN was discovered. Gastrointestinal disorders such as Crohn's disease can impair selenium absorption. Most cases of selenium depletion or deficiency are associated with severe gastrointestinal problems, such as in individuals who have had over half of their small intestines surgically removed. A physician, who will determine the need for selenium supplementation, should evaluate individuals who have gastrointestinal disease and depleted blood levels of selenium.

What Are Some Current Issues and Controversies about Selenium?

Selenium and Cancer

Some studies indicate that mortality (death) from cancer, including lung, colorectal, and prostate cancers, is lower among people with higher selenium blood levels or intake. Also, the incidence of nonmelanoma skin cancer is significantly higher in areas of the United States with low soil selenium levels.

The effect of selenium supplementation on the recurrence of these types of skin cancers was studied in seven dermatology clinics in the US from 1983 through the early 1990s. Supplementation with 200 mcg selenium daily did not affect recurrence of skin cancer, but significantly reduced total mortality and mortality from cancers. In addition, incidence of prostate cancer, colorectal cancer, and lung cancer was lower in the group given selenium supplements.

However, not all studies have shown a relationship between selenium status and cancer. In 1982, over 60,000 participants of the Nurses Health Study with no history of cancer submitted toenail clippings for selenium analysis. Toenail analysis is thought to reflect selenium status over the previous year. After three and one-half years, researchers compared the toenail selenium levels of nurses with and without cancer. They did not find any apparent benefit of higher selenium levels.

These conflicting results emphasize the need for additional research on the relationship between selenium and chronic diseases such as cancer. A study that may help answer some of the questions about the effect of selenium supplementation on cancer risk has started in France. The Supplementation en Vitamines et Mineraux AntiXydants, or SU.VI.MAX Study, is a prevention trial that is providing doses of antioxidant vitamins and minerals that are one to three times higher than recommended intakes, including a daily supplement of 100 mcg selenium. More than 12,000 men and women are being followed for eight years to determine the effect of supplementation on the incidence of chronic disease, such as cancers and cardiovascular disease.

Selenium and Heart Disease

Some population surveys have indicated an association between a lower antioxidant intake with a greater incidence of heart disease. Additional lines of evidence suggest that oxidative stress from free radicals may promote heart disease. For example, it is the oxidized form of low-density lipoproteins (LDL, often called "bad" cholesterol) that promotes plaque build-up in coronary arteries. Selenium is one of a group of antioxidants that may help limit the oxidation of LDL cholesterol and thereby help to prevent coronary artery disease. Currently there is insufficient evidence available to recommend selenium supplements for the prevention of coronary heart disease.

Selenium and Arthritis

Surveys of patients with rheumatoid arthritis, a chronic disease that causes pain, stiffness, swelling, and loss of function in joints, have indicated that they have reduced selenium levels in their blood. In addition, some individuals with arthritis have a low selenium intake.

The body's immune system naturally makes free radicals that can help destroy invading organisms and damaged tissue, but that can also harm healthy tissue. Selenium, as an antioxidant, may help control levels of free radicals and help to relieve symptoms of arthritis. Current findings are considered preliminary, and further research is needed before selenium supplements can be recommended for individuals with arthritis.

Selenium and HIV

HIV/AIDS related malabsorption can deplete levels of many nutrients. Selenium deficiency is commonly associated with HIV/AIDS, and has been associated with a high risk of death from this disease. Of 24 children with HIV who were observed for five years, those with low selenium levels died at a younger age, which may indicate faster disease progression. An examination of 125 HIV positive men and women also associated selenium deficiency with mortality. Researchers believe that selenium may be important in HIV disease because of its role in the immune system and as an antioxidant. Selenium also may be needed for the replication of the HIV virus, which could deplete host levels of selenium. Researchers are actively investigating the role of selenium in HIV/AIDS, and see a need for clinical trials that evaluate the effect of selenium supplementation on HIV disease progression.

What Is the Health Risk of Too Much Selenium?

There is a moderate to high health risk of too much selenium. High blood levels of selenium can result in a condition called selenosis. Symptoms include gastrointestinal upsets, hair loss, white blotchy nails, and mild nerve damage. Selenium toxicity is rare in the United States and the few reported cases have been associated with industrial accidents and a manufacturing error that led to an excessively high dose of selenium in a supplement. The Institute of Medicine has set a tolerable upper intake level for selenium at 400 micrograms per day for adults to prevent the risk of developing selenosis. "Tolerable upper intake levels represent the maximum intake of a nutrient that is likely to pose no risk of adverse health effects in almost al individuals in the general population."

Chapter 24

St. John's Wort

St. John's wort (*Hypericum perforatum*) is a long-living, wild-growing herb with yellow flowers that has been used for centuries to treat mental disorders as well as nerve pain. In ancient times, doctors and herbalists (herb specialists) wrote about its use as a sedative and antimalarial agent as well as a balm for wounds, burns, and insect bites. Today, the herb is a popular treatment for mild to moderate depression; it also is used to treat anxiety, seasonal affective disorder, and sleep disorders.

St. John's wort is most widely used in Germany, where doctors prescribed almost 66 million daily doses in 1994 for psychological complaints. In fact, German doctors prescribe St. John's wort about 20 times more often than Prozac, one of the most widely prescribed antidepressants in the United States.

The use of St. John's wort is growing in the United States, and several brands now are available. Extracts of the plant are sold as a nutritional supplement after being prepared with a powder or an oil; the herb is available in capsule, tea, or tincture forms. St. John's wort was among the top-selling botanical products in the United States in 1997, with industry-estimated sales of $400 million in 1998.

FDA's Role

St. John's wort is 1 of 200 plant products approved by the U.S. Food and Drug Administration (FDA) for sale to the public as a dietary

National Center for Complementary and Alternative Medicine (NCCAM), NCCAM Clearinghouse, 2000.

supplement. The FDA does not subject dietary supplements to an extensive premarket approval process, however, as it does new drugs. On the other hand, the Dietary Supplement Health and Education Act of 1994 permits the FDA to remove a supplement from the market if it determines the supplement is unsafe. Herbal products such as St. John's wort can be marketed without stating standards for dosage or evidence of safety. Often, information on specific products may be misleading or even inaccurate. For instance, when the *Los Angeles Times*, a newspaper in California, commissioned laboratory tests on 10 St. John's wort products, researchers found that the potency of the products varied dramatically from what their labels claimed.

At the same time, a St. John's wort product stating the words "standardized extract" in its label may be more likely to contain the exact amount of the specific active ingredient needed to be effective. Standardized products generally are considered the highest-quality herbal products that a consumer can buy.

Treating Depression

Depression is a common illness that strikes perhaps 1 in 15 Americans each year. A person's mood, thoughts, physical health, and behavior all may be affected. Symptoms can include a persistent sad, anxious, or "empty" feeling; loss of energy, appetite, or sexual drive; and lack of interest in socializing, work, or hobbies.

Depression can be mild, moderate, or severe. Mild depression is characterized by difficulty in functioning normally, while moderate depression may involve impaired functioning at work or in social activities. Severe depression, which may involve delusions or hallucinations, markedly interferes with a person's ability to work or otherwise function and may lead to suicide. Genetic factors may put a person at risk for developing depression, and alcohol or drug use can make the problem worse. While the public misperception persists that depression is voluntary or a "character flaw," depression is a real condition that can be treated effectively by qualified professionals.

Specific psychotherapies (such as interpersonal and cognitive-behavioral therapy) and antidepressant medications both have been found to be effective for patients with major depression. Major depression includes mild, moderate, or severe depression that is not characterized by manic-depressive mood swings or induced by a substance such as alcohol. Several antidepressant drugs have become more widely used in the past several years and been found to be effective. However, patients sometimes report unpleasant side effects such as a dry mouth, nausea, headache, diarrhea, or impaired sexual function or sleep.

In part because of these types of drug side effects, many patients with depression are turning to herbal treatments such as St. John's wort. Researchers are studying it for possibly having fewer and less severe side effects than antidepressant drugs. St. John's wort also costs far less than antidepressant medication. In addition, St. John's wort does not require a prescription.

St. John's wort is not completely free of side effects, however. Some users have complained of a dry mouth, dizziness, gastrointestinal symptoms, increased sensitivity to sunlight, and fatigue. In addition, herbal treatments often are not as potent or as quick to act as conventional treatments. Furthermore, herbal treatments may not produce the desired results and may not be as effective as conventional medicine. Still, some people turn to herbs because they prefer to use "natural" products.

Clinical depression is a serious medical disorder that, in many cases, can be treated. However, St. John's wort is not a proven therapy for clinical depression. Therefore, there is some risk in taking it to treat clinical depression.

In any case, St. John's wort should not be mixed with other standard antidepressants because side effects may result. This is one reason why it is important to tell your doctor about all medications you are taking. Check with your doctor before taking St. John's wort or any other herb or medication. Your doctor can help you weigh the risks and benefits of a particular treatment so you can make informed health care decisions.

How St. John's Wort Works

The major components in extracts of St. John's wort include flavonoids, kaempferol, luteolin, biapigenin, hyperforin, polycyclic phenols, hypericin, and pseudohypericin. Researchers believe the last three substances are the active ingredients. New research suggests that hyperforin also may play a large role in the herb's antidepressant effects. Some German manufacturers of St. John's wort have begun standardizing, not only to hypericin as most U.S. manufacturers do, but to hyperforin as well. Standardizing means that the manufacturer ensures that each individual supplement contains a uniform amount of a certain compound, in this case hypericin and hyperforin.

Recent research suggests a possible application of St. John's wort for alcoholism. Researchers from the University of North Carolina at

Chapel Hill found that St. John's wort reduced alcohol intake in laboratory animals.

Several mechanisms of action of St. John's wort have been proposed, including the following:

- Inhibition of monoamine (serotonin, dopamine, and norepinephrine) re-uptake: St. John's wort appears to reduce the rate at which brain cells reabsorb serotonin (an important neurotransmitter or chemical that aids communication between nerve cells). Low levels of serotonin in the body are associated with depression.

- Modulation of interleukin-6 (IL-6) activity: Raised levels of IL-6, a protein involved in the communication between cells in the body's immune (disease-fighting) system, may lead to increases in adrenal regulatory hormones, a hallmark of depression. St. John's wort may reduce levels of IL-6, and thus help treat depression.

More research is needed to determine precisely the active ingredients in St. John's wort and to learn how the herb works.

Clinical Trials

Clinical trials (studies of a treatment's safety and effectiveness in humans) have found a similar rate of response with St. John's wort as with standard, conventional antidepressants in treating mild to moderate depression. However, it is hard to interpret these studies as definite proof of the efficacy of St. John's wort because low doses of standard antidepressants were used and there was no placebo (a pharmacologically inactive substance) control. An analysis of 23 European clinical studies of St. John's wort that was published in the *British Medical Journal* in 1996 concluded that the herb has antidepressive effects in cases of mild to moderate depression (the dosage varied considerably among the studies). However, no studies of its long-term use have been conducted. More research is needed to explore the long-term effects and optimum safe dosage of the extract.

A new study funded by the National Institutes of Health's National Center for Complementary and Alternative Medicine (NCCAM), Office of Dietary Supplements, and the National Institute of Mental Health will provide more information about St. John's wort. This study, which is in progress, is the first large-scale controlled clinical trial in the United States to assess whether the herb has a significant therapeutic effect in patients with clinical depression.

The $4.3 million study will involve 336 patients with major depression. The Duke University Medical Center in Durham, North Carolina, is coordinating the 3-year study, which has 13 clinical sites around the country.

There are three different treatment groups in the trial. One group will receive an initial dose of 900 mg per day of St. John's wort; a second will receive a placebo; and the third will receive Zoloft (a commonly used antidepressant). Patients who respond positively to their randomly assigned treatment will be continued on it for another 4 months.

Risk of Drug Interactions with St. John's Wort

Relatively little is known about the effects of taking dietary supplements with prescription drugs. However, through rigorous research, the NIH is learning more about how several of these alternative treatments work and whether they are safe and effective.

Two new studies from the NIH suggest that a popular botanical, St. John's wort (*Hypericum perforatum*), makes several prescription medications less effective. The herb speeds up activity in a key pathway responsible for breaking these drugs down in the body. When the medications are taken with St. John's wort, the end result is that blood levels of the drugs decrease because the body breaks them down faster.

Which Drugs Are Affected?

St. John's wort especially affects Crixivan (indinavir) and other protease inhibitors used to treat HIV infection. In addition, St. John's wort has been shown to affect cyclosporine, a drug used to help prevent organ transplant rejection, and other immunosuppressant drugs. It also may reduce the effectiveness of birth control pills, cholesterol-lowering medications such as Mevacor (lovastatin), cancer medications, seizure drugs, and blood thinners such as Coumadin (warfarin). The therapeutic mechanisms of these drugs are vulnerable because the medications are broken down by the same pathway as mentioned above.

Evidence from NIH Studies

In an NIH Clinical Center study, eight healthy, HIV-negative volunteers received 800 mg of indinavir every 8 hours for a total of four doses. Serial drug-action sampling was done before and after the

235

fourth dose. For the next 14 days, participants took 300 mg of St. John's wort three times daily with food. On the last day of St. John's wort treatment, participants again took 800 mg of indinavir every 4 hours for a total of four doses, with drug-action sampling before and for 5 hours serially after the fourth dose.

In this study, St. John's wort significantly decreased plasma concentrations of indinavir, which may lead to drug resistance and treatment failure.

Another report strongly suggests that the herb causes a drop in plasma levels of cyclosporine after heart transplantation.

Dietary Supplement Dilemma

Many people are taking dietary supplements, but, scientifically speaking, not much is known about these products.

A number of herbal products, such as St. John's wort, are widely used in the United States and are available in various forms such as combination products and teas. St. John's wort is a popular herbal product sold as a dietary supplement to ease mild to moderate depression and anxiety disorders as well as seasonal-affective and sleep disorders.

In the United States, dietary supplements are not subjected to an extensive pre-market approval process, as are new drugs. Often, little is known about their safety, content, quality, and effectiveness. Frequently, information on specific products may be misleading or even inaccurate. While a few products may help some people, many may be much less effective than conventional, proven therapies. Some may not work at all, and could even be dangerous, especially if they are used instead of or along with conventional treatments.

This new information about the risk of dangerous drug interactions between St. John's wort and other drugs used to treat serious health conditions may be the tip of the iceberg. Much more rigorous scientific research is needed to see if a number of dietary supplements and other herbal products are safe and effective when taken alone or with other drugs.

Need for Consumer and Provider Awareness

Doctors and patients should be aware of these negative drug interactions that could interfere with the proper functioning of these types of drugs. Again, the drugs include certain protease inhibitors, immunosuppressant drugs, birth control pills, cholesterol-lowering medications, cancer medications, seizure drugs, and blood thinners.

It is critical that health care professionals ask their patients about simultaneous use of products that could contain St. John's wort. Health care providers also should alert their patients about these potential drug interactions to prevent loss of therapeutic effect of any drug broken down via this pathway. Equally important is the need for patients to tell their health care providers about every treatment they are taking or considering.

Reporting Adverse Effects

The U.S. Food and Drug Administration (FDA) encourages all health care professionals to report any serious adverse event associated with the concomitant use of prescription drugs and St. John's wort products to FDA's MedWatch program at 1-800-FDA-1088 (Fax: 1-800-FDA-0178). The FDA is working closely with drug manufacturers to ensure that product labeling of certain HIV treatments is revised to highlight the potential for drug interactions with St. John's wort.

Other Federal Information Resources

For more information about the St. John's wort research and potential drug interactions, you may wish to visit NCCAM's Web site http://nccam.nih.gov or the FDA Center for Drug Evaluation and Research's Web site http://www.fda.gov/cder/drug/advisory/stjwort. htm. Or, you may want to call the FDA Center for Food Safety and Applied Nutrition at 1-800-332-4010.

Chapter 25

Vitamin A and Carotenoids

Vitamin A: What Is It?

Vitamin A is a family of fat-soluble vitamins. Retinol is one of the most active, or usable, forms of vitamin A, and is found in animal foods such as liver and eggs. It can be converted to retinal and retinoic acid, other active forms of the vitamin A family. Some plant foods contain orange pigments called provitamin A carotenoids that the liver can convert to retinol. Beta-carotene is a provitamin A carotenoid found in many foods. Lycopene, lutein, and zeaxanthin are also carotenoids commonly found in food, but your body cannot convert them to vitamin A.

Vitamin A plays an important role in vision, bone growth, reproduction, cell division and cell differentiation, which is the process by which a cell decides what it is going to become. It also maintains the surface linings of your eye and your respiratory, urinary, and intestinal tracts. When those linings break down, bacteria can enter your body and cause infection. Vitamin A also helps your body regulate its immune system. The immune system helps prevent or fight off infections by making white blood cells that destroy harmful bacteria and viruses. Vitamin A may help lymphocytes, a type of white blood cell that fights infections, function more effectively. Vitamin A also may help prevent bacteria and viruses from entering your body by maintaining the integrity of skin and mucous membranes.

This text was developed by the Clinical Nutrition Service, Warren Grant Magnuson Clinical Center, in conjunction with the Office of Dietary Supplements (ODS), National Institutes of Health (NIH), January 2001.

Some carotenoids, in addition to serving as a source of vitamin A, have been shown to function as antioxidants in laboratory tests. However, this role has not been consistently demonstrated in humans. Antioxidants protect cells from free radicals, which are potentially damaging by-products of the body's metabolism that may contribute to the development of some chronic diseases.

What Foods Provide Vitamin A?

Whole eggs, whole milk, and liver are among the few foods that naturally contain vitamin A. Vitamin A is present in the fat portion of whole milk, so it is not found in fat-free milk. Most fat-free milk and dried nonfat milk solids sold in the US are fortified with vitamin A. There are many other fortified foods such as breakfast cereals that also provide vitamin A. Tables 25.2 and 25.3 suggest animal sources of vitamin A and plant sources of provitamin A carotenoids.

It is important for you to regularly eat foods that provide vitamin A or beta-carotene even though your body can store vitamin A in the liver. Stored vitamin A will help meet your needs when intake of provitamin A carotenoids or vitamin A is low.

What Is the Recommended Dietary Allowance for Vitamin A for Adults?

The Recommended Dietary Allowance (RDA) is the average daily dietary intake level that is sufficient to meet the nutrient requirements of nearly all (97-98%) healthy individuals in each life-stage and gender group. The 1989 RDAs for vitamin A for adults and children are listed in Table 25.1

Results of the third National Health and Nutrition Examination survey (NHANES III 1988-91) suggested that the dietary intake of some Americans does not meet recommended levels. The Continuing Survey of Food Intakes of Individuals (CSFII 1994) suggested that diets of many Americans provide less than 75% of recommended intake levels. These surveys highlight the importance of encouraging Americans to include dietary sources of vitamin A in their daily diets.

There is no separate RDA for beta-carotene or other carotenoids. The Institute of Medicine (IOM) report suggests that consuming 3 to 6 mg of beta-carotene daily will maintain plasma B-carotene blood levels in the range associated with a lower risk of chronic diseases. This concentration can be achieved by a diet that provides five or more servings of fruits and vegetables per day.

Table 25.1. RDAs for Vitamin A for Adults and Children

Life-Stage	Children	Men	Women	Pregnancy	Lactation
Ages 1-3	400 RE or 2000 IU*				
Ages 4-6	500 RE or 2500 IU				
Ages 7-10	700 RE or 3,500 IU				
Ages 11-18		1000 RE or 5000 IU	800 RE or 4000 IU	800 RE or 4000 IU	800 RE or 4000 IU
Ages 19 +		1000 RE or 5000 IU	800 RE or 4000 IU	800 RE or 4000 IU	800 RE or 4000 IU

*Food labels list vitamin A in International Units (IU).

When Can Vitamin A Deficiency Occur?

Vitamin A deficiency rarely occurs in the United States, but it is still a major public health problem in the developing world. It is most often associated with protein/calorie malnutrition and affects over 120 million children worldwide. It is also a leading cause of childhood blindness. In countries where immunization programs are not widespread and vitamin A deficiency is common, millions of children die each year from complications of infectious diseases such as measles.

Signs of Vitamin A Deficiency

Signs of vitamin A deficiency include night blindness, dry skin, and decreased resistance to infections. In ancient Egypt it was known that night blindness could be cured after eating liver, which was later found to be a rich source of vitamin A. Vitamin A deficiency contributes to blindness by making the eye very dry, damaging the cornea of the eye (referred to as xerophthalmia), and promoting damage to the retina of the eye. Extremely dry skin, dry hair, sloughing off of skin, and broken fingernails are other common signs of vitamin A deficiency.

Vitamin A deficiency also decreases resistance to infections. When there is not enough vitamin A, cells lining the lung lose their ability

241

to remove disease-causing microorganisms. This may contribute to the pneumonia associated with vitamin A deficiency.

There is increased interest in subclinical forms of vitamin A deficiency, described as low storage levels of vitamin A that do not cause overt deficiency symptoms. This mild degree of vitamin A deficiency may increase children's risk of developing respiratory and diarrheal infections, decrease growth rate, slow bone development, and decrease likelihood of survival from serious illness.

Children living in the United States who are considered to be at increased risk for subclinical vitamin A deficiency include:

- toddlers and preschool age children

- children living at or below the poverty level

Table 25.2. Table of Selected Animal Sources of Vitamin A

Food	IU (International Units)	%DV*
Liver, beef, cooked, 3 oz	30,325	610
Liver, chicken, cooked, 3 oz	13,920	280
Egg substitute, fortified, 1/4 c	1355	25
Fat free milk, fortified w/ vitamin A, 1 c	500	10
Cheese pizza, 1/8 of a 12" diameter	380	8
Milk, whole, 3.25% fat, 1 c	305	6
Cheddar cheese, 1 oz	300	6
Whole egg, 1 medium	280	6
Swiss cheese, 1 oz	240	4
Margarine, soft, corn oil, 1 tsp	165	4
Yogurt, fruit flavored, low fat, 1 c	120	2

*DV = Daily Value. DVs are reference numbers based on the Recommended Dietary Allowance (RDA). They were developed to help consumers determine if a food contains a lot or a little of a specific nutrient. The DV for vitamin A is 5,000 IU (1,000 RE). The percent DV (%DV) listed on the nutrition facts panel of food labels tells adults what percentage of the DV is provided by one serving. Percent DVs are based on a 2,000-calorie diet. Your Daily Values may be higher or lower depending on your calorie needs. Foods that provide lower percentages of the DV will contribute to a healthful diet.

- children with inadequate health care or immunizations
- children living in areas with known nutritional deficiencies
- recent immigrants or refugees from developing countries with high incidence of vitamin A deficiency or measles, and
- children with diseases of the pancreas, liver, intestines, or with inadequate fat digestion/absorption.

As a result of the worldwide significance of vitamin A deficiency in children, the World Health Organization (WHO) and the United Nations International Children's Emergency Fund (UNICEF) issued joint statements about vitamin A and children's health. Both agencies recommend vitamin A administration for all children diagnosed with measles in communities where vitamin A deficiency is a serious problem and where death from measles is greater than 1%. In 1994, the American Academy of Pediatrics recommended vitamin A supplementation for children 6 to 24 months of age hospitalized with measles and for hospitalized children older than 6 months who are considered to be at high-risk for subclinical vitamin A deficiency.

Who May Need Extra Vitamin A to Prevent a Deficiency?

Children with low body stores of vitamin A who have measles may require vitamin A supplementation, as discussed above. Also, individuals with chronic fat malabsorption also poorly absorb vitamin A. Fat malabsorption can occur with cystic fibrosis, sprue, pancreatic disorders, and after stomach surgery. Healthy adults usually have a one-year reserve of vitamin A stored in their livers and should not be at risk of deficiency during periods of temporary or short term fat malabsorption. Long term problems absorbing fat, however, can result in deficiency and may require vitamin A supplementation. Children may only have enough stores of vitamin A to last several weeks, so children with fat malabsorption may require immediate vitamin A supplementation.

What Is the Association between Vitamin A, Beta Carotene and Cancer?

Surveys suggest an association between diets rich in beta-carotene and vitamin A and a lower risk of many types of cancer. There is evidence that higher intake of green and yellow vegetables or food sources

243

of beta carotene and/or vitamin A decreased the risk of lung cancer. A number of studies have tested the role of beta-carotene supplements in cancer prevention. Unfortunately, recent intervention studies have not supported a protective role for beta carotene in cancer prevention. In a study of 29,000 men, incidence of lung cancer was greater in the group of smokers who took a daily supplement of beta carotene. The Carotene and Retinol Efficacy Trial, a lung cancer chemoprevention trial that provided randomized subjects with

Table 25.3. Table of Selected Plant Sources of Vitamin A (from beta-carotene) (continued on next page)

Plant sources such as beta carotene are not as well absorbed as animal sources of vitamin A.

Food	IU (International Units)	%DV*
Carrot, 1 raw (7 1/2")	20,250	410
Carrots, boiled, 1/2 c slices	19,150	380
Carrot juice, canned, 1/2 c	12,915	260
Mango, raw, without refuse, 1 fruit	8,050	160
Sweet potatoes, 1/2 c Junior mashed	7,430	150
Spinach, boiled, 1/2 c	7,370	150
Cantaloupe, raw, 1 c cubes	5,160	100
Kale, boiled, 1/2 c	4,810	100
Vegetable soup, prepared with equal volume water, 1 c	3,005	60
Pepper, sweet, red, raw, 1/2 c sliced	2,620	50
Apricots, without skin, canned in water, 1/2 c halves	2,055	40
Spinach, raw, 1 cup	2,015	40
Broccoli, frozen, chopped, boiled, 1/2 c	1,740	35
Apricot nectar, canned, 1/2 c	1,650	30
Oatmeal, instant, fortified, low sodium, dry, 1 packet	1,050	20

supplements of beta carotene and vitamin A, was stopped after re-searchers discovered that subjects receiving beta carotene had a 46% higher risk of dying from lung cancer. The IOM states that "B-carotene supplements are not advisable for the general population," although they also state that this advice "does not pertain to the possible use of supplemental B-carotene as a provitamin A source for the prevention of vitamin A deficiency in populations with inadequate vitamin A nutriture."

Table 25.3. Table of Selected Plant Sources of Vitamin A (from beta-carotene) (continued from previous page)

Plant sources such as beta carotene are not as well absorbed as animal sources of vitamin A.

Food	IU (International Units)	%DV*
Tomato juice, canned, 6 oz	1,010	20
Ready-to-eat cereal, fortified, 1 oz (15% fortification)	750	15
Peaches, canned, water pack, 1/2 c halves or slices	650	15
Peach, raw, 1 medium	525	10
Papaya, raw, 1 small	430	10
Orange, raw, 1 large	375	8
Asparagus, boiled, 4 spears	325	6
Tomato, red, ripe, raw, 1/2" thick slice	170	2

*DV = Daily Value. DVs are reference numbers based on the Recommended Dietary Allowance (RDA). They were developed to help consumers determine if a food contains a lot or a little of a specific nutrient. The DV for vitamin A is 5,000 IU (1,000 RE). The percent DV (%DV) listed on the nutrition facts panel of food labels tells adults what percentage of the DV is provided by one serving. Percent DVs are based on a 2,000-calorie diet. Your Daily Values may be higher or lower depending on your calorie needs. Foods that provide lower percentages of the DV will contribute to a healthful diet.

What Is the Health Risk of Too Much Vitamin A?

Hypervitaminosis A refers to high storage levels of vitamin A in the body that can lead to toxic symptoms. Toxicity can result in dry, itchy skin, headache, fatigue, hair loss, loss of appetite, vomiting, and liver damage. When toxic symptoms arise suddenly, which can happen after consuming very large amounts of vitamin A over a short period of time, signs of toxicity include dizziness, blurred vision, and muscular uncoordination.

Although hypervitaminosis A can occur when very large amounts of liver are regularly consumed, most cases of vitamin A toxicity result from an excess intake of vitamin A in supplements. A generally recognized safe upper limit of intake for vitamin A from diet and supplements is 1,600 to 2,000 RE (8,000 to 10,000 IU) per day. The Institute of Medicine is currently reviewing the scientific literature on vitamin A. They are considering revising the RDAs and establishing an Upper Limit (UL) of safe intake for vitamin A.

Vitamin A toxicity also can cause severe birth defects. Women of child-bearing age are advised to limit their total daily intake of vitamin A (retinol) from foods and supplements combined to no more than 1,600 RE (8,000 IU) per day.

Retinoids are compounds that are chemically similar to vitamin A. Over the past 15 years, synthetic retinoids have been prescribed for acne, psoriasis, and other skin disorders. Isotretinoin (Roaccutane or Accutane) is considered an effective anti-acne therapy. At very high doses, however, it can be toxic, which is why this medication is usually saved for the most severe forms of acne. The most serious consequence of this medication is birth defects.

It is extremely important for sexually active females who may become pregnant and who take these medications to use an effective method of birth control. Women of childbearing age who take these medications are advised to undergo monthly pregnancy tests to make sure they are not pregnant.

What Is the Health Risk of Too Many Carotenoids?

Nutrient toxicity traditionally refers to adverse health effects from a high intake of a particular vitamin or mineral. For example, large amounts of the active form of vitamin A (naturally found in animal foods such as liver but also available in dietary supplements) can cause birth defects.

Provitamin A carotenoids such as beta-carotene are generally considered safe because they are not traditionally associated with specific adverse health effects. The conversion of provitamin A carotenoids to vitamin A decreases when body stores are full, which naturally limits further increases in storage levels. A high intake of provitamin A carotenoids can turn the skin yellow, but this is not considered dangerous to health.

Recent clinical trials that suggested a greater incidence of lung cancer and total mortality (death) in current smokers who supplemented their diet with 20 mg of beta-carotene per day have raised concern about the safety of beta-carotene supplements. However, conflicting studies make it difficult to interpret the health risk. For example, the Physicians' Health Study compared the effects of taking 50 mg beta-carotene every other day to a placebo (sugar pill) in over 22,000 male physicians and found no adverse health effects. Also, a trial that tested the ability of four different nutrient combinations to inhibit the development of esophageal and gastric cancers in 30,000 men and women in China suggested that after 5 years those participants who took a combination of beta-carotene, selenium and vitamin E had a 13% reduction in cancer deaths. One point to consider is that there may be a relationship between alcohol and beta-carotene because "only those men who consumed more than 11 g per day of alcohol (approximately one drink per day) showed an adverse response to B-carotene supplementation" in the lung cancer trial.

The Institute of Medicine did not set a Tolerable Upper Intake Level (UL), the highest level of daily nutrient intake that is likely to pose no risk of adverse health effects, for B-carotene or carotenoids. Instead, they concluded that B-carotene supplements are not advisable for the general population. As stated earlier, however, they may be appropriate as a provitamin A source or for the prevention of vitamin A deficiency in specific populations.

Selected Food Sources of Vitamin A

As the 2000 Dietary Guidelines for Americans state, "Different foods contain different nutrients. No single food can supply all the nutrients in the amounts you need." The following tables suggest dietary sources of vitamin A and provitamin A carotenoids. As the tables indicate, liver, eggs and whole milk are good animal sources of vitamin A. Many orange fruits and green vegetables are good sources of provitamin A carotenoids. Including these foods in your daily diet will help you meet your daily need for vitamin A. In addition, food manufacturers fortify a wide range of products with vitamin A. Breakfast cereals, pastries, breads, crackers, cereal grain bars and other foods may be fortified with 10% to 15% of the DV for vitamin A. It is important to read the nutrition facts panel of the food label to determine whether a food provides vitamin A.

If you want more information about building a healthful diet, refer to the Dietary Guidelines for Americans and the Food Guide Pyramid.

Chapter 26

Vitamin B6

Vitamin B6: What Is It?

Vitamin B6 is a water-soluble vitamin that exists in three major chemical forms: pyridoxine, pyridoxal, and pyridoxamine. It performs a wide variety of functions in your body and is essential for your good health. For example, vitamin B6 is needed for more than 100 enzymes involved in protein metabolism. It is also essential for red blood cell metabolism. The nervous and immune systems need vitamin B6 to function efficiently, and it is also needed for the conversion of tryptophan (an amino acid) to niacin (a vitamin).

Hemoglobin within red blood cells carries oxygen to tissues. Your body needs vitamin B6 to make hemoglobin. Vitamin B6 also helps increase the amount of oxygen carried by hemoglobin. A vitamin B6 deficiency can result in a form of anemia that is similar to iron deficiency anemia.

An immune response is a broad term that describes a variety of biochemical changes that occur in an effort to fight off infections. Calories, protein, vitamins, and minerals are important to your immune defenses because they promote the growth of white blood cells that directly fight infections. Vitamin B6, through its involvement in protein metabolism and cellular growth, is important to the immune

This text was developed by the Clinical Nutrition Service, Warren Grant Magnuson Clinical Center, in conjunction with the Office of Dietary Supplements (ODS), National Institutes of Health (NIH), January 2001.

system. It helps maintain the health of lymphoid organs (thymus, spleen, and lymph nodes) that make your white blood cells. Animal studies show that a vitamin B6 deficiency can decrease your antibody production and suppress your immune response.

Vitamin B6 also helps maintain your blood glucose (sugar) within a normal range. When caloric intake is low your body needs vitamin B6 to help convert stored carbohydrate or other nutrients to glucose to maintain normal blood sugar levels. While a shortage of vitamin B6 will limit these functions, supplements of this vitamin do not enhance them in well-nourished individuals.

What Foods Provide Vitamin B6?

Vitamin B6 is found in a wide variety of foods including fortified cereals, beans, meat, poultry, fish, and some fruits and vegetables. Table 26.2 suggests many dietary sources of B6.

What Is the Recommended Dietary Allowance for Vitamin B6 for Adults?

The Recommended Dietary Allowance (RDA) is the average daily dietary intake level that is sufficient to meet the nutrient requirements of nearly all (97 to 98 percent) healthy individuals in each life-stage and gender group.

The 1998 RDAs for vitamin B6 for adults, in milligrams, are shown in Table 26.1.

Table 26.1. RDAs for Vitamin B6 for Adults

Life-Stage	Men	Women	Pregnancy	Lactation
Ages 19-50	1.3 mg	1.3 mg		
Ages 51+	1.7 mg	1.5 mg		
All ages			1.9 mg	2.0 mg

Results of two national surveys, the National Health and Nutrition Examination Survey (NHANES III1988-94) and the Continuing Survey of Food Intakes by Individuals (1994-96 CSFII), indicated that diets of most Americans meet current intake recommendations for vitamin B6.

When Can a Vitamin B6 Deficiency Occur?

Clinical signs of vitamin B6 deficiency are rarely seen in the United States. Many older Americans, however, have low blood levels of vitamin B6, which may suggest a marginal or sub-optimal vitamin B6 nutritional status. Vitamin B6 deficiency can occur in individuals with poor quality diets that are deficient in many nutrients. Symptoms occur during later stages of deficiency, when intake has been very low for an extended time. Signs of vitamin B6 deficiency include dermatitis (skin inflammation), glossitis (a sore tongue), depression, confusion, and convulsions. Vitamin B6 deficiency also can cause anemia. Some of these symptoms can also result from a variety of medical conditions other than vitamin B6 deficiency. It is important to have a physician evaluate these symptoms so that appropriate medical care can be given.

Who May Need Extra Vitamin B6 to Prevent a Deficiency?

Individuals with a poor quality diet or an inadequate B6 intake for an extended period may benefit from taking a vitamin B6 supplement if they are unable to increase their dietary intake of vitamin B6. Alcoholics and older adults are more likely to have inadequate vitamin B6 intakes than other segments of the population because they may have limited variety in their diet. Alcohol also promotes the destruction and loss of vitamin B6 from the body.

Asthmatic children treated with the medicine theophylline may need to take a vitamin B6 supplement. Theophylline decreases body stores of vitamin B6, and theophylline-induced seizures have been linked to low body stores of the vitamin. A physician should be consulted about the need for a vitamin B6 supplement when theophylline is prescribed.

What Are Some Current Issues and Controversies about Vitamin B6?

Vitamin B6 and the Nervous System

Vitamin B6 is needed for the synthesis of neurotransmitters such as serotonin and dopamine. These neurotransmitters are required for normal nerve cell communication. Researchers have been investigating the relationship between vitamin B6 status and a wide variety of neurologic conditions such as seizures, chronic pain, depression, headache, and Parkinson's disease.

Lower levels of serotonin have been found in individuals suffering from depression and migraine headaches. So far, however, vitamin B6 supplements have not proved effective for relieving these symptoms. One study found that a sugar pill was just as likely as vitamin B6 to relieve headaches and depression associated with low dose oral contraceptives.

Alcohol abuse can result in neuropathy, abnormal nerve sensations in the arms and legs. A poor dietary intake contributes to this neuropathy and dietary supplements that include vitamin B6 may prevent or decrease its incidence.

Vitamin B6 and Carpal Tunnel Syndrome

Vitamin B6 was first recommended for carpal tunnel syndrome almost 30 years ago. Several popular books still recommend taking 100 to 200 milligrams (mg) of vitamin B6 daily to treat carpal tunnel syndrome, even though scientific studies do not indicate it is effective. Anyone taking large doses of vitamin B6 supplements for carpal tunnel syndrome needs to be aware that the Institute of Medicine recently established an upper tolerable limit of 100 mg per day for adults. There are documented cases in the literature of neuropathy caused by excessive vitamin B6 taken for treatment of carpal tunnel syndrome.

Vitamin B6 and Premenstrual Syndrome

Vitamin B6 has become a popular remedy for treating the discomforts associated with premenstrual syndrome (PMS). Unfortunately, clinical trials have failed to support any significant benefit. One recent study indicated that a sugar pill was as likely to relieve symptoms of PMS as vitamin B6. In addition, vitamin B6 toxicity has been seen in increasing numbers of women taking vitamin B6 supplements for PMS. One review indicated that neuropathy was present in 23 of 58 women taking daily vitamin B6 supplements for PMS whose blood levels of B6 were above normal. There is no convincing scientific evidence to support recommending vitamin B6 supplements for PMS.

Vitamin B6 and Interactions with Medications

There are many drugs that interfere with the metabolism of vitamin B6. Isoniazid, which is used to treat tuberculosis, and L-DOPA, which is used to treat a variety of neurologic problems such as Parkinson's disease, alter the activity of vitamin B6. There is disagreement about the need for routine vitamin B6 supplementation when taking isoniazid. Acute isoniazid toxicity can result in coma and sei-zures that are reversed by vitamin B6, but in a group of children re-ceiving isoniazid, no cases of neurological or neuropsychiatric problems were observed regardless of whether or not they took a vi-tamin B6 supplement. Some doctors recommend taking a supplement that provides 100% of the RDA for B6 when isoniazid is prescribed, which is usually enough to prevent symptoms of vitamin B6 deficiency. It is important to consult with a physician about the need for a vita-min B6 supplement when taking isoniazid.

What Is the Relationship between Vitamin B6, Homocysteine, and Heart Disease?

A deficiency of vitamin B6, folic acid, or vitamin B12 may increase your level of homocysteine, an amino acid normally found in your blood. There is evidence that an elevated homocysteine level is an independent risk factor for heart disease and stroke. The evidence suggests that high levels of homocysteine may damage coronary ar-teries or make it easier for blood clotting cells called platelets to clump together and form a clot. However, there is currently no evidence avail-able to suggest that lowering homocysteine level with vitamins will reduce your risk of heart disease. Clinical intervention trials are needed to determine whether supplementation with vitamin B6, folic acid, or vitamin B12 can help protect you against developing coronary heart disease.

What Is the Health Risk of Too Much Vitamin B6?

Too much vitamin B6 can result in nerve damage to the arms and legs. This neuropathy is usually related to high intake of vitamin B6 from supplements, and is reversible when supplementation is stopped. According to the Institute of Medicine, "Several reports show sensory neuropathy at doses lower than 500 mg per day." As previously men-tioned, the Food and Nutrition Board of the Institute of Medicine has established an upper tolerable intake level (UL) for vitamin B6 of 100 mg per day for all adults. "As intake increases above the UL, the risk of adverse effects increases."

Selected Food Sources of Vitamin B6

As the 2000 *Dietary Guidelines for Americans* state, "Different foods contain different nutrients and other healthful substances. No

Table 26.2. Table of Food Sources of Vitamin B6

Food	Milligrams	%DV*
Ready-to-eat cereal, 100% fortified, 3/4 c	2.00	100
Potato, Baked, flesh and skin, 1 medium	0.70	35
Banana, raw, 1 medium	0.68	34
Garbanzo beans, canned, 1/2 c	0.57	30
Chicken breast, meat only, cooked, 1/2 breast	0.52	25
Ready-to-eat cereal, 25% fortified, 3/4 c	0.50	25
Oatmeal, instant, fortified, 1 packet	0.42	20
Pork loin, lean only, cooked, 3 oz	0.42	20
Roast beef, eye of round, lean only, cooked, 3 oz	0.32	15
Trout, rainbow, cooked, 3 oz	0.29	15
Sunflower seeds, kernels, dry roasted, 1 oz	0.23	10
Spinach, frozen, cooked, 1/2 c	0.14	8
Tomato juice, canned, 6 oz	0.20	10
Avocado, raw, sliced, 1/2 cup	0.20	10
Salmon, Sockeye, cooked, 3 oz	0.19	10
Tuna, canned in water, drained solids, 3 oz	0.18	10
Wheat bran, crude or unprocessed, 1/4 c	0.18	10
Peanut butter, smooth, 2 Tbs.	0.15	8
Walnuts, English/Persian, 1 oz	0.15	8
Soybeans, green, boiled, drained, 1/2 c	0.05	2
Lima beans, frozen, cooked, drained, 1/2 c	0.10	6

* DV = Daily Value. DVs are reference numbers based on the Recommended Dietary Allowance (RDA). They were developed to help consumers determine if a food contains a lot or a little of a specific nutrient. The DV for vitamin B6 is 2.0 milligrams (mg). The percent DV (%DV) listed on the nutrition facts panel of food labels tells you what percentage of the DV is provided in one serving. Percent DVs are based on a 2,000 calorie diet. Your Daily Values may be higher or lower depending on your calorie needs. Foods that provide lower percentages of the DV also contribute to a healthful diet.

single food can supply all the nutrients in the amounts you need." As the following table indicates, vitamin B6 is found in a wide variety of foods. Foods such as fortified breakfast cereals, fish including salmon and tuna fish, meats such as pork and chicken, bananas, beans and peanut butter, and many vegetables will contribute to your vitamin B6 intake. If you want more information about building a healthful diet, refer to the *Dietary Guidelines for Americans* and the Food Guide Pyramid.

Chapter 27

Vitamin B12

Vitamin B12: What Is It?

Vitamin B12, also called cobalamin, is important to good health. It helps maintain healthy nerve cells and red blood cells, and is also needed to make DNA, the genetic material in all cells. Vitamin B12 is bound to the protein in food. Hydrochloric acid in the stomach releases B12 from protein during digestion. Once released, B12 combines with a substance called intrinsic factor (IF) before it is absorbed into the bloodstream.

What Foods Provide Vitamin B12?

Vitamin B12 is naturally found in animal foods including fish, milk and milk products, eggs, meat, and poultry. Fortified breakfast cereals are an excellent source of vitamin B12 and a particularly valuable source for vegetarians. Table 27.2 suggests dietary sources of vitamin B12.

What Is the Recommended Dietary Allowance for Vitamin B12 for Adults?

The Recommended Dietary Allowance (RDA) is the average daily dietary intake level that is sufficient to meet the nutrient requirements

This text was developed by the Clinical Nutrition Service, Warren Grant Magnuson Clinical Center, in conjunction with the Office of Dietary Supplements (ODS), National Institutes of Health (NIH), January 2001.

of nearly all (97 to 98 percent) healthy individuals in each life-stage and gender group. The 1998 RDAs for vitamin B12 (in micrograms) for adults are shown in Table 27.1.

Table 27.1. RDAs for Vitamin B12 for Adults

Life-Stage	Men	Women	Pregnancy	Lactation
Ages 19+	2.4 mcg	2.4 mcg		
All ages			2.6 mcg	2.8 mcg

Results of two national surveys, the National Health and Nutrition Examination Survey (NHANES III-1988-91) and the Continuing Survey of Food Intakes by Individuals (CSFII 1994-96) found that most adult men and women consume recommended amounts of vitamin B12.

When Is a Deficiency of Vitamin B12 Likely to Occur?

Diets of most adult Americans provide recommended intakes of vitamin B12, but deficiency may still occur as a result of an inability to absorb B12 from food. It can also occur in individuals with dietary patterns that exclude animal or fortified foods. As a general rule, most individuals who develop a vitamin B12 deficiency have an underlying stomach or intestinal disorder that limits the absorption of vitamin B12. Sometimes the only symptom of these intestinal disorders is anemia resulting from B12 deficiency.

Characteristic signs of B12 deficiency include fatigue, weakness, nausea, constipation, flatulence (gas), loss of appetite, and weight loss. Deficiency also can lead to neurological changes such as numbness and tingling in the hands and feet. Additional symptoms of B12 deficiency are difficulty in maintaining balance, depression, confusion, poor memory, and soreness of the mouth or tongue. Some of these symptoms can also result from a variety of medical conditions other than vitamin B12 deficiency. It is important to have a physician evaluate these symptoms so that appropriate medical care can be given.

Who May Need a Vitamin B12 Supplement to Prevent a Deficiency?

Individuals with Pernicious Anemia

Pernicious anemia is a form of anemia that occurs when there is an absence of intrinsic factor, a substance normally present in the stomach. Vitamin B12 binds with intrinsic factor before it is absorbed and used by your body. An absence of intrinsic factor prevents normal absorption of B12 and results in pernicious anemia.

Anyone with pernicious anemia usually needs intramuscular (IM) injections (shots) of vitamin B12. It is very important to remember that pernicious anemia is a chronic condition that should be monitored by a physician. Anyone with pernicious anemia has to take lifelong supplemental vitamin B12.

Individuals with Gastrointestinal Disorders

Individuals with stomach and small intestinal disorders may not absorb enough vitamin B12 from food to maintain healthy body stores. Sprue and celiac disease are intestinal disorders caused by intolerance to protein in wheat and wheat products. Regional enteritis, localized inflammation of the stomach or small intestine, also results in generalized malabsorption of vitamin B12. Excess bacteria in the stomach and small intestine also can decrease vitamin B12 absorption.

Surgical procedures of the gastrointestinal tract such as surgery to remove all or part of the stomach often result in a loss of cells that secrete stomach acid and intrinsic factor. Surgical removal of the distal ileum, a section of the intestines, also can result in the inability to absorb B12. Anyone who has had either of these surgeries usually requires lifelong supplemental B12 to prevent a deficiency.

Older Adults

Vitamin B12 must be separated from protein in food before it can bind with intrinsic factor and be absorbed by your body. Bacterial overgrowth in the stomach and/or atrophic gastritis, an inflammation of the stomach, contribute to vitamin B12 deficiency in adults by limiting secretions of stomach acid needed to separate vitamin B12 from protein in food. Adults 50 years of age and older with these conditions are able to absorb the B12 in fortified foods and dietary supplements. Health care professionals may advise adults over the age of 50 to get their vitamin B12 from a dietary supplement or from foods fortified with vitamin B12 because 10 to 30 percent of older people may be unable to absorb vitamin B12 in food.

Vegetarians

Vegetarians who do not eat meats, fish, eggs, milk or milk products, or B12 fortified foods consume no vitamin B12 and are at high risk of developing a deficiency of vitamin B12. When adults adopt a vegetarian diet, deficiency symptoms can be slow to appear because it usually takes years to deplete normal body stores of B12. However, severe symptoms of B12 deficiency, most often featuring poor neurological development, can show up quickly in children and breast-fed infants of women who follow a strict vegetarian diet.

Fortified cereals are one of the few plant food sources of vitamin B12, and are an important dietary source of B12 for vegetarians who consume no eggs, milk or milk products. Vegetarian adults who do not consume plant foods fortified with vitamin B12 need to consider taking a B12-containing supplement. Vegetarian mothers should consult with a pediatrician regarding appropriate vitamin B12 supplementation for their infants and children.

Caution: Folic acid may mask signs of vitamin B12 deficiency. Folic acid can correct the anemia that is caused by vitamin B12 deficiency. Unfortunately, folic acid will not correct the underlying B12 deficiency. Permanent nerve damage can occur if vitamin B12 deficiency is not treated. Folic acid intake from food and supplements should not exceed 1,000 micrograms (mcg) daily because large amounts of folic acid can hide the damaging effects of vitamin B12 deficiency. Adults older than 50 years are advised to consult with their physician about the advisability of taking folic acid without also taking a vitamin B12 supplement.

What Is the Relationship between Vitamin B12, Homocysteine, and Heart Disease?

A deficiency of vitamin B12, folate, or vitamin B6 may increase your blood level of homocysteine, an amino acid normally found in your blood. There is evidence that an elevated blood level of homocysteine is an independent risk factor for heart disease and stroke. The evidence suggests that high levels of homocysteine may damage coronary arteries or make it easier for blood clotting cells called platelets to clump together and form a clot. However, there is currently no evidence

Table 27.2. Table of Food Sources of Vitamin B12

Food	Micrograms	%DV*
Beef liver, cooked, 3 oz	60.0	1000
Fortified breakfast cereals, (100%) fortified), 3/4 c	6.0	100
Trout, rainbow, cooked, 3 oz	5.3	90
Salmon, sockeye, cooked, 3 oz	4.9	80
Beef, cooked, 3 oz	2.1	35
Fortified breakfast cereals (25% fortified), 3/4 c	1.5	25
Haddock, cooked, 3 oz	1.2	20
Clams, breaded and fried, 3/4 c	1.1	20
Oysters, breaded and fried, 6 pieces	1.0	15
Tuna, white, canned in water, 3 oz	0.9	15
Milk, 1 cup	0.9	15
Yogurt, 8 oz	0.9	15
Pork, cooked, 3 oz	0.6	10
Egg, 1 large	0.5	8
American Cheese, 1 oz	0.4	6
Chicken, cooked, 3 oz	0.3	6
Cheddar cheese, 1 oz	0.2	4
Mozzarella cheese, 1 oz	0.2	4

* DV = Daily Value. DVs are reference numbers based on the Recommended Dietary Allowance (RDA). They were developed to help consumers determine if a food contains a lot or a little of a specific nutrient. The DV for vitamin B12 is 6.0 micrograms (mcg). The percent DV (%DV) listed on the nutrition facts panel of food labels tells adults what percentage of the DV is provided by one serving. Percent DVs are based on a 2,000 calorie diet. Your Daily Values may be higher or lower depending on your calorie needs. Foods that provide lower percentages of the DV also contribute to a healthful diet.

available to suggest that lowering homocysteine level with vitamins will actually reduce your risk of heart disease. Clinical intervention trials are needed to determine whether supplementation with vitamin B12, folic acid, or vitamin B6 can help protect you against developing coronary heart disease.

What Is the Health Risk of Too Much Vitamin B12?

Vitamin B12 has a very low potential for toxicity. The Institute of Medicine states that "no adverse effects have been associated with excess vitamin B12 intake from food and supplements in healthy individuals." The Institute recommends that adults over 50 years of age get most of their vitamin B12 from supplements or fortified food because of the high incidence of impaired absorption of B12 from unfortified foods in this population.

Selected Food Sources of Vitamin B12

As the 2000 Dietary Guidelines for Americans state, "Different foods contain different nutrients and other healthful substances. No single food can supply all the nutrients in the amounts you need." As the following table indicates, vitamin B12 is found naturally in animal foods. It is also found in fortified foods such as fortified breakfast cereals. If you want more information about building a healthful diet, refer to Dietary Guidelines for Americans and the Food Guide Pyramid.

Chapter 28

Vitamin D

Vitamin D: What Is It?

Vitamin D, calciferol, is a fat-soluble vitamin. It is found in food, but also can be made in your body after exposure to ultraviolet rays from the sun. Vitamin D exists in several forms, each with a different activity. Some forms are relatively inactive in the body, and have limited ability to function as a vitamin. The liver and kidney help convert vitamin D to its active hormone form. The major biologic function of vitamin D is to maintain normal blood levels of calcium and phosphorus. Vitamin D aids in the absorption of calcium, helping to form and maintain strong bones. It promotes bone mineralization in concert with a number of other vitamins, minerals, and hormones. Without vitamin D, bones can become thin, brittle, soft, or misshapen. Vitamin D prevents rickets in children and osteomalacia in adults, which are skeletal diseases that result in defects that weaken bones.

What Are the Sources of Vitamin D?

Food Sources

Fortified foods are the major dietary sources of vitamin D. Prior to the fortification of milk products in the 1930s, rickets (a bone disease

This text was developed by the Clinical Nutrition Service, Warren Grant Magnuson Clinical Center, in conjunction with the Office of Dietary Supplements (ODS), National Institutes of Health (NIH), January 2001.

seen in children) was a major public health problem in the United States. Milk in the United States is fortified with 10 micrograms (400 IU) of vitamin D per quart, and rickets is now uncommon in the US.

One cup of vitamin D fortified milk supplies about one-fourth of the estimated daily need for this vitamin for adults. Although milk is fortified with vitamin D, dairy products made from milk such as cheese, yogurt, and ice cream are generally not fortified with vitamin D. Only a few foods naturally contain significant amounts of vitamin D, including fatty fish and fish oils. Table 28.2 suggests dietary sources of vitamin D.

Exposure to Sunlight

Exposure to sunlight is an important source of vitamin D. Ultraviolet (UV) rays from sunlight trigger vitamin D synthesis in the skin. Season, latitude, time of day, cloud cover, smog, and suncreens affect UV ray exposure. For example, in Boston the average amount of sunlight is insufficient to produce significant vitamin D synthesis in the skin from November through February. Sunscreens with a sun protection factor of 8 or greater will block UV rays that produce vitamin D, but it is still important to routinely use sunscreen whenever sun exposure is longer than 10 to 15 minutes. It is especially important for individuals with limited sun exposure to include good sources of vitamin D in their diet.

Is There a Recommended Dietary Allowance for Vitamin D for Adults?

The Recommended Dietary Allowance (RDA) is the average daily dietary intake level that is sufficient to meet the nutrient requirements

Table 28.1. RDAs for Vitamin D for Adults

Life-Stage	Men	Women
Ages 19-50	5 mcg* or 200 IU	5 mcg* or 200 IU
Ages 51-69	10 mcg* or 400 IU	10 mcg* or 400 IU
Ages 70 +	15 mcg* or 600 IU	15 mcg* or 600 IU

*1 mcg vitamin D = 40 International Units (IU)

of nearly all (97-98%) healthy individuals in each life-stage and gender group. There is insufficient evidence to establish a RDA for vitamin D. Instead, an Adequate Intake (AI), a level of intake sufficient to maintain healthy blood levels of an active form of vitamin D, has been established. The 1998 AIs for vitamin D for adults, in micrograms (mcg) and International Units (IUs) are shown in Table 28.1.

Estimates of vitamin D intake in the United States are not available because dietary surveys do not assess vitamin D intake. Dietary intake of vitamin D is largely determined by the intake of fortified food.

When Can Vitamin D Deficiency Occur?

A deficiency of vitamin D can occur when dietary intake of vitamin D is inadequate, when there is limited exposure to sunlight, when the kidney cannot convert vitamin D to its active form, or when someone cannot adequately absorb vitamin D from the gastrointestinal tract.

The classic vitamin D deficiency diseases are rickets and osteomalacia. In children, vitamin D deficiency causes rickets, which results in skeletal deformities. In adults, vitamin D deficiency can lead to osteomalacia, which results in muscular weakness in addition to weak bones.

Who May Need Extra Vitamin D to Prevent a Deficiency?

Older Americans (greater than age 50) are thought to have a higher risk of developing vitamin D deficiency. The ability of skin to convert vitamin D to its active form decreases as we age. The kidneys, which help convert vitamin D to its active form, sometimes do not work as well when people age. Therefore, some older Americans may need vitamin D from a supplement.

It is important for individuals with limited sun exposure to include good sources of vitamin D in their diets. Homebound individuals, people living in northern latitudes such as in New England and Alaska, women who cover their body for religious reasons, and individuals working in occupations that prevent exposure to sunlight are at risk of a vitamin D deficiency. If these individuals are unable to meet their daily dietary need for vitamin D, they may need a supplement of vitamin D.

Individuals who have reduced ability to absorb dietary fat (fat malabsorption) may need extra vitamin D because it is a fat soluble vitamin. Some causes of fat malabsorption are pancreatic enzyme deficiency, Crohn's disease, cystic fibrosis, sprue, liver disease, surgical removal of part or all of the stomach, and small bowel disease. Symptoms of fat malabsorption include diarrhea and greasy stools.

Vitamin D supplements are often recommended for exclusively breast-fed infants because human milk may not contain adequate vitamin D. The Institute of Medicine states that "With habitual small doses of sunshine breast- or formula-fed infants do not require supplemental vitamin D." Mothers of infants who are exclusively breastfed and have a limited sun exposure should consult with a pediatrician on this issue. Since infant formulas are routinely fortified with vitamin D, formula fed infants usually have adequate dietary intake of vitamin D.

What are Some Current Issues and Controversies about Vitamin D?

Vitamin D and Osteoporosis

It is estimated that over 25 million adults in the United States have, or are at risk of developing osteoporosis. Osteoporosis is a disease characterized by fragile bones. It results in increased risk of bone fractures. Having normal storage levels of vitamin D in your body helps keep your bones strong and may help prevent osteoporosis in elderly, non-ambulatory individuals, in post-menopausal women, and in individuals on chronic steroid therapy.

Researchers know that normal bone is constantly being remodeled (broken down and rebuilt). During menopause, the balance between these two systems is upset, resulting in more bone being broken down (resorbed) than rebuilt. Estrogen replacement, which limits symptoms of menopause, can help slow down the development of osteoporosis by stimulating the activity of cells that rebuild bone.

Vitamin D deficiency, which occurs more often in post-menopausal women and older Americans, has been associated with greater incidence of hip fractures. A greater vitamin D intake from diet and supplements has been associated with less bone loss in older women. Since bone loss increases the risk of fractures, vitamin D supplementation may help prevent fractures resulting from osteoporosis.

In a group of women with osteoporosis hospitalized for hip fractures, 50 percent were found to have signs of vitamin D deficiency. Treatment of vitamin D deficiency can result in decreased incidence of hip fractures, and daily supplementation with 20 mcg (800 IU) of vitamin D may reduce the risk of osteoporotic fractures in elderly populations with low blood levels of vitamin D. Your physician will discuss your need for vitamin D supplementation as part of an over-all plan to prevent and/or treat osteoporosis when indicated.

Vitamin D and Cancer

Laboratory, animal, and epidemiologic evidence suggest that vitamin D may be protective against some cancers. Some dietary surveys have associated increased intake of dairy foods with decreased incidence of colon cancer. Another dietary survey associated a higher calcium and vitamin D intake with a lower incidence of colon cancer. Well-designed clinical trials need to be conducted to determine whether vitamin D deficiency increases cancer risk, or if an increased intake of vitamin D is protective against some cancers. Until such trials are conducted, it is premature to advise anyone to take vitamin D supplements to prevent cancer.

Vitamin D and Steroids

Corticosteroid medications are often prescribed to reduce inflammation from a variety of medical problems. These medicines may be essential for a person's medical treatment, but they have potential side effects, including decreased calcium absorption. There is some evidence that steroids may also impair vitamin D metabolism, further contributing to the loss of bone and development of osteoporosis associated with steroid medications. For these reasons, individuals on chronic steroid therapy should consult with their physician or registered dietitian about the need to increase vitamin D intake through diet and/or dietary supplements.

Vitamin D and Alzheimer's Disease

Adults with Alzheimer's disease have increased risk of hip fractures. This may be because many Alzheimer's patients are home-bound, and frequently sunlight deprived. Alzheimer's disease is more prevalent in older populations, so the fact that the ability of skin to convert vitamin D to its active form decreases as we age also may contribute to increased risk of hip fractures in this group. One study of women with Alzheimer's disease found that decreased bone mineral density was associated with a low intake of vitamin D and inadequate sunlight exposure. Physicians evaluate the need for vitamin D supplementation as part of an overall treatment plan for adults with Alzheimer's disease.

What Is the Health Risk of Too Much Vitamin D?

There is a high health risk associated with consuming too much vitamin D. Vitamin D toxicity can cause nausea, vomiting, poor appetite, constipation, weakness, and weight loss. It can also raise blood levels of calcium, causing mental status changes such as confusion. High blood levels of calcium also can cause heart rhythm abnormalities. Calcinosis, the deposition of calcium and phosphate in soft tissues like the kidney can be caused by vitamin D toxicity.

Consuming too much vitamin D through diet alone is not likely unless you routinely consume large amounts of cod liver oil. It is much more likely to occur from high intakes of vitamin D in supplements. The Food and Nutrition Board of the Institute of Medicine considers an intake of 25 mcg (1,000 IU) for infants up to 12 months of age and 50 mcg (2,000 IU) for children, adults, pregnant, and lactating women to be the tolerable upper intake level (UL). A daily intake above the UL increases the risk of adverse health effects and is not advised.

Selected Food Sources of Vitamin D

As the 2000 *Dietary Guidelines for Americans* state, "Different foods contain different nutrients. No single food can supply all the nutrients in the amounts you need." The following table suggests dietary sources of vitamin D. As the table indicates, fortified foods are a major source of vitamin D. Breakfast cereals, pastries, breads, crackers, cereal grain bars and other foods may be fortified with 10% to 15% of the DV for vitamin D. It is important to read the nutrition facts panel of the food label to determine whether a food provides vitamin D.

If you want more information about building a healthful diet, refer to the *Dietary Guidelines for Americans* and the Food Guide Pyramid.

Table 28.2. Table of Selected Food Sources of Vitamin D

Food	International Units	%DV *
Cod Liver Oil, 1 Tbs.	1,360 IU	340
Salmon, cooked, 3 1/2 oz	360 IU	90
Mackerel, cooked, 3 1/2 oz	345 IU	90
Sardines, canned in oil, drained,3 1/2 oz	270 IU	70
Eel, cooked, 3 1/2 oz	200 IU	50
Milk, nonfat, reduced fat, and whole, vitamin D fortified, 1 c	98 IU	25
Margarine, fortified, 1 Tbs.	60 IU	15
Cereal grain bars, fortified w/ 10% of the DV, 1 each	50 IU	10
Pudding, 1/2 c prepared from mix and made with vitamin D fortified milk	50 IU	10
Dry cereal, Vit D fortified w/10%* of DV, 3/4 c * Other cereals may be fortified with more or less vitamin D	40-50 IU	10
Liver, beef, cooked, 3 1/2 oz	30 IU	8
Egg, 1 whole (vitamin D is present in the yolk)	25 IU	6

* DV = Daily Value. DVs are reference numbers based on the Recommended Dietary Allowance (RDA). They were developed to help consumers determine if a food contains very much of a specific nutrient. The DV for vitamin D is 400 IU. The percent DV (%DV) listed on the nutrition facts panel of food labels tells adults what percentage of the DV is provided by one serving. Percent DVs are based on a 2,000-calorie diet. Your Daily Values may be higher or lower depending on your calorie needs. Foods that provide lower percentages of the DV will contribute to a healthful diet.

Chapter 29

Vitamin E

Vitamin E: What Is It?

Vitamin E is a fat-soluble vitamin that exists in eight different forms. Each form has its own biological activity, the measure of potency or functional use in the body. Alpha-tocopherol is the most active form of vitamin E in humans, and is a powerful biological antioxidant. Antioxidants such as vitamin E act to protect your cells against the effects of free radicals, which are potentially damaging by-products of the body's metabolism. Free radicals can cause cell damage that may contribute to the development of cardiovascular disease and cancer. Studies are underway to determine whether vitamin E might help prevent or delay the development of those chronic diseases.

What Foods Provide Vitamin E?

Vegetable oils, nuts, and green leafy vegetables are the main dietary sources of vitamin E. Fortified cereals are also an important source of vitamin E in the United States. Table 29.2 suggests foods that contain vitamin E.

This text was developed by the Clinical Nutrition Service, Warren Grant Magnuson Clinical Center, in conjunction with the Office of Dietary Supplements (ODS), National Institutes of Health (NIH), January 2001.

What Is the Recommended Dietary Allowance for Vitamin E for Adults?

The Recommended Dietary Allowance (RDA) is the average daily dietary intake level that is sufficient to meet the nutrient requirements of nearly all (97-98%) healthy individuals in each life-stage and gender group. The 2000 RDAs for vitamin E for adults, in milligrams (mg) and International Units (IUs) are presented in Table 29.1.

Table 29.1. RDAs for Vitamin E for Adults

Life-Stage	Men and Women	Pregnancy	Lactation
Ages 19+	15 mg* or 22 IU		
All ages		15 mg* or 22 IU	19 mg* or 28 IU

*1 mg alpha-tocopherol equivalents = 1.5 IU

The RDA for vitamin E is based on the alpha-tocopherol form because it is the most active, or usable, form. Unlike other vitamins, the form of alpha-tocopherol made in the laboratory and found in supplements is not identical to the natural form, and is not quite as active as the natural form.

Results of two national surveys, the National Health and Nutrition Examination Survey (NHANES III 1988-91) and the Continuing Survey of Food Intakes of Individuals (1994 CSFII) indicated that the dietary intake of most Americans does not provide the recommended intake for vitamin E. However, a 2000 Institute of Medicine (IOM) report on vitamin E states that intake estimates of vitamin E may be low because energy and fat intake is often underreported in national surveys and because the kind and amount of fat added during cooking is often not known. The IOM states that most North American adults get enough vitamin E from their normal diets to meet current recommendations. However, they do caution individuals who consume low fat diets because vegetable oils are such a good dietary source of vitamin E. "Low-fat diets can substantially decrease vitamin E intakes if food choices are not carefully made to enhance alpha-tocopherol intakes."

When Can Vitamin E Deficiency Occur?

Vitamin E deficiency is rare in humans. There are three specific situations when a vitamin E deficiency is likely to occur. It is seen in persons who cannot absorb dietary fat, has been found in premature, very low birth weight infants (birth weights less than 1500 grams, or 3 1/2 pounds), and is seen in individuals with rare disorders of fat metabolism. A vitamin E deficiency is usually characterized by neurological problems due to poor nerve conduction.

Who May Need Extra Vitamin E to Prevent a Deficiency?

Individuals who cannot absorb fat may require a vitamin E supplement because some dietary fat is needed for the absorption of vitamin E from the gastrointestinal tract. Anyone diagnosed with cystic fibrosis, individuals who have had part or all of their stomach removed, and individuals with malabsorptive problems such as Crohn's disease may not absorb fat and should discuss the need for supplemental vitamin E with their physician. People who cannot absorb fat often pass greasy stools or have chronic diarrhea.

Very low birth weight infants may be deficient in vitamin E. These infants are usually under the care of a neonatologist, a pediatrician specializing in the care of newborns, who evaluates and treats the exact nutritional needs of premature infants.

Abetalipoproteinemia is a rare inherited disorder of fat metabolism that results in poor absorption of dietary fat and vitamin E. The vitamin E deficiency associated with this disease causes problems such as poor transmission of nerve impulses, muscle weakness, and degeneration of the retina that can cause blindness. Individuals with abetalipoproteinemia may be prescribed special vitamin E supplements by a physician to treat this disorder.

What are Some Current Issues and Controversies about Vitamin E?

Vitamin E and Heart Disease

Preliminary research has led to a widely held belief that vitamin E may help prevent or delay coronary heart disease. Researchers are fairly certain that oxidative modification of LDL-cholesterol (sometimes called "bad" cholesterol) promotes blockages in coronary arteries that may lead to atherosclerosis and heart attacks. Vitamin E may help prevent or delay coronary heart disease by limiting the oxidation of LDL-cholesterol. Vitamin E also may help prevent the formation of blood clots, which could lead to a heart attack. Observational studies have associated lower rates of heart disease with higher vitamin E intake. A study of approximately 90,000 nurses suggested that the incidence of heart disease was 30% to 40% lower among nurses with the highest intake of vitamin E from diet and supplements. The range of intakes from both diet and supplements in this group was 21.6 to 1,000 IU (32 to 1,500 mg), with the median intake being 208 IU (139 mg). A 1994 review of 5,133 Finnish men and women aged 30-69 years suggested that increased dietary intake of vitamin E was associated with decreased mortality (death) from heart disease. But even though these observations are promising, randomized clinical trials raise questions about the role of vitamin E supplements in heart disease. The Heart Outcomes Prevention Evaluation (HOPE) Study followed almost 10,000 patients for 4.5 years who were at high risk for heart attack or stroke. In this intervention study the subjects who received 265 mg (400) IU of vitamin E daily did not experience significantly fewer cardiovascular events or hospitalizations for heart failure or chest pain when compared to those who received a sugar pill. The researchers suggested that it is unlikely that the vitamin E supplement provided any protection against cardiovascular disease in the HOPE study. This study is continuing, to determine whether a longer duration of intervention with vitamin E supplements will provide any protection against cardiovascular disease.

Vitamin E and Cancer

Antioxidants such as vitamin E help protect against the damaging effects of free radicals, which may contribute to the development of chronic diseases such as cancer. Vitamin E also may block the formation of nitrosamines, which are carcinogens formed in the stomach from nitrites consumed in the diet. It also may protect against the development of cancers by enhancing immune function. Unfortunately, human trials and surveys that tried to associate vitamin E with incidence of cancer have been generally inconclusive.

Some evidence associates higher intake of vitamin E with a decreased incidence of prostate cancer and breast cancer. There is evidence that vitamin E may reduce the size of cysts in women with fibrocystic breast disease, which is a risk factor for breast cancer. However, an examination of the effect of dietary factors, including vitamin E, on incidence of postmenopausal breast cancer in over 18,000 women from New York State did not associate a greater vitamin E intake with a reduced risk of developing breast cancer.

A study of women in Iowa provided evidence that an increased dietary intake of vitamin E may decrease the risk of colon cancer, especially in women under 65 years of age. On the other hand, vitamin E intake was not statistically associated with risk of colon cancer in almost 2,000 adults with cancer who were compared to controls without cancer. At this time there is limited evidence to recommend vitamin E supplements for the prevention of cancer.

Vitamin E and Cataracts

Cataracts are growths on the lens of the eye that cloud vision. They increase the risk of disability and blindness in aging adults. Antioxidants are being studied to determine whether they can help prevent or delay cataract growth. Observational studies have found that lens clarity, which is used to diagnose cataracts, was better in regular users of vitamin E supplements and in persons with higher blood levels of vitamin E. A study of middle aged male smokers, however, did not demonstrate any effect from vitamin E supplements on the incidence of cataract formation. The effects of smoking, a major risk factor for developing cataracts, may have overridden any potential benefit from the vitamin E, but the conflicting results also indicate a need for further studies before researchers can confidently recommend extra vitamin E for the prevention of cataracts.

What Is the Health Risk of Too Much Vitamin E?

The health risk of too much vitamin E is low. A recent review of the safety of vitamin E in the elderly indicated that taking vitamin E supplements for up to four months at doses of 530 mg or 800 IU (35 times the current RDA) had no significant effect on general health, body weight, levels of body proteins, lipid levels, liver or kidney function, thyroid hormones, amount or kinds of blood cells, and bleeding time. Even though this study provides evidence that taking a vitamin E supplement containing 530 mg or 800 IU for four months is safe, the long term safety of vitamin E supplementation has not been tested. The Institute of Medicine has set an upper tolerable intake level for vitamin E at 1,000 mg (1,500 IU) for any form of supplementary alpha-tocopherol per day because the nutrient can act as an antico-agulant and increase the risk of bleeding problems. Upper tolerable intake levels "represent the maximum intake of a nutrient that is likely to pose no risk of adverse health effects in almost all individuals in the general population."

Table 29.2. Table of Food Sources

Food	International Units	%DV*
Wheat germ oil, 1 Tb	26.2	90
Almonds, dry roasted, 1 oz	7.5	25
Safflower oil, 1 Tb	4.7	15
Corn oil, 1 Tb	2.9	10
Soybean oil, 1 Tb	2.5	8
Turnip greens, frozen, boiled, 1/2 c	2.4	8
Mango, raw, without refuse,1 fruit	2.3	8
Peanuts, dry roasted, 1 oz	2.1	8
Mixed nuts w/ peanuts, oil roasted, 1 oz	1.7	6
Mayonnaise, made w/ soybean oil, 1 Tb	1.6	6
Broccoli, frozen, chopped, boiled, 1/2 c	1.5	6
Dandelion greens, boiled, 1/2 c	1.3	4
Pistachio nuts, dry roasted, 1 oz	1.2	4
Spinach, frozen, boiled, 1/2 c	0.85	2
Kiwi, 1 medium fruit	0.85	2

* DV = Daily Value. DVs are reference numbers based on the Recommended Dietary Allowance (RDA). They were developed to help consumers determine if a food contains a lot or a little of a specific nutrient. The DV for vitamin E is 30 International Units (or 20 mg). The percent DV (%DV) listed on the nutrition facts panel of food labels tells adults what percentage of the DV is provided by one serving. Percent DVs are based on a 2,000-calorie diet. Your Daily Values may be higher or lower depending on your calorie needs. Foods that provide lower percentages of the DV will contribute to a healthful diet.

Table of Selected Food Sources of Vitamin E

As the 2000 *Dietary Guidelines for Americans* state, "Different foods contain different nutrients. No single food can supply all the nutrients in the amounts you need." The following table lists selected sources of vitamin E. As the tables indicate, vegetables oils, nuts, and green leafy vegetables are good dietary sources of vitamin E. Including these foods in your diet will help you meet your daily need for vitamin E, but it is still important to moderate total fat intake as recommended by the Dietary Guidelines for Americans.

Food manufacturers fortify many foods with vitamins and minerals. It is important to read the nutrition facts panel of the food label to determine whether a food provides vitamin E. If you want more information about building a healthful diet, refer to the *Dietary Guidelines for Americans* and the Food Guide Pyramid.

Chapter 30

Zinc

Zinc: What Is It?

Zinc has been known for more than 50 years to be an essential mineral. It is found in almost every cell in the body and is contained within more than 200 enzymes, substances needed for biochemical reactions. Zinc is important for a healthy immune system, for healing cuts and wounds, and for maintaining your sense of taste and smell. Zinc also supports normal growth and development during pregnancy, childhood, and adolescence.

What Foods Provide Zinc?

Meat and poultry provide the majority of zinc in the American diet. Other food sources include beans, nuts, and dairy products. Oysters are the food containing the most zinc by weight, but beef is a more common source in the U.S. diet. The zinc found in meat and oysters is easily absorbed by the body. Dietary phytates, which are found in whole grain cereals and unleavened bread, may significantly decrease the body's absorption of zinc. Table 30.2 suggests many dietary sources of zinc.

This text was developed by the Clinical Nutrition Service, Warren Grant Magnuson Clinical Center, in conjunction with the Office of Dietary Supplements (ODS), National Institutes of Health (NIH), January 2001.

What Is the Recommended Dietary Allowance for Zinc?

The Recommended Dietary Allowance (RDA) is the average daily dietary intake level that is sufficient to meet the nutrient requirements of nearly all (97-98%) individuals in each life-stage and gender group. The 1989 RDAs for zinc for adults, in milligrams (mg), are presented in Table 30.1.

Results of two national surveys, the National Health and Nutrition Examination Survey (NHANES III 1988-91) and the Continuing Survey of Food Intakes of Individuals (1994 CSFII) indicated that the diets of many adults, especially older Americans and women, do not provide the recommended amounts of zinc.

When Can Zinc Deficiency Occur?

Zinc deficiency can occur when zinc intake is inadequate, when there are increased losses of zinc from the body, or when the body's requirement for zinc increases. There is no specific deficiency disease associated with zinc. Instead, many general signs of zinc deficiency can appear, including poor appetite, weight loss, delayed healing of wounds, taste abnormalities, and mental lethargy. As body stores of zinc decline, these symptoms worsen and are accompanied by diarrhea, hair loss, recurrent infection, and a form of dermatitis, a skin disorder. Zinc deficiency has also been linked to poor growth in childhood.

Who May Need Extra Zinc?

There is no single laboratory test available to determine zinc nutritional status. Instead, dietary intake is typically used to estimate the risk of a zinc deficiency. People who may benefit from a zinc

Table 30.1. RDAs for Zinc for Adults

Life-Stage	Men	Women	Pregnancy	Lactation
Ages 19 +	15 mg	12 mg		
All ages			15 mg	19 mg (first six months)
				16 mg (second six months)

supplement include those who do not consume enough calories, vegetarians, the elderly, pregnant and lactating women, and people who suffer from alcoholism or digestive diseases that cause diarrhea.

Anyone with a low caloric intake is at higher risk for having a low zinc intake and for developing a zinc deficiency. Vegetarians who consume a variety of legumes and nuts will probably meet their zinc requirement, but otherwise a vegetarian diet may be inadequate in zinc. Since the zinc from plant sources is absorbed less readily, this increases the concern about zinc status in vegetarians who do not consume legumes and nuts.

Dietary surveys suggest that many Americans aged 51 and older, pregnant women and breastfeeding mothers do not consume recommended amounts of zinc. Therefore, to decrease their risk for developing a zinc deficiency, it is important for individuals in these groups to include sources of zinc in their daily diet. Zinc supplementation has been found to improve the growth rate in children with mild zinc deficiency and mild to moderate growth failure. Maternal zinc deficiency can delay fetal growth, and mothers who give birth to small for gestational age babies have been found to have lower zinc intakes during pregnancy. Breastfeeding increases the risk of depleting nutritional zinc status when dietary zinc intake is chronically low because of the greater need for zinc during lactation.

Zinc deficiency is frequently associated with alcoholism, which is often due to a lower intake of food. The need for a supplement as part of an overall treatment plan is usually evaluated by a physician in this situation.

Diarrhea causes a loss of zinc. Therefore, digestive diseases or gastrointestinal surgery that result in diarrhea are often associated with zinc deficiency. Individuals who experience chronic diarrhea should make sure they include sources of zinc in their daily diet. A medical doctor can evaluate the need for a zinc supplement if diet alone fails to maintain normal zinc levels in the body.

What are Some Current Issues and Controversies about Zinc?

Zinc, Infections, and Wound Healing

The immune system is adversely affected by even moderate degrees of zinc deficiency. People who are zinc-deficient have a more difficult time resisting infections. T-cell lymphocytes, white blood cells that help fight infection, do not function efficiently when zinc stores are

Table 30.2. Table of Food Sources of Zinc

Food	Milligrams	%DV*
Oysters, 6 medium	76.4	510
Beef shank, lean only, cooked 3 oz	8.9	60
Beef chuck, lean only, cooked, 3 oz	7.4	45
Beef tenderloin, lean only, cooked, 3 oz	4.8	30
Pork shoulder, lean only, cooked, 3 oz	4.7	25
Pork tenderloin, lean only, cooked, 3 oz	2.2	15
Chicken leg, cooked, 3 oz	2.4	15
Baked beans, canned, 1/2 c	1.8	10
Cashews, dry roasted w/out salt, 1 oz	1.6	10
Pecans, dry roasted w/out salt, 1 oz	1.6	10
Raisin bran, 1 oz	1.5	10
Almonds, dry roasted, unblanched, w/out salt, 1 oz	1.4	9
Chickpeas, mature seeds, canned, 1/2 c	1.3	9
Mixed nuts, dry roasted w/peanuts, w/out salt, 1 oz	1.1	5
Chicken breast, cooked, 3 oz	1.1	5
Bran muffin, 1 medium	1.1	5
Walnuts, black, dried, 1 oz	1.0	5
Milk, 1 c	1.0	5
Yogurt, 1 c	1.0	5
Kidney beans, 1/2 c cooked	0.9	5
Cheese, cheddar, 1 oz	0.9	5
Peas, green, boiled, 1/2 c	0.8	5
Oatmeal, instant, 1 packet	0.8	5
Flounder/sole, cooked, 3 oz	0.5	5

DV = Daily Value. DVs are reference numbers based on the Recommended Dietary Allowance (RDA). They were developed to help consumers determine if a food contains very much of a specific nutrient. The DV for zinc is 15 milligrams (mg). The percent DV (%DV) listed on the nutrition facts panel of food labels tells adults what percentage of the DV is provided by one serving. Even foods that provide lower percentages of the DV will contribute to a healthful diet.

low. When zinc supplements are given to individuals with low zinc levels, the numbers of T-cell lymphocytes circulating in the blood increase and the ability of lymphocytes to fight infection improves. Studies show that poor, malnourished children in India, Africa, South America, and Southeast Asia experience shorter courses of infectious diarrhea after taking zinc supplements. Zinc supplements are often used to treat skin ulcers or bed sores, but they do not increase rates of wound healing when zinc levels are normal.

Zinc and the Common Cold

A study of over 100 employees of the Cleveland Clinic indicated that zinc lozenges decreased the duration of colds by one-half. Some of the participants reported fewer days of congestion and nasal drainage, but no differences were seen in how long their fevers lasted or in the level of muscle aches they experienced. However, this study has been criticized by some researchers who believe that since zinc lozenges often have a bad taste, the participants may have known the difference between the supplement and placebo, which would compromise the results. Also, since other studies have shown no benefit the debate continues on the true value of zinc supplements for cold symptoms.

Zinc and Iron Absorption

Iron deficiency anemia is considered a serious public health problem in the world today. Iron fortification programs were developed to prevent this deficiency and they have been credited with improving the iron status of millions of women, infants, and children. Some researchers, however, have raised concern about the effects of iron fortification on other nutrients, including zinc. Iron taken in solution can inhibit the absorption of zinc, but foods fortified with iron do not.

What Is the Health Risk of Too Much Zinc?

The health risk of taking too much zinc is moderate to high. Zinc toxicity has been seen in both acute and chronic forms. Intakes of 150 to 450 mg of zinc per day have been associated with low copper status, altered iron function, reduced immune function, and reduced levels of high-density lipoproteins (the good cholesterol). One case report cited severe nausea and vomiting within 30 minutes after the person ingested four grams of zinc gluconate (570 mg elemental zinc).

The 1989 RDA committee stated that "chronic ingestion of zinc supplements exceeding 15 mg/day is not recommended without adequate medical supervision." The National Academy of Sciences is currently reviewing recent research and considering new recommendations on zinc intake and risk.

Chapter 31

Detoxification

So many problems in our Western society come from excessive use of foods and drugs. Abuses and addictions touch almost every person's life. This chapter deals with many of the dietary and substance abuses and ways to heal them.

What Is Detoxification?

Detoxification is the process of clearing toxins from the body or neutralizing or transforming them, and clearing excess mucus and congestion. Many of these toxins come from our diet, drug use, and environmental exposure, both acute and chronic. Internally fats, especially oxidized fats and cholesterol, free radicals, and other irritating molecules act as toxins. Functionally, poor digestion, colon sluggishness and dysfunction, reduced liver function, and poor elimination through the kidneys, respiratory tract, and skin all add to increased toxicity.

Detoxification involves dietary and lifestyle changes that reduce intake of toxins and improve elimination. Avoidance of chemicals, from food or other sources, refined food, sugar, caffeine, alcohol, tobacco, and many drugs helps minimize the toxin load. Drinking extra water

Excerpted from *The Detox Diet: A How-to and When-to Guide for Cleansing the Body,* © 1996 by Elson M. Haas, M.D., and from *Staying Healthy with Nutrition,* © 1992 by Elson M. Haas, M.D. Reprinted by permission of the author and Celestial Arts, Berkeley, CA. Text reviewed by author January 2002. Complete information about Elson Haas, M.D. is included at the end of this chapter.

(purified) and increasing fiber by including more fruits and vegetables in the diet are steps in the detoxification process. Moving from a more to a less congesting diet will help us to move along the detox road.

Detoxification therapy, as fasting, is the oldest treatment known to humans and is a completely natural process; and in many cases, as we listen to our inner guidance as animals do, we may apply this process to many illnesses and states of health and life. Many authorities claim the detox process helps clear wastes and old or dead cells and revitalizes the body's natural functions and healing capacities.

Table 31.1. Specific Detoxification Programs

General Detoxification and Cleansing
Drug Detoxification
Alcohol Detoxification
Caffeine Detoxification
Nicotine Detoxification
Fasting
Immortality and Beyond

General Detoxification and Cleaning

It is somewhat difficult to separate the concepts and practices of detoxification from those of fasting. Fasting, or the avoidance of solid food is one method of detoxification, probably the most effective, yet extreme, form. There are many other ways to detoxify.

Toxicity is of much greater concern in the twentieth century than ever before. There are many new and stronger chemicals, air and water pollution, radiation and nuclear power. We ingest new chemicals, use more drugs of all kinds, eat more sugar and incidence of many toxicity diseases has increased as well. Cancer and cardiovascular disease are two of the main ones. Arthritis, allergies, obesity, and many skin problems are others. In addition, a wide range of symptoms, such as headaches, fatigue, pains, coughs, gastrointestinal problems, and from immune weakness, can all be related to toxicity.

Toxicity occurs on two basic levels—external and internal. We can acquire toxins from our environment by breathing them, by ingesting them, or through physical contact with them. We all are exposed to toxins daily. We eat them, drink them and impose them upon ourselves repeatedly and regularly. Most drugs, food additives, and allergens can create toxic elements in the body. In fact, any substance can have toxicity—water, sodium, and almost all nutrients can be a problem in certain circumstances.

On the internal level, our body produces toxins through its normal everyday functions. Biochemical, cellular, and bodily activities generate substances that need to be eliminated. Free radicals are biochemical toxins. When these substances/molecules/toxins are not eliminated, they can cause irritation or inflammation of the cells and tissues, blocking normal functions on a cellular, organ, and whole-body level. Microbes of all kinds—intestinal bacteria, foreign bacteria, yeasts, and parasites—produce metabolic waste products that we must handle. Our thoughts and emotions, and stress itself, generate increased biochemical toxicity. The proper level of elimination of these toxins is essential to health. Clearly, a normal functioning body was created to handle certain levels of toxins; the concern is with excess intake or production of toxins or a reduction in the process of elimination.

A toxin is basically any substance that creates irritating and/or harmful effects in the body, undermining our health or stressing our biochemical or organ functions. This may result from drugs which have side effects, or from patterns of physiology that are different from our usual functioning. Recreational drugs also have some harmful effects. The free radicals irritate, inflame, age, and cause degeneration of body tissues. Negative "ethers," psychic and spiritual influences, thought patterns, and negative emotions all can be toxins as well—both as stressors and by changing the normal physiology of the body and possibly producing specific symptoms.

Toxicity occurs in our body when we take in more than we can utilize and eliminate. Homeostasis means that our body functions are in balance. This balance is disturbed when we feed ourselves more than we can utilize or partake of specific substances that are toxic. Toxicity may depend on the dosage, frequency, or potency of the toxin. A toxin may produce an immediate or rapid onset of symptoms, as many pesticides and some drugs do; possibly, even more commonly, it may cause some long-term negative effect, such as asbestos exposure leading to lung cancer.

Of course, if our body is working well, with good immune and eliminative functions, we can handle our basic everyday exposure to toxins. The purpose of this chapter is to discuss ways to support the elimination of toxins, excessive mucus, congestion, and disease and to prevent, on a day-to-day basis, the buildup of toxicity. Through detoxification, we clear and filter toxins and wastes and allow our body to work on enhancing its basic functions.

Table 31.2. Our General Detoxification Systems

Respiratory—lungs, bronchial tubes, throat, sinuses, and nose
Gastrointestinal—liver, gallbladder, colon, and whole GI tract
Urinary—kidneys, bladder, and urethra
Skin and dermal—sweat and sebaceous glands and tears
Lymphatic—lymph channels and lymph nodes

Our body handles toxins by either neutralizing, transforming, or eliminating them. As examples, many of the antioxidant nutrients may neutralize free-radical molecules. The liver helps transform many toxic substances into harmless agents, while the blood carries wastes to the kidney; the liver also dumps wastes through the bile into the intestines, where much waste is eliminated. We also clear toxins through sweating, from exercise or heat. Our sinuses and skin may also be accessory elimination organs whereby excess mucus or toxins can be released, as with sinus congestion or skin rashes, respectively.

Detoxification occurs on many other levels as well. Physically, this process can help clear congestions, illnesses, and disease potential. It can improve energy. Many "detox" processes can help rejuvenate us and prevent degeneration. Mental detoxification is also important. Cleansing our minds of negative thought patterns is essential to health; the physical detoxification also helps this mental process. Emotionally, detoxification helps us uncover and express feelings, especially hidden frustrations, anger, resentments, or fear, and replace them with forgiveness, love, joy, and hope. On a spiritual level, many people experience new clarity and/or an enhancement of their purpose of life during cleansing processes. A light detox over a couple of days can help us feel better, while a longer process and deeper commitment to a new way of life, such as eliminating certain abusive habits and eating a better diet, will help us really change our whole life.

Detoxification is part of a transformational medicine that instills change on many levels. Change and evolution are keys to healing. Enhancing elimination helps us deal with and clear problems from our past, from childhood and parental patterns to recent job or relationship stress. When our body has eliminated much of its toxic buildup, we feel lighter and are able to really experience the moment and be open for the future.

Detoxification is a relative term. Anything that supports our elimination can be said to help us detoxify. Doing nothing more than drinking an extra quart of water a day will usually help us eliminate more toxins. Eating more fruits and vegetables—the high-water-content, cleaning foods—and less meat and milk products will create less congestion and more elimination. There are many levels of the progressive detoxification diets, from these simple changes to complete fasting.

Some people go to extremes with fasting, laxatives, enemas, colonics, diuretics, and even exercise and begin to lose essential nutrients from their body. A negative balance can be created in this manner, such as protein or vitamin-mineral deficiencies though congestion from overintake and underelimination is a more common problem in this culture. The best and simplest way to look at symptoms and disease is in terms of excess (congestion) and deficiency; this is the basis of the traditional Oriental philosophy.

Who Is Best Suited for Detoxification?

Almost everyone needs to detox, cleanse themselves, and rest their body functions at times. Cleansing or detoxification is one part of the trilogy of nutritional action, the others being building, or toning, and balance, or maintenance. With a regular, balanced diet, devoid of excesses, we will need less intensive detoxification. Our body has a daily elimination cycle, mostly carried out at night and in the early morning, up until breakfast. However, when we eat a congesting diet higher in fats, meats, dairy products, refined foods, and chemicals, detoxification becomes more necessary. Who needs to detoxify, and when, is based in part on individual lifestyle and needs.

More common toxicity symptoms include headache, fatigue, mucus problems, aches and pains, digestive problems, "allergy" symptoms, and sensitivity to environmental agents such as chemicals, perfumes, and synthetics. People who experience these and others may benefit from diet changes or avoidance of the drug or agent that may be influencing the symptom. It may be important to differentiate allergic symptoms from those of toxicity to determine the appropriate medical care. The diet and detox program is often helpful in reducing allergic symptoms. Fasting can be extremely beneficial for people with allergies. Of course, there may be subtle characteristics of toxicity that differentiate it from other health concerns.

Many common acute and chronic illnesses may be alleviated by a program of detoxification/cleansing, as they are basically created by

Table 31.3. Signs and Symptoms of Toxicity

Headaches	Frequent colds	Mood changes
Joint pains	Irritated eyes	Anxiety
Cough	Immune weakness	Depression
Wheezing	Environmental sensitivity	Fatigue
Sore throat	Sinus congestion	Skin rashes
Tight or stiff neck	Fever	Hives
Angina pectoris	Runny nose	Nausea
Circulatory deficits	Nervousness	Indigestion
High blood fats	Sleepiness	Anorexia
Backaches	Insomnia	Bad breath
Itchy nose	Dizziness	Constipation

Table 31.4. Problems Related to Congestion/Stagnation/Toxicity

Acne	Thrombophlebitis	Kidney disease
Abscesses	Gout	Stroke
Boils	Obesity	Prostate disease
Eczema	Infections by:	Menstrual problems
Allergies	Bacteria	Vaginitis
Arthritis	Virus	Varicose veins
Asthma	Fungus	Diabetes
Constipation	Parasites	Peptic ulcers
Colitis	Worms	Gastritis
Hemorrhoids	Uterine fibroid tumors	Pancreatitis
Diverticulitis	Cancer	Mental illness
Cirrhosis	Cataracts	Multiple sclerosis
Hepatitis	Colds	Alzheimer's disease
Fibrocystic breast disease	Bronchitis	Senility
Artherosclerosis	Pneumonia	Parkinson's disease
Heart disease	Sinusitis	Drug addiction
Hypertension	Emphysema	Tension headaches
	Kidney stones	Migraine headaches
		Gallstones

short- and long-term congestive patterns. People with addictions to any substance may benefit from a detox program, even if it is only the temporary avoidance of the addictive agent or agents. Withdrawal symptoms that commonly occur with many drugs, including sugar, caffeine, and over-the-counter medications, are precipitated by detoxification. Many of the poisons (toxins) that we ingest or make are stored in the fatty tissues. Obesity is almost always associated with toxicity. When we lose weight, we reduce our fat and thereby our toxic load. However, during weight loss we release more toxins, and thus need protection through greater intake of water, fiber, and the antioxidant nutrients, such as vitamins C, E, and beta-carotene, selenium, and zinc. With exercise we can also turn fat into muscle (not literally) and help further detoxification.

Of course, not all of these problems are solely problems of toxicity or completely cured by detoxification. Most of these diseases, and the majority of those factors, have to do with abuses, especially on a nutritional level. Often, these problems are alleviated by eliminating the related toxins and following a detox program.

When Is the Best Time to Cleanse/Detoxify?

We need to incorporate nature's cycles with our own cycles. We may notice regular periods of congestion, and we may reduce or prevent these by following a more detoxifying program. Whenever we feel congested, our first step is to follow detox procedures, many of which we can fine-tune in time with our experience of what works for us.

Each of us has a natural cleansing time when our body wants a lighter diet, more liquids, and greater elimination than intake. This occurs daily, usually in the night until midmorning; it may occur weekly buy more commonly for a few days a month. Women, in particular, are aware of this natural cleansing time with their female cycle. In fact, many women do much better premenstrually and during their periods of the follow a cleansing program—more juices, greens lighter foods, herbs, and so on—in the week before their menstruation.

The seasonal cycle is really the most important in regard to natural detoxification periods. If we can harmonize with these, we can do much to stay healthy.

To summarize here, the seasonal changes are the key stress times in nature and the times where we most need to lighten up our outer demands and consumptions and turn more within to listen to our inner world that mirrors the natural cycles. Spring is the key time for detoxification; autumn is also important.

The sample yearly program following is designed for a basically healthy person who eats well. It would not be appropriate for those with deficiency problems such extreme fatigue, underweight people, those who experience coldness, or those with heart weakness. There are even more contraindications for fasting, which releases more toxins than this program does. Releasing too much toxicity can make many sick people sicker; if that happens, they will need to increase fluids and eat again until they feel better. People with cancer need to be very careful about how they detoxify. Prior to or just after surgery is not a good time to detoxify. Pregnant or lactating women should not do any heavy detoxification, though they can usually handle mild programs.

Sample Year-Long Detox Program

Spring

For 7-21 days between March 10 and April 15, use one or more of the following plans:

- Fruits, vegetables, greens
- Juices of fruits, vegetables, and greens
- Herbs with any of the above
- These plans can be alternated and even include a 3-5 day supervised water fast
- Remember to take time (about half as long as the fast) for the transition back to the regular diet
- Elimination and food testing can be done at this time

Mid-Spring

- 3-day cleanse at new moon time in May as a reminder and enhancer of food awareness.

Summer

- One week of fruits and vegetables and/or fresh juices to usher in the warm weather some time between June 10 and July 4.

Late Summer

- 3-day cleanse of fruit and vegetable juices around the new moon time in August.

Autumn

7-10 day cleanse between September 11 and October 5 such as:

- Grape fast—whole and juiced—grapes, all fresh
- Apple and lemon juice together, diluted
- Fresh fruits and vegetables, raw and cooked
- Fruit and vegetable juices—fruit in the morning, vegetables in the afternoon
- Juices plus spirulina, algae, or other green chlorophyll powders
- Whole grains, cooked squashes and other vegetables (a lighter detox)
- Mixture of the above plans
- Basic low-toxicity diet with herbal programs
- Colon detox with fiber (psyllium, pectin, and so on) along with enemas or colonics
- Preparing and planning new autumn diet, enhancing positive dietary habits

Mid-Autumn

- 3-day cleanse on juices or in-season produce around new moon in late October/early November.

Winter

A lighter diet in preparation for the holidays (can be done between December 10 and January 5):

- Avoidance of toxins and treats, with a very basic wholesome diet
- One week of brown rice, cooked vegetables, miso broth, and seaweed. Ginger and cayenne pepper can be used in soups
- Saunas or steams and massage—you deserve it.
- Hang on until spring!

Where Can We Detoxify?

During basic, simple detox plans, most of us can maintain our normal life functions. In fact, energy, performance, and health often improve. For some though, detox may produce symptoms such as headaches, fatigue, irritability, mucous congestions, or aches and pains.

For many, especially those new to detoxification or inexperienced, it is wise to begin any special programs, diet, or lifestyle changes with a few days at home. In time, experienced will show what is best. Most can maintain a regular work schedule during a cleanse or detox program, but it may be easier to begin a program on a Friday, as the first few days are usually the hardest. This is because some people may be more sensitive during cleansing to their work environment or to chemical exposures, for example. Also, certain individuals may be faced with temptations or the influence of other workers or family members challenging their decisions, and for this, knowing and trusting what they are doing and having the support of a professional or group will add to their comfort and willpower.

At the end of the first day, at around dinnertime, symptoms may begin to appear, with headache and fatigue the most common, and it is good to be able to rest and spend time in familiar surroundings without a lot of outer demands. By the third day, people usually feel pretty stable and ready for work life. However, many people like to start new programs on Monday and just know that they will do fine, using willpower and visualization to see it through. People often feel better than ever and are able to accomplish tasks and meet challenges more easily than usual. Preparation and projection, clearing doubts and fears, and keeping a daily journal are all useful during this vital process and are crucial to any successful undertaking.

Why Detoxify?

We detoxify/cleanse for many reasons, mainly to do with health, vitality, and rejuvenation—to clear symptoms, treat disease, and prevent further problems. A cleansing program is ideal for helping us to reevaluate our lives, to make changes, or to clear abuses or addictions. It takes us through our withdrawal and reduces cravings fairly rapidly, and if we are ready, we can begin a new life without the addictive habits or drugs.

Many people detox/cleanse—or, more commonly, fast on water or juices—for spiritual renewal and to feel more alive, awake, and aware. Christ, Paramahansa Yoganada, and many other religious figures and teachers have advocated fasting for health and for spiritual attunement. It really does help move our energies from our lower centers of digestion and elimination up into our heart, mind, and consciousness centers.

Detoxification can be helpful for weight loss, though it is not a primary reduction plan; I think it is more important as a transition. However, anyone eating 4,000 calories a day of a fatty, sweet, and poorly balanced diet who begins to eat 2,000-2,500 calories of more wholesome foods will definitely experience detoxification, weight loss, and improved health.

We also cleanse/detoxify to rest our overloaded organs of digestion and our liver, gallbladder, and kidneys and allow them to catch up on past work. Most often our energy is increased and more steady. There are many reasons why we may want to cleanse.

Table 31.5. Reasons for Cleansing

Prevent disease	To be more:
Reduce symptoms	Organized
Treat disease	Creative
Cleanse body	Motivated
Rest organs	Productive
Purification	Relaxed
Rejuvenation	Energetic
Weight loss	Clear
Clear skin	Conscious
Slow aging	Inwardly attuned
Improve flexibility	Spiritual
Improve fertility	Environmentally attuned
Enhance the senses	Relationship focused

How Do We Detoxify/Cleanse?

Ways to detoxify have been discussed; the remainder is a discussion of general and specific diet plans, other activities, and supplements, including vitamins, minerals, amino acids, and herbs, to aid us in this healing process.

There are many levels to this part of the program. The first is to eat a nontoxic diet. If we do this regularly, we have less need for cleansing. If we have not been eating this way, we should detoxify first and then make permanent changes.

Another aspect of the nontoxic diet is avoiding drugs—over-the-counter, prescription, and recreational types—and substituting natural remedies, such as nutrients, herbs, and homeopathic medicines, all of which have fewer side effects. Other natural therapies, such as acupuncture, massage, and chiropractic may help in treating some problems so that we will not need drugs for them. Avoiding or minimizing exposure to chemicals as home and work is also important. This lessens our total toxic load. Substituting natural cleansers, cosmetics, and clothes is helpful.

The effects of the detoxification diet may vary. Even mild changes from our current plan may produce some responses, while more dramatic dietary shifts will produce a profound cleansing. Shifting from the most congesting foods to the least—eating more fruits, vegetables, grains, nuts and legumes and less baked goods, sweets, refined foods, fried foods and fatty foods—will help most of us detoxify somewhat and bring us into better balance, with more vitalized cells, organs, and body.

Maintaining the same diet but adding certain supplements can also stimulate detoxification. Fiber, vitamin C, other antioxidants, chlorophyll, and glutathione, mainly as amino acid L-cysteine, will all help. Herbs such as garlic, red clover, Echinacea, or cayenne may also induce some detoxification. Saunas, sweats, and niacin therapy have been used to cleanse the body. Simply increasing liquids and decreasing fats will shift the balance strongly toward improved elimination and less toxin buildup. Increased consumption of filtered water, herb

Table 31.6. The Nontoxic Diet

- Eat organic food whenever possible
- Drink filtered water
- Rotate foods, especially common allergens, such as milk products, eggs, wheat, and yeast foods
- Practice food combining
- Eat a natural, seasonal cuisine
- Include fruits, vegetables, whole grains, legumes, nuts and seeds, and, for omnivarians, some low-fat dairy products, and fresh fish (not shellfish) and organic poultry
- Cook in iron, stainless steel, glass, or porcelain
- Avoid or minimize red meats, cured meats, organ meats, refined foods, canned foods, sugar, salt, saturated fats, coffee, alcohol, and nicotine

teas, fruits, and vegetables and reducing fats, especially most fried food, red meats, and milk products will also help detoxification. This is a more structured, basic diet, but for most average Westerners, it will be a major shift to a cleaner diet. A vegetarian diet would also be a healthful step toward detoxification for those with some congestive problems. In general, moving from an acid-generating diet to a more alkaline one will aid the process of detoxification. Acid-forming foods, such as meats, milk products, breads and baked goods, and especially the refined sugar and carbohydrate products, will increase body acidity and lead to more mucus production and congestion to attempt to balance the body chemistry, whereas the more alkaline, wholesome vegetarian foods enhance cleansing and clarity in the body. The right balance of acid and alkaline foods for each of us is, of course, the key.

A deeper level of the detox diet is one made up exclusively of fresh fruits, fresh vegetables, either raw and cooked, and whole grains, both cooked and sprouted; however, no breads or baked goods, animal foods and dairy products, alcohol, or nuts are used. This diet keeps fiber and water intake up and helps colon detoxification. Most people can handle this well and make the shift from their regular diet with a few days transition. Some people do well on a brown rice fast (a more macrobiotic plan), usually for a week or two, eating three to four bowls of rice daily along with liquids such as teas.

The next level of detoxification involves a diet consisting solely of fruits and vegetables, all cleansing foods. The green vegetables, especially the chlorophyllic and high-nutrient leafy greens, are very cleansing and supportive for purification of the gastrointestinal tract and the whole body. Ann Wigmore and her staff at the Hippocrates, or Optimum, Health Institute guides people in wheatgrass and sprout cleansing program that is a wonderfully rejuvenating experience for many.

A raw foods diet is fulfilling for many people, very high in energy and nutrition. It contains lots of sprouted greens from seeds and grains such as wheat, buckwheat, sunflower, alfalfa, and clover; sprouted beans; soaked or sprouted raw nuts; and fresh fruits and vegetables. Cooking food is not allowed with this diet; eating foods raw maintains the highest concentrations of vitamins, minerals and important enzymes, and allows them to find their way into our body and cells. Many people feel that this is the best of diets; it can be health supportive over quite some time if it is balanced properly.

Other specialized detox diets include macrobiotics and diets that treat certain problems, such as yeast overgrowth or allergies. Treating these problems properly allows the body to reduce its irritating reactions and to heal.

Beyond the fruit and vegetable diet are the liquid cleanses or fasts. Juices, vegetable broths, and teas can be used to purify our body and life. Miso, a paste of fermented soybean, can be used during fasting. It provides many nutrients and supports colon function and the intestinal bacteria, which help detoxification. Spirulina, an algae powder, can also be helpful to many fasters when added to juices. It provides protein to meet body needs and may aid those who experience some fatigue with fasting. Consuming fresh, diluted juices from various fruits and vegetables is safe and helpful for many conditions. Fasting experts believe that it actually works better than a straight water fast, as it helps to eliminate wastes and old or dead cells while restoring and building new tissue with the easily accessible nutrients from the juices. Water fasting is more intense, often resulting in more sickness and less energy, than fasting with juices. Paavo Airola, one of the pioneers of fasting in America, states in *How to Get Well* and other books, that "systematic undereating and periodic fasting are the two most important health and longevity factors." Dr. Airola lists fruits and vegetable juices that cleanse and help in the healing of specific organs.

A key to proper treatment at the proper time is to work with detoxification individually. It does take a sensitive person or a sensitive practitioner to find the right path. Detoxification experiences can range from subtle to intense. We have to look at a person's general health, physiological balance, energy level, and current life activities in order to set up the right program. There are a lot of possibilities. If unsure, start with your basic diet and move along the changes toward juice fasting and see how you feel. Take a couple of days for each step, and, if you feel fine, move to the next level, as described.

Table 31.7. Levels of Dietary Detoxification

- Basic Diet
- Eliminate toxins daily from more congesting to less; for example, drugs, sugar, fried foods, meats, dairy, etc. Take one to seven days.
- Fruits, vegetables, whole grains, nuts, seeds and legumes
- Raw foods
- Fruits and vegetables
- Fruit and vegetable juices
- Specific juices, Master Cleanser, apple, carrot-greens, etc.
- Water

Some Important Components of Detoxification

Colon cleansing is one of the most important parts of detoxification. Much toxicity comes out of the large intestine, and sluggish functioning of this organ can rapidly produce general toxicity. During a detox program, most people will work on some level with their colon. There are entire programs for colon detoxification available, such as Dr. Robert Gray's *Colon Cleansing* program, which includes a book and special supplements, found mainly in health food store. A series of colonic water irrigations, best performed by a trained professional can be the focal point of detox program, usually along with some cleansing diet and fiber supplements for toning and cleaning the colon. During a basic dietary detox program, other, more subtle colon stimuli are usually used to enhance colon action. These may include herbal or pharmaceutical laxatives, fiber and colon detox supplements, such as psyllium seed husks alone or mixed with other agents, for example, aloe vera powder, betonite clay, and acidophilus culture. Enemas using water, herbs, or even diluted coffee (stimulates liver cleansing) may also be used.

To improve elimination through the skin, regular exercise is important to stimulate sweating. Exercise also improves our general metabolism and helps overall with detoxification. Regular aerobic exercise is a key to maintaining a nontoxic body, especially when we are a little abusive of various substances. On the other hand, exercise increases the production of toxins in the body, so it must be accompanied by adequate fluids, antioxidants, vitamin and mineral replenishment, and other detoxifying principles already discussed.

Regular bathing is essential to cleanse the skin of the toxins it has released and to open the pores to eliminate more. Saunas and sweats are commonly used to help purify the body through enhanced skin elimination. Dry brushing the skin with an appropriate skin brush before bathing is usually suggested, especially during detox programs, to cleanse the skin of old cells and invigorate it. Massage therapy, especially lymphatic and even deeper massage, is very useful in supporting our detox program. It stimulates elimination and body functions and promotes relaxation. Clearing tensions, worries, and other mental messes also makes for a more complete detoxification.

Resting, relaxation, and recharging are important to this rejuvenation process. During detox, we may need more rest, quiet time, and sleep, although more commonly we have more energy and function better on less sleep. Relaxation exercises help our body rebalance as our mind and attitudes stop interfering with our natural homeostasis.

Practicing yoga combines quiet, yet powerful exercises with breathing awareness and regulation, allowing increased flexibility and relaxation. It may be appropriate for many to help balance more active and/or more contractive exercise programs, especially during detox and transition times.

Certain supplements may be used during most of these detoxification programs. Potassium, extra fiber with olive oil to clear toxins from the colon, sodium alginate from seaweeds to bind heavy metals, and apple cider vinegar in water (1 tablespoon of vinegar in 8 ounces hot water) to help reduce mucus are among these. With weight loss, toxins stored in the fat will need to be mobilized and cleared. More water, fiber, and antioxidants can help handle this.

The supplement program used for general detoxification is outlined in Table 31.11 at the end of this section. It includes a low-dosage multiple vitamin/mineral to fulfill the basic requirements during the transitional diet. The B vitamins, particularly niacin, are important, as are minerals such as zinc, calcium, magnesium, and potassium. The antioxidant nutrients are also important. These include basic levels of beta-carotene, vitamin a and zinc, and vitamin E and selenium, with special focus on vitamin C, probably our main detox vitamin. Some authorities believe that higher amounts of vitamin A (50,000 IUs), vitamin C (8-12 grams), and vitamin E (1,000-1,200 IUs) are helpful in detoxification.

The liver is our most important detox organ because of its many metabolic functions. Certain authorities suggest liver-supportive nutrients and even a liver glandular during general detoxification. The liver needs water and glycogen (glucose storage) as glucuronic acid for many of its detoxification functions. A higher starch or carbohydrate diet with lower levels of protein and fats is helpful. The B vitamins, especially B3 and B6, vitamins A and C, zinc, calcium, vitamin E and selenium, and L-cysteine are all also needed to support liver detoxification.

Several amino acids are helpful in detoxification, particularly the sulfer-containing ones, cysteine and methionine. L-cysteine supplies sulfhydryl groups which help to prevent oxidation and to bind heavy metals, especially mercury (vitamin C and selenium also help with this). Cysteine is the precursor of glutathione, our most important detoxifier, and thus helps to counter many chemicals and carcinogens. Glutathione is part of detoxification enzymes, specifically glutathione peroxidase and reductase, which work to prevent peroxidation of lipids and to decrease many toxins, such as smoke, radiation, auto exhaust, chemicals and drugs, and many other carcinogens.

Glycine is a secondary helper. An amino acid that supports glutathione synthesis, it also decreases the toxicity of substances such as phenols or benzoic acid, the latter used as a food preservative. Other amino acids that may have mild detoxifying effects include methionine, tyrosine, and taurine. For more information on amino acid metabolism and uses, I suggest a book by Eric R. Braverman and the late Dr. Carl C. Pfeiffer entitled *The Healing Nutrients Within: Facts, Findings and New Research on Amino Acids.*

As mentioned earlier, another detoxification supporter is fiber, as psyllium seed husks, often combined with other detox nutrients, such as pectin, aloe vera, alginates, and/or colon herbs. This helps cleanse mucus along the small intestine, create bulk in the colon, and pull toxins from the gastrointestinal tract. When fiber is combined with one or two tablespoons of olive oil to help detoxify. Acidophilus bacteria in the colon help neutralize some toxin, reduce the metabolism of other microbes, and lessen colon toxicity. Supplemental acidophilus is often added to a detox program.

Remember, water should always be used during any type of detox program to help dilute and eliminate toxin accumulations. It is likely the most important detoxifyer. It helps clean us through our skin and kidneys, and it improves our sweating with exercise. Eight to ten glasses a day (depending on our size and activity level) of clean, filtered water are suggested.

A special elimination process has been developed and used in some clinics to help in the detoxification of chemicals, especially pesticides and even pharmaceutical drugs. This program usually involves several weeks at a center with a therapy including a high-fluid and juice diet, exercise, and large amounts of niacin (vitamin B3) with sauna therapies. The saunas are extended and may last for several hours daily, with breaks to drink fluids. The idea is to cleanse the hidden chemicals from the fat through juice cleansing, weight loss, niacin therapy, exercise, and sweats. Niacin is a vasostimulator and vasodilator, aiding circulation.

This "niacin-sauna" program is interesting and definitely has possibilities as an intense, medically supervised detoxification process. However, it is still experimental and does entail risks. Preliminary results are good, especially for people with symptoms caused by exposure to pesticides, such as Agent Orange, yet there are some drawbacks. Besides the cost and time required, the extreme detox can cause losses of nutrients, especially minerals, creating depletions from which it could take months to recover. Special attention must be given to ensuring proper nutrient restoration during and after this therapy. This program, even short versions of it, can be used to help detoxify from most drugs, especially the recreational types, and daily abuses of alcohol and nicotine. Many of us can do a modified version on our own with the use of a sauna, a few days' juice fast, regular exercise, and supplemental niacin, beginning at 100-200 mg and moving up to 2-3 grams daily. Be sure to replenish fluids and minerals. If there are medical problems, weakness, or fatigue, I would not suggest doing this without the advice and supervision of a physician.

Many herbs can support or even create detoxification. In fact, this area is really the strength, of herbal medicine. There are hundreds of possible herbs to be used for blood cleansing and cleaning the tissues or strengthening the function of specific organs. The old term for blood cleansers is "alteratives," which is the term used in many standard herbal texts. Table 31.8 includes some of the more important ones.

Table 31.8. Cleansing Herbs

Garlic—blood cleanser, lowers blood fats, natural antibiotic

Red clover blossoms—blood cleanser, good during convalescence and healing

Echinacea—lymph cleanser, improves lymphocyte and phagocyte actions

Dandelion root—liver and blood cleanser, diuretic, filters toxins, a tonic

Chaparral—strong blood cleanser, with possibilities for use in cancer therapy

Cayenne pepper—blood purifier, increases fluid elimination and sweat

Ginger root—stimulates circulation and sweating

Licorice root—"great detoxifier," biochemical balancer, mild laxative

Yellow dock root—skin, blood, and liver cleanser, contains vitamin C and iron

Burdock root—skin and blood cleanser, diuretic and diaphoretic, improves liver function, antibacterial and antifungal properties

Sarsaparilla root—blood and lymph cleanser, contains saponins, which reduce microbes and toxins

Prickly ash bark—good for nerves and joints, anti-infectious

Oregon grape root—skin and colon cleanser, blood purifier, liver stimulant

Parsley leaf—diuretic, flushes kidneys

Goldenseal root—blood, liver, kidney, and skin cleanser, stimulates detoxification

Table 31.9. A General Classification of Herbs Useful in Detoxification*

Blood Cleansers
Echinacea
Red clover
Dandelion
Burdock
Yellow dock
Oregon grape root

Laxatives
Cascara sagrada
Buckthorn
Dandelion
Yellow dock
Rhubarb root
Senna leaf
Licorice

Diuretics
Parsley
Yarrow
Cleavers
Horsetail
Corn silk
Uva ursi
Juniper berries

Skin Cleansers—Diaphoretics
Burdock
Oregon grape
Yellow dock
Goldenseal
Boneset
Elder flowers
Peppermint
Cayenne pepper
Ginger root

Antibiotics
Garlic
Myrrh
Prickly ash
Wormwood
Echinacea
Propolis
Clove
Eucalyptus

Anticatarrhals**
Echinacea
Boneset
Goldenseal
Sage
Hyssop
Garlic
Yarrow

* Not usually for fasting or juice cleansing, but mainly for dietary detoxification—using herbs alone may be the most productive in some detoxification programs. Consult a naturopathically oriented doctor.

** anticatarrhals help eliminate mucus

Table 31.10. Sample Detox Formula

Echinacea
Goldenseal root
Yellow dock root
Cayenne pepper
Garlic
Parsley leaf
Licorice root

Obtain powders (or ground herb), equal amounts of all of these herbs except half the cayenne, and put this mixture into 00 capsules. Take two capsules two or three times daily between meals.

General Detoxification Nutrient Program

Table 31.11 is a list of supplements tying together many aspects of the detoxification process. The specific supplements to be used should take into account individual circumstances. The program can be carried out for varying lengths of time, from one week to one or two months. Remember to work on all the levels of detoxification and listen within for your true healing information.

The Detox Diet Daily Menu Plan

Upon Rising

Two glasses of water (filtered or spring), one glass with half a lemon squeezed into it.

Breakfast

One piece of fresh fruit (at room temperature), such as an apple, pear, banana, a citrus fruit, or some grapes. Chew well, mixing each bite with saliva.

Fifteen to thirty minutes later: One bowl of cooked whole grains—specifically millet, brown rice, amaranth, quinoa, or buckwheat.

For flavoring, use two tablespoons of fruit juice for sweetness, or use the Better Butter, made by mixing a quarter cup of cold-pressed canola oil into a soft (room temperature) quarter-pound of butter; then place in dish and refrigerate. Use about one teaspoon per meal or maximum of 3 teaspoons daily.

Table 31.11. General Detoxification Nutrient Program

Water	2 ½-3 qt.		
Fiber	20-40 g.		
Vitamin A	5,000 IUs	Calcium	600-850 mg.
Beta-carotene	15,000 IUs	Chromium	200 mcg.
Vitamin D	200 IUs	Copper	2 mg.
Vitamin E	400-800 IUs	Iodine	150 mcg.
Vitamin K	200 mcg.	Iron	10-18 mg.
Thiamine (B1)	10-25 mg.	Magnesium	300-500 mg.
Riboflavin (B2)	10-25 mg.	Manganese	5-10 mg.
Niacinamide (B3)	50 mg.	Molybdenum	300 mcg.
Niacin (B3)	50-2,000 mg.*	Potassium	300-500 mg.
Pantothenic acid (B5)	250 mg.	Selenium	300 mcg.
Pyridoxine (B6)	10-25 mg.	Silicon	100mg.
Cobalamin (B12)	50-100 mcg.	Vanadium	300 mcg.
Folic acid	400-800 mcg.	Zinc	30 mg.
Biotin	200 mcg.		
Vitamin C	1-4 g.		
Bioflavonoids	250-500 mg.		

Optional:

L-amino acids	500-1,000 mg.
L-cysteine	250-500 mg.
DL-methionine	250-500 mg.
L-glycine	250-500 mg.
Psyllium seed	4-8 g.
Flaxseed oil	1-2 teaspoons
Olive oil	3-6 teaspoons
Liquid chlorophyll	2-4 teaspoons
Apple cider vinegar	1-2 tablespoons
Acidophilus culture	1-2 billion organisms
Detox formula herbs:	4-6 capsules

    Echinacea, yellow dock,
    goldenseal, garlic, parsley,
    licorice, cayenne pepper

*May be used for special detox programs.

Lunch

(Noon-1 PM) One to two medium bowls of steamed vegetables; use a variety, including roots, stems, and greens. For example, potatoes or yams, green beans, broccoli or cauliflower, carrots or beets, asparagus, kale, chard, and cabbage. Be sure to chew well.

Dinner

(5-6 PM) Same as lunch.

Special Drinks

(11 AM and 3 PM) One to two cups veggie water, saved from the steamed vegetables. Add a little sea salt or kelp and drink slowly, mixing each mouthful with saliva.

Before Retiring

Consume no additional foods after dinner. Drink only water and herbal teas, such as peppermint, chamomile, pau d'arco, or blends.

About Dr. Haas

Dr. Elson M. Haas is a practicing physician of Integrated Medicine for over 25 years. He is the Founder and Medical Director of the Preventive Medical Center of Marin in San Rafael. Dr, Haas is also the author of the classic preventive medicine text *Staying Healthy With the Seasons* (1981, now in its 26th printing and 21st anniversary with a revised 2002 edition) and *Staying Healthy With Nutrition* (1992). Other books by Celestial Arts in Berkeley, CA, include his diet and recipe book, *A Cookbook For All Seasons* (2000), *The Detox Diet*: (1997), and *The Staying Healthy Shopper's Guide: Feed Your Family Safely* (1999). Further recent books are *Vitamins for Dummies* and *The False Fat Diet* (2000, Ballantine Books). Dr. Haas speaks nationally, is on radio and TV shows, and appears in many national magazine articles.

See http://www.elsonhaas.com for more information on a wide variety of health topics.

Chapter 32

Fasting

Fasting is the single greatest natural healing therapy. It is nature's ancient, universal "remedy" for many problems. Animals instinctively fast when ill. When I first discovered fasting, 15 years ago, I felt as if it had saved my life and transformed my illnesses into health. My stagnant energies began flowing, and I became more creative and vitally alive. I still find fasting both a useful personal tool and an important therapy for many medical and life problems.

Of course, most of the problems for which I recommend fasting as treatment are ones that result from overnutrition rather than malnutrition. Dietary abuse problems, more common in the Western world than in Third World countries, generate many chronic degenerative diseases; these include atherosclerosis, hypertension and heart disease, allergies, diabetes, and cancer. Fasting is therapeutic and, more importantly, preventive for many of these conditions and more.

Fasting, as used here, is the avoidance of solid food and the intake of liquids only (true fasting would be the total avoidance of anything by mouth). The most stringent form of fasting is taking only water; more liberally, fasting includes the use of fresh juices made from fruits and vegetables as well as herbal teas. All of these limited diets generate varying degrees of detoxification—that is, elimination of toxins from the body. Individual experiences with fasting depend on the

From *Staying Healthy with Nutrition,* © 1992 by Elson M. Haas, M.D. Reprinted with permission of the author and Celestial Arts, Berkeley, CA. Text reviewed by author January 2002. Complete information about Dr. Elson Haas in included at the end of this chapter.

condition of the body (also mind and attitude). Detoxification might be intense and temporarily increase sickness or might be immediately helpful and uplifting.

Juice fasting is commonly used (rather than water alone) as a mild and effective cleansing plan; this is suggested by myself and other doctors and authors and by many of the European fasting clinics. Fresh juices are easily assimilated and require minimum digestion, while they supply many nutrients and stimulate our body to clear its wastes. Juice fasting is also safer than water fasting, because it supports the body nutritionally while cleansing and probably even produces a better detoxification and quicker recovery.

Fasting (cleansing, detoxification) is one part of the triology of nutrition; balancing and building (toning) are the others. I believe that fasting is the "missing link" in the Western diet. Most people overeat, eat too often, and eat a high-protein, high-fat, rich-food, building and congesting diet more consistently than they need. If we regularly eat a more balanced and well-combined diet, we will have less need for fasting and toning plans, although both would still be required at certain intervals throughout the year.

In a sense, detoxification is an important corrective and rejuvenative process in our cycle of nutrition. It is a time when we allow our cells and organs to breathe out, become current, and restore themselves. We do not necessarily need to fast to experience some cleansing, however. Minor shifts in the diet such as including more fluids, more raw foods, and fewer congesting foods will allow for better detoxification; for a carnivore, for example, a vegetarian or macrobiotic diet will be cleansing and purifying. The general process of detoxification is discussed in Chapter 31; here we focus on fluid fasting—its history, therapeutic use, benefits, contraindications, and, of course, how to do it, along with other aspects of lifestyle that support fasting.

Fasting is a time-proven remedy. Its use goes back many thousands of years, really to the beginning of life forms. As a healing process and spiritual/religious process, it has continued to be more intelligently applied, we hope, in the last several thousand years.

Voluntary abstinence from food has been a tradition in most religions and is clearly a spiritual purification rite. Many religions, including Christianity, Judaism, and the Eastern religions, have encouraged fasting for a variety of reasons, such as penitence, preparation for ceremony, purification, mourning, sacrifice and union with God, and the enhancement of knowledge and powers. From Moses, Elijah, and Daniel to Christ, the Bible is filled with fasters, who employed it to assist their purification and communion with God. Fasts as long as 40 days were employed to cleanse people of sins and the "devil."

The Essenes, authors of the Dead Sea Scrolls, also advocated fasting to purify themselves and commune with God. This was one of their primary healing methods. *The Essene Gospel of Peace*, transcribed by Edmond Bordeaux Szekely from the third-century Aramaic manuscript, suggests that Satan, his evil spirits, and his plagues will be cast out of our being by fasting and prayer. The Essenes believed that disease came from Satan (they claimed that it took three days without food to starve Satan) and from sins upon our body—the temple, which must be purified for God to reside there. To bring God into our life more completely, we would fast on water and "go to the waters (stream, lake) and find a hollow reed, insert it in our rear ends and flush the evils from our bowels."

For many philosophers, scientists, and physicians, fasting was an essential part of life, health, and the healing process needed to recreate health where there was sickness. Socrates, Plato, Aristotle, Galen, Paracelsus, and Hippocrates all used and believed in fasting therapy. Most spiritual teachers also recommend fasting as a useful tool. In a booklet from the 1947 lecture entitled "Healing by God's Unlimited Power," Paramahansa Yogananda suggested that fasting is a way to increase our natural resistance to disease, stating that "Fasting is a natural method of healing. When animals or savages are sick, they fast." He continued, "Most diseases can be cured by judicious fasting. Unless one has a weak heart, regular short fasts have been recommended by the yogis as an excellent health measure." Yogananda referred to an Armenian doctor, Grant Sarkisyan, who had treated many patients successfully with fasting therapy for such disorders as asthma, skin diseases, digestive problems, and early stages of atherosclerosis and hypertension.

Throughout the centuries, many doctors have treated a variety of patients and maladies with fasting, acknowledging that ignorance (of how to live in accordance with nature) may be our greatest disease. Knowledge, not necessarily from books, but our inherent and experienced knowing of how to live according to the natural laws and spiritual truth, leads to the sacred wisdom of life and subsequent good health. Knowing when and how long to fast is part of this knowledge. Through fasting, we can turn our energies inward, where we can use them for healing, clarity, and change.

Physicians with a spiritual orientation tend to be more inclined than others to employ fasting, both personally and medically. Many of my life transitions were acknowledged, stimulated, and supported through fasting. In *Spiritual Nutrition and the Rainbow Diet*, Gabriel Cousens, M.D., a California physician and spiritual teacher, includes an excellent chapter on fasting in which he describes his concepts of fasting and his own 40-day fast. According to Dr. Cousens, . . . fasting in a larger context, means to abstain from that which is toxic to mind, body, and soul. A way to understand this is that fasting is the elimination of physical, emotional, and mental toxins from our organism, rather than simply cutting down on or stopping food intake. Fasting for spiritual purposes usually involves some degree of removal of oneself from worldly responsibilities. It can mean complete silence and social isolation during the fast, which can be a great revival to those of us who have been putting our energy outward.

From a medical point of view, I believe that fasting is not utilized often enough. We go on vacations from work to relax, recharge, and to gain new perspectives on our life; why not take occasional breaks from food? Or, for that matter, we might consider fasts from phones, cars, computers, talking, or from whatever activity/consumption we feel is excessive. Most people cannot break out of the conditioned pattern of eating three meals daily. Eating is a habit, an addiction. Most of us do not need nearly the amounts (and types) of food we consume. I have discussed allergy-addiction; in a sense, eating itself is an allergy-addiction. When we stop and let our stomach remain empty, our body goes into an elimination cycle, and most people, especially when toxicity exists, will experience some "withdrawal" symptoms, such as headaches, irritability, or fatigue (only pure hunger is a clear sign of need for food). When they eat again, their withdrawal symptoms subside, and they feel better. This situation is worse when it involves allergic people eating allergenic foods.

I believe that fasting is one of the best overall healing methods because it can be applied to so many conditions and people. Those who are acid, sympathetic, or yang types, who tend to develop congestive symptoms and diseases rather than those of deficiency, do better on fasting than do other types. Some acid conditions, including colds, flus, bronchitis, mucus congestion, and constipation, can lead to headaches, other intestinal problems, skin conditions, and many other ailments. Those who follow a basic, wholesome, and balanced diet have less need to fast or detoxify, although on occasion it is a good idea for anyone, provided that they are not undernourished. Most of us living in Western, industrialized nations are mixed types, with both overnutrition and undernutrition. We may take in excessive amounts of potentially toxic nutrients, such as fats and chemicals, and inadequate amounts of many essential vitamins and minerals. Juice fasting supplies some of these needed nutrients and allows the elimination of toxins. Excess mucus and clogging of the eliminative systems constitute the basic process of congestive diseases; deficiency problems result from poor nourishment or ineffective digestion/assimilation.

A number of symptoms and diseases of toxicity can be alleviated by detoxification. Juice fasting is mentioned as part of the treatment plan as well. It can be used to detoxify from drugs or whenever we want to embark on a new plan or life transition, provided that there are no contraindications to fasting (discussed later in this chapter). Fasting is very versatile and generally fairly safe; however, when it is used in the treatment of medical conditions, proper supervision should be employed, including monitoring of physical changes and biochemistry values. Many doctors, clinics, acupuncturists, nutritionists, and chiropractors feel comfortable overseeing people during fasting.

The use of fasting to treat fevers is controversial. Eastern medicine thinks of fasting as increasing body fire, so that it might worsen fever. In actuality, when we consume liquids, we generate less heat, so this really helps to cool the body. With fever, we need more liquids than usual; with high temperatures and sweating, we need even more.

Some cases fatigue will respond well to fasting, particularly when the fatigue results from congested organs and energy. With fatigue that results from chronic infection, nutritional deficiency, or serious disease, more nourishment is probably needed, rather than fasting.

Back pains that are due to muscular tightness and stress rather than from bone disease or osteoporosis are usually alleviated with a lighter diet or juice fasting. Many tight muscles and sore areas along the back may result from referred pain from colon or other organ congestion. In my experience, poor bowel function and constipation are fairly commonly associated with back pains.

Table 32.1. Conditions for which Fasting May Be Beneficial

colds	constipation	environmental allergies
atherosclerosis	diabetes	mental illness
flus	indigestion	asthma
coronary artery disease	fever	obesity
bronchitis	diarrhea	insomnia
angina pectoris	fatigue	cancer
headaches	food allergies	skin conditions
hypertension	back pains	epilepsy

Many patients with mental illness, from anxiety to schizophrenia, may be helped by fasting. The purpose of fasting in this case, however, is not to cure these problems but to help understand the relationship of foods, chemicals, or drugs to the mental difficulties. Allergies and hypersensitive environmental reactions are not at all uncommon in people with mental illness. Care must be exercised with the use of fasting in mental patients as the toxicity or lack of nourishment may worsen their problems. If, however, the patient is strong and congested, fasting may be indicated.

Obesity can be remedied by fasting. Obesity is the problem for which fasting is currently most often used (mainly protein drinks) in the traditional medical system, although it is not the best use of this healing technique. Fasting is not even a good treatment for those who are overweight; it is too temporary and may generate feasting reactions in people coming off the fast. Better would be a change of diet and a longer-term weight-release plan; something that will allow new dietary habits and food choices to replace the old ones. A short fast, perhaps of five to ten days, can be useful as a motivator and catalyst for making these necessary dietary changes and new commitments and to help release a pound or two daily.

Some very obese patients have been monitored by doctors while on water fasts done in hospitals for months at a time to shed weights of a hundred pounds or more. With other patients, the jaws have been wired shut so that they can take in only fluids drunk through straws. Newer fasting programs substitute a variety of protein-rich powders for meals. These are usually medically supervised programs for people who are at least 30-50 pounds overweight and make use of a prepackaged, low-calorie powder, such as Optifast or Medifast. This high-protein, low-calorie diet allows patients to burn more fat. These programs are not nearly as healthful as vital juice fasts, but they are nutritionally supportive over a longer time period and can be used on an outpatient basis fairly safely if people are monitored regularly. They provide all the needed vitamins, minerals, and amino acids to sustain life and help many obese people to lower their weight, blood fats, blood pressures, and blood sugars. However, as with any weight-loss program, if it does not motivate the participants to change their diets and habits, they then may stay in the "yo-yo" syndrome (weight going up and down and up), which may actually be more harmful than just remaining overweight.

A balanced, low-calorie diet with lots of exercise is still the best way to reduce and maintain a good weight and figure. Many obese people are also deficient in nutrients because they eat a highly refined, fatty, sweet diet. Often, these obese people are fatigued, and they need to be nourished first before they will do well on any fast.

Fasting to treat cancer is also a controversial topic. Many alternative clinics outside the United States use fasting in the treatment of cancers. Since cancer can be a devitalizing, debilitating disease, this may not be wise. Possibly with early cancer, and definitely as a cancer preventive to reduce toxicity, juice fasting may be helpful. Anyone with cancer needs adequate nourishment, and adding fresh juices to an already wholesome diet can help induce a mild detoxification and enhance vitality.

The Process and Benefits of Fasting

Although the process of fasting may generate various results, depending on the individual condition of the faster, there are clearly a number of common metabolic changes and experiences. First, fasting is a catalyst for change and an essential part of transformational medicine. It promotes relaxation and energization of the body, mind and emotions, and supports a greater spiritual awareness. Many fasters feel a letting go of past actions and experiences and develop a positive attitude toward the present. Having energy to get things done and clean up old areas, both personal and environmental, without the usual procrastination is also a common experience. Fasting clearly improves motivation and creative energy; it also enhances health and vitality and lets many of the body systems rest.

In other words, fasting is a multidimensional experience. Physiologically, refraining from eating minimizes the work done by the digestive organs, including the stomach, intestines, pancreas, gallbladder, and liver. Most important here is that our liver, our body's large production and metabolic factory, can spend more time during fasting cleaning up and creating its many new substances for our use. Breakdown of stored or circulating chemicals is the basic process of detoxification. The blood and lymph also have the opportunity to be cleaned of toxins as all the eliminative functions are enhanced with fasting. Each cell has the opportunity to catch up on its work; with fewer new demands, it can repair itself and dump its waste for the garbage pickup. Most fasters also experience a new vibrancy of their skin and clarity of mind and body.

Initially, the reduction of calories allows the liver to convert glycogen stores to glucose and energy. Body fat can be used for energy (ATP) but it cannot generate or reform glucose; although many cells can metabolize fatty acids for energy, the brain and central nervous

313

system need direct glucose. Proteins can be broken down into amino acids; of these, alanine and serine can be used to produce glucose. With fasting, some protein breakdown occurs, less if calories are provided by juices. When there is no stored glycogen left, our body will convert protein to amino acids and to energy. Fatty acids can also be a fair source of energy, usually after being converted to ketones.

With total fasting, ketosis occurs as an adaptation by the body to prevent protein loss by burning fats. Still, protein and fats can be used to provide energy for brain cell function. With juice fasting, there is less ketosis, and the simple carbohydrates in the juices are easily used for energy and cellular function. The high-protein diets and fasts do burn fat and generate ketosis and weight loss, but they also add more toxin buildup in the body from the foods or powders used. Also, they do not rest and cleanse the digestive tract and other organs as well.

Fasting increases the process of elimination and the release of toxins from the colon, kidneys and bladder, lungs and sinuses, and skin. This process can generate discharge such as mucus from the gastrointestinal tract, respiratory tract, sinuses, or in the urine. This is helpful to clear out the problems that have arisen from overeating and a sedentary lifestyle. Much of aging and disease, I believe, results from "biochemical suffocation," where our cells do not get enough oxygen and nutrients or cannot adequately eliminate their wastes. Fasting helps us decrease this suffocation by allowing the cells to eliminate and clear the old products.

Table 32.2. Some Benefits of Fasting

Purification	Inspiration
More energy	Creativity
Rejuvenation	Reduction of allergies
Better sleep	New ideas
Revitalization	Weight loss
More relaxation	Clearer planning
Rest for digestive organs	Drug detoxification
Better attitude	Change of habits
Clearer skin	Better resistance to disease
More clarity, mentally and emotionally	Diet changes
Antiaging effects	Spiritual awareness
Improved senses—vision, hearing, taste	Right use of will

This physiological rest and concentration on cleanup can also generate a number of toxicity symptoms. Hunger is usually present for two or three days and then departs, leaving many people with a surprising feeling of deep abdominal peace; yet, others may feel really hungry. It is good to ask ourselves, "What are we hungry for?" Fasting is an excellent time to work on our psychological connections to consumption.

As far as fasting symptoms, headache is not at all uncommon during the first day or two. Fatigue or irritability may arise at times, as may dizziness or lightheadedness. Our sensitivity is usually increased. Common sounds like television, music, refrigerators may irritate us more now. The sense of smell is also exaggerated, both positively and negatively; I have had whole meals of smells while fasting. The tongues of most people will develop a thick white or yellow fur coating, which can be scraped or brushed off. Bad breath and displeasing tastes in the mouth or foul-smelling urine or stools may occur. Skin odor or skin eruptions such as small spots or painful boils, may also appear, depending on the state of toxicity. Digestive upset, mucusy stools, flatulence, or even nausea and vomiting may occur during fasting. Some people experience insomnia or bad dreams as their body releases poisons during the night. The mind may put up resistance, with doubt or lack of faith or a fear that the fasting is not right. (This can be influenced even more by listening to other people's fears.) Most of these symptoms, however, will occur early if they do appear and are usually transient. The general energy level is usually good during fasting, although there can be ups and downs. Every two or three days, as the body goes into a deeper level of dumping wastes, the energy may go down, and resistance and fears as well as symptoms may arise. Between these times, we usually feel cleaner, better, and more alive.

The natural therapy term for periods of cleansing and symptoms is "crisis," or "healing crisis." During these times, old symptoms or patterns from the past may arise, usually transiently, or new symptoms of detoxification may appear. This "crisis" is not predictable and is thus often accompanied with some question by the fasters as well as their practitioners—is this some new problem arising or is it part of the healing process? Usually only time will tell, yet if it is associated with the fasting and one or more of the common symptoms, it is likely a positive part of detoxification. We should use the maxim of healing, Hering's Law of Cure, to guide us—it states that healing happens from the inside out, the top down, from more important organs to less important ones, and from the most recent to the oldest symptoms. Most healing crises pass within a day or two, although some cleansers experience several days of "cold" symptoms or sinus congestion. If any symptom lasts longer than two or three days, it should be considered as a side effect or a new problem possibly unrelated to cleansing. If there is a problem that worsens or is severe and causes concern, such as fainting, heart arrhythmias, or bleeding, the fast should be stopped and a doctor consulted.

A doctor or knowledgeable practitioner should supervise anyone for whom fasting is questionable—that is, anyone in poor health or without fasting experience. If the fast is extended for more than three to five days, regular monitoring, including physical examination and blood work should be done, probably about weekly. Fasting may reduce blood protein levels and will definitely lower blood fats. Uric acid levels may rise secondary to protein breakdown, while levels of some minerals, such as potassium, sodium, calcium, or magnesium, may drop. Iron levels are usually lower, and the red blood count may also drop during this time.

Hazards of Fasting

If fasting is overused, it may create depletion and weakness, lower resistance, and allow diseases to begin. Certain people are not good candidates for fasting or cleansing. Others may enjoy fasting so much that they overindulge in it and take it beyond the limits of normal elimination, resulting in protein and other nutritional deficits, reduced immunity, and loss of energy. While fasting allows the organs, tissues, and cells to rest, clean house, and handle excesses, the body needs the nourishment provided by food to function after it has used its stores.

Many people of the world are involuntary fasters, while those of the Western nations are more likely to be feasters. In Third World countries, many starvation deaths result from the disease of protein deficiency, termed kwashiorkor, and protein-calorie malnutrition, known as marasmus. What happens to these people is what happens with chronic fasting—loss of muscle mass, weight, and energy, and finally swelling and death.

Malnourished people should definitely not fast, nor should some overweight people who are undernourished. Others who should not fast include people with fatigue resulting from nutrient deficiency, those with chronic degenerative disease of the muscles or bones, or those who are underweight. Diseases associated with clogged or toxic organs respond better to fasting. Sluggish men or women who retain water or whose weight is concentrated in their hips and legs often do poorly with fasting. Those with low daytime energy and more vitality at night (more yin or alkaline types) may not enjoy fasting, either.

I do not suggest fasting for pregnant or lactating women. People who have weak hearts, such as those with congestive heart failure, or who have weakened immunity usually are not good candidates for fasting. Before or after surgery is not a good time to fast, as the body then needs its nourishment to handle the stress and healing demands of surgery. Although some of the nutritional therapies for cancer include fasting, I do not recommend fasting for cancer patients, especially those with advanced problems. Ulcer disease is not something for which I usually suggest fasting, either, although fasting may be beneficial for other conditions present in a patient whose ulcer is under control.

As with any therapy that has some physiological effect and benefit, fasting also may have some hazards. The potential for the development of these problems is maximized with lengthy, noncaloric or water fasts and minimized with juice fasting of reasonable length, such as one to two weeks. Clearly, excessive weight loss and nutritional deficiencies may occur, again more marked with water fasts (juices provide calories and nutrients, although they do not provide complete nutrition). Weakness may occur, or muscle cramps may result from mineral deficits. Sodium, potassium, calcium, magnesium, and phosphorus losses occur initially but diminish after a week. Blood pressure drops, and this can lead to episodes of dizziness, especially when changing position from lying to sitting or sitting to standing. Uric acid levels may rise, which may result in acute gout attacks or a uric acid kidney stone, although this is rare. This problem is minimized with adequate fluid intake.

Some research reports have described hormone level changes with fasting. Initially, the level of thyroid hormone falls, but it rises again in association with protein-sparing ketosis. Female hormone levels fall, possibly as a result of protein malnutrition, and this can lead to

Table 32.3. Contraindications for Fasting

Underweight	Alkaline type	Low blood pressure
Pregnancy	Pre- and post surgery	Peptic ulcers
Fatigue	Low immunity	Cardiac arrhythmias
Nursing	Mental illness	Nutritional deficiencies
Fatigue	Weak heart	Cold weather
Nursing	Cancer	

loss of menstrual flow; that is, secondary amenorrhea. This cessation of the periods in women is also seen in longtime vegetarians, especially those who engage in extensive exercise programs.

Cardiac problems, such as abnormal rhythms (arrhythmias), can occur more easily with prolonged fasting and/or with subclinical preexisting problems. Extra beats, both ventricular and atrial, have been seen, and there have been deaths from serious ventricular arrhythmias, such as ventricular tachycardia, most often occurring during long water fasts. Similar problems have occurred recently in people using the nutrient-deficient protein powders that have been freely sold; many unhealthy weight reducers have been put at risk by using these powders over extended periods on unmonitored fasts. This risk is minimized with juice fasting (up to two weeks) or when basic minerals, mainly potassium, calcium, and magnesium, are supplemented during water fasts. Having our progress followed medically through physical exams, blood tests, and even electrocardiograms is a way to protect ourselves from the potential hazards of fasting.

Another side effect of fasting involves its transformative aspects and how they relate to personal life changes. Often we maintain certain relationships and attitudes toward other people or our careers by resisting inner guidance, feelings, and desires to do something new. Divorce, job changes, and moves are all more likely after fasts, because fasting often stimulates self-realization and change, enhances our potential, and leads us to focus on where we are going, rather than where we have been. During fasting transitions, many people question all aspects of their lives and make new plans for the future. They also have new sensitivity to and awareness of their job, mate, home, and so on.

How to Fast

The general plan for fasting works progressively, from a moderate approach for new fasters and unhealthy subjects to a stricter program for the more experienced. It is important to take the proper time with this potentially powerful process and not jump into a water fast from an average American carnivorous diet. Although many people do fine even if they make such extreme changes, it clearly maximizes the risks of fasting.

A sensible daily plan is one where fasting is mixed with eating. Each day can include a 12-14 hour period of fasting in the evening and during sleep before awakening and getting ready for the day. (Breakfast was given that name to denote the time where we break the fast of the night.) Many people eat very lightly or not at all in the early morning to extend their daily fast. This is more important if dinner or snacking tends to be extended into the later evening, though this is not ideal. On the other hand, if we eat a decent, not excessive, meal in the early evening and awaken hungry, a good breakfast can be consumed after water intake and some exercise.

In preparation for our first day of fasting, we may want to take a few days to eliminate some foods or habits from our diet. When many self-indulgent habits exist, longer preparations may be indicated. Eliminating alcohol, nicotine, caffeine, and sugar if possible is very helpful, although some people choose to wait until their actual fast days to clear these. Red meats and other animal foods, including milk products and eggs, could be avoided for a day or two before fasting. Intake of most nutritional supplements can also be curtailed the day before fasting; these are usually not recommended during a fast. Many people do well by preparing for their fasts with three or four days of consuming only fruit and vegetable foods. These nourish and slowly detoxify the body so that the actual fasting will be less intense.

The first one-day fast (actually 36 hours, including the nights— from 8 p.m. one night until 8 a.m. the following day) gives us a chance to see what a short fast can be like, to see that it is not so very difficult and does not cause any major distress. Most people will feel a little hungry at times and may experience a few mild symptoms (such as a headache or irritability) by the end of the day, usually around late afternoon or dinnertime, but this depends on the individual and the state of toxicity. In actuality, the first two days are the hardest for most people. Feeling great usually begins around day three, so longer juice fasts are really needed for the grand experience.

One of the problems with fasting is that it can be the most difficult for those who need it the most, such as the regular three-square-meals-plus-snacks consumers who eat whatever and whenever they want. Often such people must start with more subtle diet changes and prepare even more slowly for fasting. A transition plan that can be used before even going on the one-day fast is the one-meal-a-day plan. The one daily meal is usually eaten around 3 p.m. Water, juices, and teas and even some fresh fruit or vegetable snacks can be eaten at other times. The one wholesome meal is not excessive or rich. It can be a protein-vegetable meal, such as fish and salad or steamed vegetables, or a starch-vegetable meal, such as brown rice and mixed steamed greens, carrots, celery, and zucchini. People on this plan start to detox slowly, lose some weight, and after a few days feel pretty sound. The chance of any strong symptoms developing, as might occur with fasting, is minimal with this type of transition, and the actual fast, when begun, will be handled more easily, also.

The goal, then, is to move into a one-day fast and then a few two- and three-day fasts with one or two days between them when light foods and more raw fruits and vegetables are consumed, and also provide fluids, juices, soups, and a generally alkaline cleansing diet. This way, we can build up to a five- to ten-day fast. When the transition is made this slowly, even a water fast can be less intense and more profound for those wishing a powerful personal and spiritual experience. With a water fast, however, I strongly suggest medical monitoring and retreating from usual daily life.

A juice fast, which I usually recommend, can be longer and is much easier for most people. The fresh juices of raw fruits and vegetables are what most fasting clinics and practitioners recommend. They provide calories and nutrients on which to function and build new cells, and also provide the inherent enzymes contained in these vital foods. (Food enzyme theories, discussed throughout this century, have recently been described in books such as *Enzyme Nutrition* by Dr. Edward Howell.) Raw foods are considered the healing force in our diet because they contain active enzymes, which are broken down when foods are cooked. Many health enthusiasts consider a raw-food diet the most healing and most nutritious diet.

For the inexperienced faster, it is best to go slowly through the various steps and to avoid being excessive or impatient so that we learn about ourselves in the process. To do this, we need to make a plan and put it into effect, observing or "listening" to our body and even keeping notes in a journal. Get to know yourself. Then, once we have fasted successfully, we could continue to do one-day fasts weekly or a three-day fast every month if we need them. This helps to reconnect us with a better diet and to remotivate us toward our goal of optimum health.

In a more adventurous mode, many people, even some who have never fasted, begin with a seven- to ten-day or even longer fast on fresh juices. I recommend this for most people who have any of the indications and none of the contraindications discussed in this program. People planning these longer fasts, especially inexperienced fasters who have been eating a random diet, should spend a period about equal in length to the planned fast preparing for it. During this preparatory period we can follow some of the previous suggestions, such as eliminating sugar and refined foods, fatty foods, chemicals, and drugs from the diet and reducing consumption of meats and other acid-forming foods, and then moving into several days of consuming primarily fruits and vegetables and more fluids. This will lead into an easier and more energizing fast.

For any cleansing period, it is essential to plan times to meditate, exercise, get fresh air and sunshine, clear our intestines, get massages, take baths, clean our house, brush our skin, and more. Maybe you thought you were going to sit back and relax and have juice delivered to your room? With less shopping, food preparation, and eating time, we have more hours in the day to take care of ourselves in other ways. These supportive aspects of cleansing are discussed further below.

Timing of Fasts

The two key times for natural cleansing are the times of transition into spring and autumn. In Chinese medicine, the transition time between the seasons is considered to be about ten days before and after the equinox or solstice. For spring, this period is about March 10 through April 1; for autumn, it is from about September 11 through October 2. In cooler climates, where spring weather begins later and autumn earlier, the fasting can be scheduled appropriately, as it is easier to do in warmer weather. With fasting, the body tends to cool down. As discussed in Chapter 31, The General Detoxification program, there is also a complete yearly cycle for cleansing with a variety of ideas and options. For spring, I usually suggest lemon and/or greens as the focus of the cleansing. Diluted lemon water, lemon and honey, could be used.

Table 32.4. Spring Master Cleanser

2 Tablespoons fresh lemon or lime juice
1 Tablespoon pure maple syrup
1/4 teaspoon cayenne pepper
8 ounces spring water

Mix and drink 8-12 glasses a day. Eat or drink nothing else except water, laxative herb tea, and peppermint or chamomile tea.

Fresh fruit or vegetable juices diluted with an equal amount of water will also provide a good cleansing. Some vegetable choices are carrots, celery, beets, and lots of greens. Soup broths can also be used. Juices with blue-green algae, such as spirulina or chlorella, mixed in can provide more energy, as these are high-protein plants and easily assimilable.

Autumn is the second most important cleansing time, when we prepare for a new health program, focus on our career or school year, and let go of the fun and games of summer. At this time, a fast of at least three to five days can be done, using water or a variety of juices, apples and/or grapes (usually mixed with a little lemon and water to reduce sweetness), vegetable juices, and warm broths.

How do we know how long to fast? We may use a certain time plan, such as discussed previously. Ideally, though, we should follow our own individual cycles and our body's needs. As we gain some fasting experience, we should become attuned to when we need to strengthen or lighten our diet and when we need to cleanse. Usually, if we are under stress or have been overindulging or develop some congestive symptoms, we want to lighten our diet to balance this. If more changes are needed, a more cleansing, raw-food diet or a fast can be begun.

Table 32.5. Autumn Rejuvenation Ration

3 cups spring water
1 Tablespoon ginger root, chopped
1-2 Tablespoons miso paste
1-2 stalks green onion, chopped
cilantro, to taste, chopped
1-2 pinches cayenne pepper
2 teaspoons olive oil
juice of 1/2 lemon

Boil water. Add ginger root. Simmer 10 minutes. Stir in miso paste to taste. Turn off fire. Then add green onion, some cilantro, cayenne, olive oil, lemon juice. Remove from burner and cover to steep for 10 minutes. May vary ingredient portions to satisfy flavors. Enjoy.

Breaking a Fast

When to stop fasting and make a transition back into eating also takes some inner attunement. Things to watch for include energy level, weight, detox symptoms, tongue coating, and degree of hunger. If our energy is up and then falls for more than a day or if our weight gets too low, these may be signs that we should come off the fast. If symptoms are intense or if any suddenly appear, it is possible that we need food. Generally, the tongue is a good indicator of our state of toxicity or cleansing and clarity. With fasting, the tongue usually becomes coated with a white, yellow, or gray film. This represents the body's cleansing, and it will usually clear when the detox cycle is complete. Tongue observation is not a foolproof indicator, however. Some people's tongues may coat very little, while others will remain coated. In this case, if we were to wait until it totally cleared, we may overextend our cleanse. If in doubt, it is better to make the transition back to foods and then cleanse again later. Hunger is another sign of readiness to move back into eating. Often during cleansing times, hunger is minimal. Occasionally, people are very hungry throughout a fast, but most lose interest in food from day three to day seven or ten and then experience real, deep-seated hunger again. This is a sign to eat (carefully).

It is important to make a gradual transition into a regular diet, rather than just going out to dinner after a week-long fast. Breaking a fast must be planned and done slowly and carefully to prevent creating symptoms and sickness. It is suggested that we take several days, or half of our total cleansing time, to move back into our diet, which is hopefully a newly planned, more healthful diet. Our digestion has been at rest, so we need to go slowly and chew our foods very well. If we have fasted on water alone, we need to prepare our digestive tract with diluted juices, perhaps beginning with a few teaspoons of fresh orange juice in a glass of water and progressing to stronger mixtures throughout the day. Diluted grape or orange juice will stimulate the digestion. Arnold Ehret, a European fasting expert and proponent of the "mucusless" diet, suggests that fruits and fruit juices should not be used right after a meat eater's first fast because they may coagulate intestinal mucus and cause problems. More likely, a meat eater's colon bacteria are different than a vegetarian's; with fruit sugars, the active gram-positive anaerobic bacteria in the meat eater will produce more toxins. Initially, a transition from meats to more vegetable foods will then allow a smoother fast, mainly with vegetable juices and broths. They could also take extra acidophilus to begin to shift their colon ecology.

With juice fasting, it is easier to make the transition back into foods. A raw or cooked low-starch vegetable, such as spinach or other greens, can be used. A little sauerkraut, a fermented cabbage, helps to stimulate the digestive function. A laxative-type meal, such as grapes, cherries, or soaked or stewed prunes, can also be used to initiate eating, as it is important to keep the bowels moving. Some experts say that the bowels should move within an hour or two after the first meal. If not, take an enema. Some people may do a saltwater flush (drinking a quart of water with 2 teaspoons of sea salt dissolved in it) before their first day of food.

However you make the transition, go slowly, chew well, and do not overeat or mix too many foods at a meal. Simple vegetable meals, salads, or soups can be used to start. Fruit should be eaten alone. Soaked prunes or figs are helpful. Well-cooked brown rice or millet is handled well by most people by the second day. From there, progress slowly through grains and vegetables. Some nuts, seeds, or legumes can be added, and then richer protein foods if these are desired. Coming back into foods is a crucial time for learning individual responses or reactions to them. You may even wish to keep notes, following such areas as energy level, intestinal function, sleep patterns, and food desires. If you respond poorly to a food, avoid it for a while, perhaps a week, and then eat it alone to see how it feels.

Juice Specifics

Some juices work better for certain people or conditions. In general, diluted fresh juices of raw organic fruits and vegetables are best. Canned and frozen juices should be avoided. Some bottled juice may be used, but fresh squeezed is best, as long as it is used soon after squeezing.

Water and other liquids are what primarily cleanse our system, increasing waste elimination-rather like squeezing out a dirty sponge in clean water. Lemon tends to loosen and bring out mucus and is useful for liver cleansing. Diluted lemon juice, with or without a little honey, can loosen mucus fast, so if this is used, we need to cleanse the bowels regularly to prevent getting sick. Most vegetable juices are a little milder than lemon juice.

Each juice has a certain nutritional composition and probably certain physiological actions, although these have not been studied extensively. We can think of fresh juices as natural vitamin pills with a very high assimilation percentage, and we do not need to do the work of digesting them. In general, some juices are more caloric than others and might be used less if more weight loss is desired. The juices of apples, grapes, oranges, and carrots are good cleansing juices but might be minimized for weight loss. More grapefruit, lemon, cucumber, and greens, such as lettuce, spinach, or parsley, may be more helpful in this situation. Also, a variety of juices can be used in a fast with different ones squeezed daily.

Table 32.6. Fruit Juices

Lemon—liver, gallbladder, allergies, asthma, cardiovascular disease (CVD), colds

Citrus—CVD, obesity, hemorrhoids, varicose veins

Apple—liver, intestines

Pear—gallbladder

Grape—colon, anemia

Papaya—stomach, indigestion, hemorrhoids, colitis

Pineapple—allergies, arthritis, inflammation, edema, hemorrhoids

Watermelon—kidneys, edema

Black cherry—colon, menstrual problems, gout

Table 32.7. Vegetable Juices

Greens—CVD, skin, eczema, digestive problems, obesity, breath

Spinach—anemia, eczema

Parsley—kidneys, edema, arthritis

Beet greens—gallbladder, liver, osteoporosis

Watercress—anemia, colds

Wheat grass—anemia, liver, intestines, breath

Cabbage—colitis, ulcers

Comfrey—intestines, hypertension, osteoporosis

Carrots—eyes, arthritis, osteoporosis

Beets—blood, liver, menstrual problems, arthritis

Celery—kidneys, diabetes, osteoporosis

Cucumber—edema, diabetes

Jerusalem artichokes—diabetes

Garlic—allergies, colds, hypertension, CVD, high fats, diabetes

Radish—liver, high fats, obesity

Potatoes—intestines, ulcer

These juices may be helpful for particular organs or illnesses, based on my experience as well as information contained in Paavo Airola's *How to Get Well*. To prepare juices, we obviously want to start with the freshest and most chemical-free fruits and vegetables possible. They should be cleaned or soaked and stored properly. If there is a question of toxicity, sprays, or parasites, a chlorine bleach bath can be used. If not organic, they should be peeled, especially if they are waxed. With root vegetables such as carrots or beets, the above-ground ends should be trimmed. Some people like to drop their vegetables into a pot of boiling water for a minute or so for cleansing as well.

The best juicers are the compressors, such as the Norwalk brand, but these are very expensive. The rotary-blade juicers, such as the Champion, are good at squeezing the juice with minimum molecular irritation. The centrifuge juicers are also fine, but they waste juice left in the pulp. Blenders are not really juicers; what they make is more like liquid salads. These are high in fiber.

Other Aspects of Healthy Fasting

- Fresh air—plenty is needed to support cleansing and oxygenation of the cells and tissues.

- Sunshine—also needed to revitalize our body; avoid excessive exposure.

- Water—bathing is very important to cleanse the skin at least twice daily. Steams and saunas are also good for giving warmth as well as supporting detoxification.

- Skin brushing—with a dry, soft brush prior to bathing; this will help clear toxins from the skin. This is a good year-round practice as well.

- Exercise—very important to support the cleansing process. It helps to relax the body, clear wastes, and prevent toxicity symptoms. Walking, bicycling, swimming, or other usual exercises can usually be done during a fast, although more dangerous or contact sports might be avoided.

- No drugs—none should be used during fasts except mandatory prescription drugs. Particularly, avoidance of alcohol, nicotine, and caffeine is wise.

- Vitamin supplements—these are not used during fasting; thus, no program of nutrients will follow at the end of this section. Some supplemental fiber, such as psyllium husks, can be part of a colon detox program. Special chlorophyll foods, such as green barley, chlorella, and spirulina, may also be vitality enhancers and purifiers during cleanses. Occasionally, some mineral support, especially potassium, calcium, and magnesium, or vitamin C will be suggested, usually in powdered or liquid forms (pills are not suggested) to help in preventing cramps, if there is a lot of physical activity, sweating, and fluid and mineral losses, or for an extended fast. Some people even use amino acid powders and other vitamin powders with some benefit during cleanses. In general, most of these supplemental nutrients are best used with foods.

- Colon cleansing—an essential part of healthy fasting. Some form of bowel stimulation is recommended. Colonic irrigations with water are the most thorough. These can be done at the beginning, midpoint, and end of the fast. It is suggested that enemas be used at least every other day if these are the primary colon cleansing. Fasting clinics often suggest that enemas be used daily, even up to several times a day. With these, usually water alone is used to flush the colon of toxins. It may be helpful for an enema or laxative preparation to be used the day before the fast begins to lessen initial toxicity. Herbal laxatives are commonly taken orally during fasting, and many formulas are available, as capsules or for making teas. These include cascara sagrada, senna leaves, licorice root, buckthorn, rhubarb root, aloe vera, and the LB formula of Dr. Christopher. Laci LeBeau tea is also very effective. The saltwater flush, or internal bath, recommended by Stanley Burroughs, is useful for those who can tolerate it. A solution of 2 teaspoons of sea salt is dissolved in a quart of warm purified water (not distilled) and is drunk first thing in the morning on alternate days throughout the fast to flush the entire intestinal tract, an advantage of this cleansing formula. It does not, however, work well for everyone. For example, it is not recommended for salt-sensitive or water-retaining people, or for hypertensives. Whatever colon cleansing method is used, keep in mind that regular cleansing of the intestines and colon is a key component to healthy and stress-free fasting.

- Work and be creative—and make plans for your life. Staying busy is helpful in breaking our ties to food. We also need time for ourselves. Most fasters experience greater work energy and more creativity and, naturally, find lots to do.

- Cleanup—a motto during fasting. As we clean our body, we want to clean our room, desk, office, closet, and home—just like "spring cleaning." It clearly brings us into harmony with the cleansing process of nutrition. If we want to get ready for the new, we need to make space by clearing out the old.

- Joining others in fasting can generate strong bonds and provide an added spiritual lift. It opens up new supportive relationships and new levels of existing ones. It will also provide support if we feel down or want to quit. Most people feel better as their fast progresses—more vital, lighter, less blocked, more flexible, clearer, and more spiritually attuned. For many, it is nice to have someone with whom to share this.

- Avoid the negative influence of others who may not understand or support us. There are many fears and misconceptions about fasting, and they may affect us. We need to listen to our own inner guidance and not to others' limitations, but we also need to maintain awareness and insight into any problems should they arise. Being in contact with fasters will provide us with the positive support we need.

- The economy of fasting allows us to save time, money, and future health care costs. While we may be worried about not having enough, we may already have too much. Many of us are inspired to share more of ourselves when we are freed from food.

- Meditation and relaxation are also an important aspect of fasting to help attune us to deeper levels of ourselves and clear the stresses that we have carried with us.

- Spiritual practice and prayer will affirm our positive attitude toward ourselves and life in general. This supports our meditation and relaxation and provides us with the inner fuel to carry on our life with purpose and passion.

Conclusion

Fasting can easily become a way of life and an effective dietary practice. Over a period of time (different for each of us), through newly gained clarity, we can go from symptom cleansing to prevention fasting.

Ideally, we should fast at specific times to treat symptoms and/or to enhance our vitality and spiritual practice.

Otherwise, we should support ourselves regularly with a balanced, wholesome diet. This diet may change somewhat through the year as we experience different needs, and occasional fasting or feasting may be valuable. We also must maintain good digestion and elimination.

Fasting is needed more frequently by those who have abused themselves with foods or other agents so readily available these days. We all need to return to the cycle of a daily fast of 12-14 hours overnight until our morning "break-fast," and then find our own natural pattern of food consumption. This usually means one main meal and two lighter ones. For low-weight, high-metabolism people, two larger or three moderately sized meals are probably needed. If we eat a heavier evening meal, we need only a light breakfast, and vice versa. Through awareness and experience, we can find our individual nutritional needs and listen to that inner nutritionist, our body.

Choosing healthful foods, chewing well, and maintaining good colon function minimize our need for fasting. However, if we do get out of balance, we can employ the oldest treatment known to us, the instinctive therapy for many illnesses, nature's doctor and knifeless surgeon, the great therapist and tool for preventing disease—fasting!

About Dr. Haas

Dr. Elson M. Haas is a practicing physician of Integrated Medicine for over 25 years. He is the Founder and Medical Director of the Preventive Medical Center of Marin in San Rafael. Dr, Haas is also the author of the classic preventive medicine text *Staying Healthy with the Seasons* (1981, now in its 26th printing and 21st anniversary with a revised 2002 edition) and *Staying Healthy with Nutrition* (1992). Other books by Celestial Arts in Berkeley, CA, include his diet and recipe book, *A Cookbook For All Seasons* (2000), *The Detox Diet*: (1997), and *The Staying Healthy Shopper's Guide: Feed Your Family Safely* (1999). Further recent books are *Vitamins for Dummies* and *The False Fat Diet* (2000, Ballantine Books). Dr. Haas speaks nationally, is on radio and TV shows, and appears in many national magazine articles.

See http://www.elsonhaas.com for more information on a wide variety of health topics.

Part Five

Other Alternative Therapies

Chapter 33

Alexander Technique

We are often unaware of habits that cause us stress and interfere with our ability to respond effectively to the stimuli in our daily lives. How can we change our habits so that we can respond more effectively and achieve better functioning? This fundamental problem is addressed and dealt with in the Alexander Technique, a method that has been recognized for 100 years as a unique and remarkably effective technique of mind-body reeducation.

A Brief History

F. Matthias Alexander (1869-1955) was an Australian actor and teacher. He originally developed the Alexander Technique as a method of vocal training for singers and actors in the 1890s. While Alexander was developing his method of voice training, he realized that the basis for all successful vocal education was an efficiently and naturally functioning respiratory mechanism. So, in teaching voice, Alexander focused primarily on helping the breathing mechanism to function more effectively. Because of his focus on "reeducating" the breathing mechanism, some of Alexander's students, who had come to him for vocal training, found that their respiratory difficulties also improved. These improvements were recognized by medical doctors who began referring their patients with respiratory ailments to Alexander for

"The F.M. Alexander Technique," by Marian Goldberg, © 1995 Marian Goldberg, for further information go to http://www.alexandercenter.com. Reprinted with permission.

help. In this way, F.M. Alexander's technique of vocal training developed into a technique he termed "respiratory re-education."

Alexander had also made the discovery that breathing and vocalization are part and parcel of how the body functions as a whole. Habitual breathing and vocal patterns are parts of habitual patterns of general coordination. In fact, many problems we see as involving just one particular part of the body, e.g. lower back pain and "RSI," are often symptoms of larger habitual patterns of malcoordination.

Just as people had found Alexander's "vocal" technique helped them with their breathing problems, so a number of his students found his method of respiratory re-education helped them with other physical difficulties. Basically, Alexander had evolved a method for learning how to consciously change maladaptive habits of coordination. (Coordination includes movement, posture, breathing, and tension patterns.) He had come to the understanding that the mind and body function as an integrated entity, a rather unusual realization for that time. Alexander found that habits, whether "physical" habits or "mental" habits, are all psychophysical in nature. He observed that how we think about our activities determines how we coordinate ourselves to do those activities, and, equally, how long-held habits of excessive tension and inefficient coordination affect how we feel and think. In a relatively short period of time, Alexander evolved his technique from a method of vocal training into a method of breathing re-education and then into a comprehensive technique of psychophysical reeducation. His technique deals with the psychophysical coordination of the whole person, or what he termed more concisely as "the use of the self."

Try This

Try to breathe from high up in your chest or from low down in your abdomen. Try walking or moving your arms while you breathe in one of these ways. Do you walk or move your arms differently when you change your breathing? Or make a conscious effort to change the way you walk or the way you hold your neck, or try clenching your arms: Do these efforts affect your breathing or your voice? What if these were habitual efforts—efforts which you made all the time but you were unaware that you were making them? We do make habitual excessive efforts most of the time, but we are generally unaware of making them. Excessive stress in one part of the body is usually part of a larger pattern of habitual malcoordination.

How Habits Affect Our Functioning

How do habits develop? We can see how habits develop by observing the movements of a child. Babies are usually born with an overall fundamental pattern of coordination "programmed" into their nervous systems. This primary pattern works efficiently and easily with the human structure. An example of this natural efficiency of the human mechanism can be seen with a baby who spontaneously sits up by himself. Generally, a baby of 12 months sits very upright naturally. In fact, it is far easier and more natural for a baby to sit upright than for the typical adult who slouches into a supposedly "relaxed" movement/postural pattern. As a child grows, he usually starts to imitate the mannerisms of those around him, such as parents, peers, and teachers. These "imitations" often become permanent and the child will probably lose any conscious awareness that he is doing them. The child may also experience injuries or other uncomfortable experiences which lead to fixed, inefficient habits. These habits can become a constant interference with his natural fundamental coordination. This on-going interference can affect how his muscles develop, including the development of excessive tension, how he moves, how he breathes, and how his alignment and posture develop. Most importantly, the child's (and adult's) senses of movement (kinesthetic sense) and balance can become skewed by relying on long-term, fixed habits. These senses are then unable to function as reliable guides for efficient coordination. Though the child or adult may eventually sense that something is wrong with his movement, posture, or other aspects of his functioning, his senses involved in coordination (proprioception) have become so altered by his habits that he finds he can't rely on these senses when he tries to make changes and improvements.

The on-going interference of his habits may be causing him excessive and constant stress but the child or adult finds it difficult to "stop" his habits because they feel familiar and "right" to him. Maladaptive habits alter our general sensory feedback. They alter our perceptions of what feels "right": These altered perceptions and concomitant feelings affect everything we do which involves our coordination. And all activities, whether "physical" or "mental," involve coordination, or the way we use ourselves.

Learning the Alexander Technique

What one learns in Alexander Technique lessons is a unique and practical means of stopping and changing habits. This learning process allows one's sense of coordination to regain its natural "perspective." The Alexander Technique teacher takes the student through basic movements giving gentle hands-on guidance. Through this guidance, the student experiences more natural and easy coordination without the on-going interference of habits. Repeating these experiences of natural, fundamental movement stimulates the student's internal coordination feedback mechanisms to become more accurate. This develops his/her ability to choose better coordinated and non-stressful responses to stimuli. The student is able to make lasting habit changes.

The Alexander Technique does not involve exercises, forms of psychotherapy, or spiritual healing techniques. It is also unlike the manipulations of bodywork or manual healing techniques: Rather than looking at the body as a set of separate "parts" or pressure points to be individually "worked on," a skilled teacher guides a student through movement, observing and working with whole patterns of coordination, which include tension and postural patterns, how a student thinks about moving, and active movement itself. The student actively participates in this process, learning to apply his own intelligence to effectively change habits.

Benefits

This learning process can have many benefits, including easier movement, improved alignment, more natural breathing, and, most importantly, the development of skills to deal with habits on a general basis. The fundamental improvement in the reliability of sensory appreciation/feedback that occurs with Alexander Technique lessons can have significant, positive effects on a wide range of behaviors and skills, including the ability to learn.

The Technique can be very helpful for people dealing with chronic pain, excessive stress, or injury. It is also used by performing artists to enhance performing techniques. A number of universities and conservatories incorporate the Alexander Technique into their regular curriculum. John Dewey, the American philosopher, studied the technique for over 35 years and expressed a strong wish that the Alexander Technique be incorporated into the educational system. Charles Sherrington, the Nobel laureate in physiology, stated of Alexander's work, "Mr. Alexander has done a service to the subject by insistently treating each act as involving the whole integrated individual, the whole psychophysical man."

Lessons and Classes

Alexander Technique lessons are taught on an individual basis. Private lessons give the student the opportunity to make in-depth and lasting improvements and to develop substantive skills in changing habits. Students of the Alexander Technique usually take a number of private lessons.

F.M. Alexander recommended a course of 30 private lessons although there are no minimum or maximum requirements for the number of lessons one can have. Depending on the teacher, lessons can last from one-half hour to an hour. Generally, it's better to have lessons one or more times a week than to have lessons less frequently over a longer period of time. Wearing comfortable clothing to lessons is helpful but it isn't necessary to wear any special type of exercise clothes.

In recent years, there have been attempts to teach the Alexander Technique in group classes and workshops. Workshops can serve as an introduction to the Technique. They can be convenient and can offer some helpful hints. However, as classes and workshops attempt to teach the Alexander Technique in a group setting, there are some basic problems with them: they lack sufficient experience in the hands-on guidance integral to learning the Technique; they encourage end-gaining as people tend to become too self-conscious in a group and try too hard to succeed in a limited period of time, and at best they offer a cursory presentation of the Technique.

Dramatic improvement can occur during an Alexander Technique lesson. However, because people tend to become strongly habituated to certain patterns, there is only so much change that can occur at any one time. To provide sufficient individual attention and the time to make substantive and lasting improvement, the Alexander Technique is generally learned through private studies over a substantial period of time.

At times the Alexander Technique has also been presented in combination with various therapeutic, movement, or other kinds of methods, often in an effort to provide a short-cut to learning the Technique. The result is usually a diluted version of the Alexander Technique which may have little in common with the Technique's fundamentals. In order to gain the most benefit from the Alexander Technique, it's important to take the time to learn it thoroughly with a qualified teacher.

Alexander Technique Teacher Training

As with learning the Alexander Technique for oneself, teacher training in the Technique is a unique process. Trainees attend class four to five times each week for a period of three or more years for a total of 1600 or more hours of training. Much of this daily training is an intensification of the learning process that takes place with private instruction. Standard criteria for training were established over 60 years ago by F. M. Alexander. Alexander Technique teacher-training programs do vary based on different interpretations of the Technique.

Finding and Choosing a Teacher

Qualified teachers have completed full-time, three-year training programs as described above. Alexander Technique teachers have different interpretations of the Technique and teaching approaches vary. It can be helpful to try lessons with several teachers before making a decision about with whom to study.

A helpful gauge for deciding on a teacher can be one's own experiences of improvement during an introductory lesson(s). However, depending on circumstances, it can take several lessons before a student notices any changes.

People often come to the Alexander Technique with some misconceptions about what efficient and easy movement and/or posture should look like. Therefore, observing the way the teacher moves or holds himself/herself is not a particularly helpful gauge for judging a teacher. Students of the Technique often find that their understanding of efficient and comfortable movement, breathing, and posture changes as they go through a series of lessons and experience improvement in their own coordination.

F. M. Alexander used to tell prospective students to read his books before starting lessons. Reading about the Alexander Technique can also be helpful in making an informed choice concerning a teacher with whom to study. Some good introductory books are listed below.

Recommended Introductory Reading

Freedom to Change by Frank Pierce Jones. London: Mouritz, 1997. (First published under the title, *Body Awareness in Action*, 1976.) Available from Mornum Time Press, 381 Bush Street, Suite 500, San Francisco, CA 94104 and the Society of Teachers of the Alexander Technique.

A comprehensive account of the Alexander Technique.

Indirect Procedures: A Musician's Guide to the Alexander Technique by Pedro de Alcantara with foreword by Sir Colin Davis. Oxford:

338

Clarendon Press, 1997. ISBN 0-19-816568-4 [0-19-816569-2, paperback]. Available from Amazon Books and STAT Books.

Although this book explains the Alexander Technique from the perspective of music-making, it is an excellent introduction for anyone interested in learning about the technique. There are a few errors in the technical descriptions of two of Alexander's procedures, otherwise it is probably the best book on the technique currently available, apart from F.M. Alexander's own works.

The Alexander Technique by Chris Stevens. Rutland, Vermont: Charles E. Tuttle Company, Inc., 1987, 1994. ISBN 0-8048-3006-1. Available from STAT Books and Amazon.

A brief, easy-to-read introduction. The *British Medical Journal* wrote: "It [the Alexander Technique] is difficult to explain without practical experience, but Chris Stevens provides an excellent introduction."

Chapter 34

Aromatherapy

Aromatherapy is the inhalation and application of volatile essential oils from aromatic plants to restore or enhance health, beauty and well-being. The basic intention of Aromatherapy is to bring together the scientific achievements of man with his intuitive understanding for the treatment of illnesses with the most effective and useful natural essential oils. Conforming with the laws of nature, the principle of Aromatherapy is to strengthen the self-healing processes by preventative methods and indirect stimulation of the immune system. Their field of activity is quite wide, ranging from deep and penetrating therapeutic actions to the extreme subtlety of unique fragrance. Simply put, essential oils can be used to enhance health as well as the quality of life. Aromatherapy is an ancient yet timely and stunningly modern approach to total well-being that is in tune with nature.

What Are Essential Oils?

Essential oils are the highly concentrated volatile extract of flowers herbs, grasses, shrubs and trees. These tiny droplets are present in particular glands, hairs or specific structures of the plant and contain some (but not all) of the active principles of the plant. Similar to herbal therapy principles, essential oils are phytochemicals with particular biological properties. Non-oily in texture, these highly concentrated

"Aromatherapy—Frequently Asked Questions," © 2001 Atlantic Institute of Aromatherapy (Tampa, FL); reprinted with permission.

substances are obtained by steam distillation, peel pressure, and solvent extraction methods. Only the utmost quality of essential oils should be used in aromatherapy. The majority of essential oils produced in the world market are used in the food flavor and fragrance industry, so essential oils are often found on the market adulterated with similar essential oils, chemicals and synthetics, as well as extenders such as dipropylene glycol. Unfortunately, even the type used in food can be adjusted with chemicals from a natural source and still legally be called natural. Therefore, it is wise to purchase only from a reputable aromatherapy source.

How Do Essential Oils Work?

Essential oils work in harmony with the body to normalize and balance. They produce certain effects that we can count on, but can also adapt to the needs of different people. Used for their undisputed anti-microbial and antiseptic effects, essential oils are not only less toxic than synthetic antibiotics but also support life (eubiotic) by working with the body's own natural healing abilities (through which the only true healing occurs). Certain oils, such as Roman chamomile, have cytophylactic (cell regeneration), antiseptic, and wound healing effects as well as anti-fungal and anti-inflammative properties making them the ultimate active principles for holistic natural skin-care.

What Are the Effects?

Oils can directly or indirectly affect the body's physiological systems. For instance, a couple of drops of peppermint taken orally can aid digestion and inhalations of mucolytic oils can relieve respiratory symptoms. Used topically for their antiseptic and soothing effects, essential oils can successfully treat minor skin conditions. It has been demonstrated that the application of certain essential oils to the skin can produce vaso-dilation which in turn causes warming of underlying muscles, however this is an indirect effect of the oil acting on the superficial tissues, it is not a pharmacological effect produced as a result of the oil entering the systemic circulation via the skin. In addition, because of the effect of relaxation on the brain and the subsequent sedating or stimulating of the nervous system, essential oils can also indirectly raise and lower blood pressure and possibly aid in normalization of hormonal secretion.

Because of olfaction's direct connection to the brain, sending electrical messages directly into the limbic system, essential oils can have effects on emotions and mental states. Perception of odors can have a major impact on memory, learning, emotions, thinking and feeling. As therapeutic agents, essential oils work similarly to tranquilizers but in a subtle organic way. Most scents uplift spirits and calm the nervous system. For example, lavender is calming and sedative; basil, rosemary and peppermint are uplifting and stimulating; and jasmine and ylang-ylang are exciting or euphoric.

How Are Essential Oils Used?

Direct inhalation of the oils can have psychological effects through olfactory links with the limbic system that can then stimulate or sedate body systems or organs. In addition, physiological effects are possible because this is the fastest route into the bloodstream. Inhalation is most useful for respiratory symptoms and can be done by sniffing drops on a tissue or by inhaling near a diffuser with glass nebulizer. Local application of diluted oils (2-10% in a vegetable oil base) on various points (spinal nerves, chakras, meridians) is effective for certain conditions. As well, full-body massage is quite effective, providing relaxation as well as a physiological action through the nervous system. Although it is claimed in the literature that many physiological systemic effects are due to essential oils entering the bloodstream via skin application, little evidence backs this up as a major route of absorption. In addition, many of the therapeutic claims are "borrowed" from herbalism, or are really the effect of ingesting the herbal extract. Nevertheless, aromatherapy does work for topical application and relaxation, we are just not sure how it works for some other conditions. Common sense and education should accompany essential oil applications for particular medicinal results. Safety data is mandatory knowledge for anyone using essential oils on the skin, as many are irritating or sensitizing as well as photo-toxic.

Aromatherapy provides health and body care on a completely natural basis, and the subtle qualities of the oils lend themselves best to a gradual experience. The combination of factual information from reference books now being offered coupled with a developed intuition make one capable of generating spectacular successes in self-healing. At first, using essential oils is pleasant; this experience then grows into a heightened awareness of increased health as a consequence of external use of essential oils. Money-wise, aromatherapy can cut your health care and cosmetic bills.

Therefore, using a diffuser, scent pot, or spraying the air (5-8 drops to one ounce of water), wearing as perfume (diluted in jojoba) or used in baths (5-10 drops), inhalations (2-5 drops), and massage treatments (15 drops in ounce of vegetable oil), essential oils can enhance health and well-being in a natural way.

Chapter 35

Art Therapy

Art therapists work with individuals of all ages, races, and ethnic backgrounds who have developmental, medical, or psychological impairments.

What Is Art Therapy?

Art therapy is a human service profession which utilizes art media, images, the creative art process and patient/client responses to the created art productions as reflections of an individual's development, abilities, personality, interests, concerns, and conflicts. Art therapy practice is based on knowledge of human developmental and psychological theories which are implemented in the full spectrum of models of assessment and treatment including educational, psychodynamic, cognitive, transpersonal, and other therapeutic means of reconciling emotional conflicts, fostering self-awareness, developing social skills, managing behavior, solving problems, reducing anxiety, aiding reality orientation, and increasing self-esteem.

Art therapy is an effective treatment for the developmentally, medically, educationally, socially or psychologically impaired; and is practiced in mental health, rehabilitation, medical, educational, and forensic institutions. Populations of all ages, races, and ethnic backgrounds are served by art therapists in individual, couples, family, and group therapy formats.

Educational, professional, and ethical standards for art therapists are regulated by the American Art Therapy Association, Inc. (AATA). The Art Therapy Credentials Board, Inc. (ATCB), an independent organization, grants postgraduate registration (ATR) after reviewing documentation of completion of graduate education and postgraduate supervised experience. The Registered Art Therapist who successfully completes the written examination administered by the ATCB is qualified as Board Certified (ATR-BC), a credential requiring maintenance through continuing education credits.

How Did Art Therapy Begin?

Although visual expressions have been basic to humanity throughout history, art therapy did not emerge as a distinct profession until the 1930's. At the beginning of the 20th Century, psychiatrists became interested in the art work done by patients, and studied it to see if there was a link between the art and the illness of their patients. At this same time, art educators were discovering that the free and spontaneous art expression of children represented both emotional and symbolic communications. Since then, the profession of art therapy has grown into an effective and important method of communication, assessment, and treatment with many populations.

Where Do Art Therapists Work?

Art therapists work in private offices, art rooms, or meeting rooms in facilities such as:

- hospitals—both medical and psychiatric
- out-patient facilities
- clinics
- residential treatment centers
- halfway houses
- shelters
- schools
- correctional facilities
- elder care facilities

- pain clinics
- universities
- art studios

The art therapist may work as part of a team which includes physicians, psychologists, nurses, rehabilitation counselors, social workers, and teachers. Together, they determine and implement a client's therapeutic, school, or mental health program. Art therapists also work as primary therapists in private practice.

What Are the Requirements to Become an Art Therapist?

Personal Qualifications: An art therapist must have sensitivity to human needs and expressions, emotional stability, patience, a capacity for insight into psychological processes, and an understanding of art media. An art therapist must also be an attentive listener, a keen observer, and be able to develop a rapport with people. Flexibility and a sense of humor are important in adapting to changing circumstances, frustration, and disappointment.

Educational Requirements: One must complete the required core curriculum as outlined in the AATA Education Standards to qualify as a professional art therapist. Entry into the profession of art therapy is at the master's level. Avenues of completion offered by graduate level art therapy programs include: a Master's degree in art therapy, a Master's degree with an emphasis in art therapy and twenty-one (21) semester units in art therapy with a Master's degree in a related field.

Registration and Board Certification Requirements: The ATR and ATR-BC are the recognized standards for the field of art therapy, and are conferred by the ATCB. In order to qualify as a registered art therapist (ATR), in addition to the educational requirements, an individual must complete a minimum of 1,000 direct client contact hours. One hour of supervision is required for every ten hours of client contact.

Chapter 36

Bioenergetic Medicine

The Electrodermal Screening Test

According to traditional Chinese medicine, a form of bodily energy called chi is generated in internal organs and circulates throughout the body, forming paths near the surface of the skin called meridians. This whole-body network is called the meridian system.

Acupuncture points are points on the skin, usually located on meridians, where the circulation of chi can be manipulated.

By stimulating an acupuncture point on the skin through pressure, suction, heat, or needle insertion, the circulation of chi is affected, which in turn affects related internal organs. But this is not the only way to take advantage of the meridian system. The meridian energy flow also carries with it information about internal organs that can be used in diagnosis. This is the basis of the electrodermal screening test (EDST). The device used in the EDST is the electrodermal screening device, or EDSD, which works by measuring electrical resistance and polarization at acupuncture points and meridians. Through these safe, skin-level measurements, it is possible to analyze the bio-energy and bio-information produced by internal organs and systems.

The predecessors to the EDST and EDSD were invented in the 1950's by the German doctor Reinhold Voll whose name is given to

"Basic Explanation of the Electrodermal Screening Test and the Concepts of Bio-Energetic Medicine," an undated document, cited December 2001, © American Association of Acupuncture and Bio-Energetic Medicine; reprinted with permission.

another title of this treatment modality, EAV or Electro Acupuncture according to Voll. Dr. Voll originally developed a system of acupuncture point electro-therapeutics, but he soon discovered that when an internal organ's function or structure changes, the performance of the related meridian and acupuncture points also changed, and that this change could be measured using a device. Voll used a device called the Dermatron, but all similar devices can be used for diagnosis and medicine testing. The core of the EDSD is an ohm meter designed to deliver approximately 10-12 microamperes of direct electrical current at 1-1.25 volts, a very small and perfectly safe amount of energy. On the majority of the devices the meter is calibrated to read from 0 to 100 such that the standard skin resistance of 100 kilo-ohms reads 50.

There are two cables coming out of the EDSD, one positive and one negative. The positive lead is attached to a stylus with an electrode tip. The doctor holds the stylus by the insulated handle and presses the tip against one of the patient's acupuncture points. The patient holds a hand electrode in their free hand. During the measurement the patient and the EDSD form a closed circuit, allowing energy and information to flow from the EDSD to the probe, through the patient to the hand electrode, and back to the EDSD. The EDSD reading is a measurement of how much energy makes it through the circuit (the lower the resistance the higher the reading). A reading taken with the EDSD is usually described using two values, the initial reading (generally the highest value) and the indicator drop (ID). An initial reading of approximately 50 followed by little or no indicator drop is considered "good." Initial readings below 45 or above 60 and substantial IDs are all considered bad signs. After the initial stimulus (the initial reading) two things occur: cells become polarized, which increases resistance, and the affected cells work to maintain their natural, unpolarized state. An ID is the result of the polarization of cells that are weakened and can not maintain their own balance.

A typical examination with the EDSD begins with the four quadrant measurements (hand to hand, foot to foot, right hand to foot, and left foot to foot) which are measurements of whole-body energy levels. These are followed by a check of the 40 control measurement points (CMPs), one for each of the 40 meridians located on the hands and feet, some of which are traditional and some of which were discovered by Voll. The CMPs show the general condition of everything associated with that meridian, and the 40 hand and foot meridians cover virtually every body part and function, so an examination of 40 CMPs alone offers the doctor a very good overview of a patient's condition. The other points along a meridian are called branch points and are checked if the CMP reading is bad. They offer more specific information than the CMP. For example, the branch points on the two heart meridians include the aortic valve, mitral valve, pulmonary valve, tricuspid valve, conduction system, and coronary arteries. A problem in the coronary arteries would probably affect the circulation CMP and the coronary arteries branch point, but not other points.

Medicine Testing

When a point is located that reads below 50, above 60, or has an ID, various reagents can be tested in a process called medicine testing. In 1945, Reinhold Voll discovered by accident that a medicine placed in contact with a patient's body effects the readings of an electro-dermal screening device (EDSD).

"I diagnosed one colleague as having chronic prostatitis and advised him to take a homeopathic preparation called Echinaceae 4x. He replied that he had this medication in his office and went to get it. When he returned with the bottle of Echinaceae in his hand, I tested the prostate measurement point again and made the discovery that the point reading which previously was up to 90 had decreased to 64, which was an enormous improvement of the prostate value. I had the colleague put the bottle aside and the previous measurement value returned. After holding the medication in his hand the measurement value went down to 64 again, and this pattern repeated itself as often as desired."

While checking branch points can be used to specify more refined locations of the disturbance, medicine testing serves to specify etiology and selection of medications for treatment. Medicine testing is performed on any abnormal points that are not balanced. The doctor's goal is to find one or a combination of reagents that will balance the point, i.e. cause the point tested to exhibit a "good" reading and to not have an ID.

Reagent samples are usually sealed in glass containers. The medicine or biological compound to be tested is placed in the circuit of the EDSD measurement. This can be done by placing it on an aluminum plate or container attached to the negative lead of the EDSD or simply by having the patient hold the sample. All matter, including medicine, has a vibratory signal which is distinct from all other types of matter. This signal enters the patient with the current and reacts with the signals within the patient, often changing the reading. A reagent that balances the reading will probably have a positive effect and can be considered for use as a medicine or dietary supplement.

351

No response implies that the reagent would have no effect, and a worsening response implies a negative effect. For example, pancreas CMP readings of a person with diabetes will become balanced when the proper dose of insulin is placed within the circuit and will show a larger ID if refined sugar is put there. In this way medicines and dosages can be tried out without the medicine actually being ingested. This process can also be used to test for the presence of contaminants and allergies.

A good example of this is Voll's description of the case of a patient with chronic pyelitis. Another doctor had prescribed 2 different types of antibiotics, terramycin and aureomycin, and Dr. Voll was curious to see if both were necessary and what side effects there might be.

"I began testing and saw that the terramycin only affects the right kidney and the aureomycin only the left kidney and not vice versa. At the same time I discovered that when the patient first held the terramycin capsules and the aureomycin capsules, indicator drops for the small intestine and colon occurred as a sign of a disturbed intestinal flora caused by the medications. Furthermore the entire values of the endocrine system, i.e., the values of the Triple Heater meridian, decreased below 50. This explained to me why fatigue occurs again and again after antibiotic treatment since this sort of treatment renders the entire hormonal system temporarily insufficient."

A theoretical model for medicine testing's mechanism of action has been developed by the Physicist Kuo-Gen Chen. All matter has a vibrational signal, including medicines, other biological reagents, and the organs and tissues of the body. When the DC current passes through the potential space of the medicine, it becomes phase modulated, carrying the vibrational signal of the medicine with it into the body. This vibrational information then reacts with vibrational patterns already existing within the body, resulting in quasi phase matching with constructive or destructive resonance, which in turn brings about an instantaneous change in the subtle energetic properties of the point being measured.

Medicine testing can be used to test any medicine or supplement administered to patients, including allopathic, homeopathic, nutritional and herbal medicines. Most physicians use the EDSD as an adjunct to their practice. Homeopathic preparations, however, appear to be particularly useful. They are made by diluting and shaking an original substance in a process called "potentization," often to the point where not a single molecule of the original substance remains in the preparation.

What remains is the vibrational signature of the original substance stored in water. Homeopathic remedies seem to work extremely well in the EDST because they are distilled samples of vibrational information with an information content that is clearer than other medicines. Though it can not yet be substantiated, medicine testing suggests that there is a similarity between the information in homeopathic remedies and the biological information that circulates through the body, primarily through the meridian system. Research in this direction may eventually lead to the verification of homeopathy's mechanism of action.

The two types of homeopathic preparations used most often in the EDST are standard remedies which are made mostly from plant matter, and nosodes, a type of remedy which is made from diseased tissue samples. Standard remedies were selected because they elicit in healthy people the same symptoms as the condition they are supposed to treat. For example, Allium Cepa, a homeopathic remedy for the common cold, causes a sore throat, runny nose, tearing, and congestion in a healthy individual. Nosodes often work similarly to standard remedies in that they cause a set of symptoms in the healthy but can counteract disease in the ill. Nosodes and standard remedies often have a similar effect during medicine testing. For example, in a person with the cold, there is a good chance that either a cold virus nosode or the remedy Allium Cepa will balance points on effected meridians.

Nosodes are particularly useful in determining many pathological illnesses. For example, if a point responds positively when tested with an Epstein Bar nosode, then that virus, at least in a latent form, is affecting the system associated with that measurement point. When a new virus, bacteria, or any other disease that takes a physical form is discovered, one can easily prepare nosodes for screening and energetic treatment. A nosode, remedy, or combinations, identified by medicine testing can be taken directly, or one can make a "recording" of their vibrational information in pure water or normal saline solution. The effect of original and recorded nosodes is usually very similar, though doctors generally prefer the originals.

One will often find that a medicine that balances one point will balance others as well. It would be optimal to find one medicine that would adequately balance all unbalanced points. Unlike classical homeopathy which emphasizes single remedy treatments however, it is common practice in EDST medicine testing and treatment to combine various homeopathic preparations. Nonetheless, the goal should be to prescribe as few remedies for the patient as possible.

Allergy Testing

One of the most popular and effective uses of medicine testing is allergy testing. The results of EDST allergy testing have been compared to standard diagnostic modalities (RAST, serum IGE, intra-dermal allergy skin testing, food rechallenge testing, and allergy history analysis). EDST medicine testing of allergies was shown to be as accurate and effective as any of these. EDST results were similar to food rechallenge testing, which is widely considered the most effective of the standard methods.

Vegatest Method of Medicine Testing

The Vegetative Reflex Test (VRT) or Vegatest testing method is a form of biological function diagnosis developed by Helmut Schimmel of West Germany. The Vegatest varies from the standard EAV-based EDST in important ways, including device design, measured response range, utilization of fewer measurement points, and richer applications of medicine testing. The Vegatest device includes a signal amplifier called the test point regulator which is inserted between the meter input and the meter itself. Meter sensitivity can then be adjusted such that a normal reading (a mid-scale reading on standard EDSDs) reaches the top of the scale. With this arrangement, small changes in impedance indicating increased resistance at the measurement point will show wider scale reading differences, which greatly increases the device's sensitivity to impedance changes near normal reading values.

In the Vegatest, very few points are used, but a larger repertoire of homeopathic testing solutions are used. Medicine testing is used to determine both the location and cause of imbalances. In general, an entire examination is done using only one point, most often allergy (1), connective tissue degeneration (1), triple warmer (1 right), or triple warmer (1 left). Proponents claim that the Vegatest is just as thorough and dependable as the standard EDST, though much less time-consuming. Drawbacks to the Vegatest system include the cost and space required by the large selection of testing solutions.

EAV and Dentistry

In his research, Dr. Voll found that every tooth relates to different organs and tissues within the body. For example, the canine tooth was found to be related to the eye, liver, and gall bladder, and the front teeth to the bladder and reproductive organs. So if, for example, someone were to have a root canal in one of the front teeth, that tooth may affect the ovary or uterus and it may in fact be the underlying problem. It is a two way street in that problems in the organs can affect the teeth, and problems in the teeth can affect the organs. So when dental work is done on specific teeth the underlying organ needs to be supported. EAV also is used before and after the removal of amalgam. Silver fillings in the mouth which are fifty percent mercury are a very great problem.

Mercury leaches into all parts of the body from the mouth. Studies have shown that the amount of mercury in the brain of autopsied patients directly correlates to the amount found in the mouth. EAV can be used to screen for heavy metals, including mercury toxicity. It can also be used to check the effect that root canals are having on the corresponding organs. EAV is the best way to find a cavitation or a hole remaining in the bone after removal of a tooth. Cavitations become a focus for problems in corresponding organs. Dr. Voll felt that 80% of all health problems had major causes in the oral cavity. So this means that the dentist is an integral part of the healing process.

Conclusion

In conclusion, the EDST is one of the most thorough, powerful, and promising modern, holistic medical/diagnostic methodologies. The EDST succeeds at addressing the body holistically for a number of reasons:

1. A standard EDST examination enables the doctor to quickly and safely collect information on 40 different individual systems. In other words, all of the body's individual parts are covered in an examination.

2. The bio-information signal read by the EDSD is a very direct and true description of the condition of the body because it is created by the body.

3. The meridian network regulates or at least participates in every type of bodily function, so naturally it is a very good means by which to monitor the function of the whole body.

4. Medicine testing allows the doctor to test any and every type of medication on the individual patient, including those made from herbs, metals, nosodes, or sarcodes. This allows the doctor

to explore all types of available treatment and determine possible side effects with no risk to the patient.

Chapter 37

Chelation

A half century of research in structural chemistry, much of it focusing on the ability of some amino acids to form constant, stable bonds with metal ions, preceded the rapid development in the 1930s and 1940s of a new range of compounds, initially applied to industrial, and then increasingly to medical, uses.

First in Germany and then in the USA, different methods were developed for the production of chelating substances for specific industrial use, such as the prevention of calcium in hard water from causing staining or other problems in textile printing. Citric acid was commonly used for this purpose until first a compound known as NTA, and then EDTA (ethylenediaminetetraacetic acid), were developed and patented to do the job more efficiently.

During the Second World War research was carried out on sodium salts of EDTA in order to establish whether these would be useful as an antidote to poison gas. Earlier chelating compounds which had been used in this role, such as BAL (British antiLewisite), had proved effective when either externally applied or used systemically in neutralizing the arsenic in poison gas, but had themselves been found to be severely toxic in other ways.

A compound of sodium citrate was used in 1941 to chelate lead from the bodies of people poisoned by this heavy metal and later research

"The History of EDTA," an undated document by Leon Chaitow, N.D., D.O., M.R.O., cited December 2001, © Leon Chaitow, N.D., D.O., M.R.O.; reprinted with permission. Dr. Chaitow is Editor-in-chief, *Journal of Therapeutic Bodywork*, and a senior lecturer at the University of Westminster, London.

established that EDTA contained a highly effective antidote to heavy metal toxicity (lead poisoning, for example), since it chelated just as well with lead as it did with calcium when it was infused into the bloodstream, and without any side effects.

It was at Georgetown University that Dr. Martin Rubin (who had studied under Frederick Bersworth, the major American pioneer researcher into EDTA) conducted the first research into the biological effects of EDTA on humans. These studies showed its effects on lowering calcium levels, although this had not been the objective of the work, which had focused on discovering its degree, or lack, of toxicity.

According to Dr. Rubin, who was the chief researcher into EDTA's applications in treatment of humans at that time, a Dr. Geschikter was the first to use an EDTA compound for treatment of a human. This work was also done at Georgetown University, using the chelating ability of EDTA to assist in the carrying into a patient of the heavy metal nickel with which it had been chemically bound in a vain attempt to treat an advanced tumor. There were sadly no benefits to the patient, but perhaps more importantly from the viewpoint of the benefits later seen with EDTA usage, there were no harmful effects either: all of the nickel EDTA complex which was put into the patient was found to be excreted via the urine, unchanged.

It was in the early 1950s that EDTA was first used in the treatment of lead poisoning, with pleasantly surprising and often dramatically unexpected results. Workers in battery factories frequently developed lead poisoning, as did sailors in the U.S. Navy who painted ships with lead based paint. Intravenous infusions of EDTA successfully dealt with this problem, and indeed to this day the Food and Drug Administration (FDA) in the USA suggests EDTA chelation as the ideal method of treating not only lead poisoning but also as the emergency treatment for hypercalcaemia. It was found that there was often a marked improvement in the circulatory status of patients with chronic lead poisoning, who also had atherosclerotic (atheromatous deposits in the arteries) conditions and who were being treated by EDTA infusion.

It is worth considering that it is not just these naval personnel who are at risk from lead toxicity. The degree of general human body contamination with lead is now at five hundred times the level of people living just two hundred years ago. Lead has many toxic effects on the body, one of the more serious being its ability to prevent the body's natural control of free radical activity which itself can result in circulatory incompetence as well as many other problems.

Research studies by doctors such as Belknap, Butler, Spencer, Foreman, Clarke, Dudley, Bechtel, Jick, Surawicz, Boyle, Perry, Kitchell and many more, published in the early and middle 1950s, all relate to aspects of the treatment of arterial disease using EDTA.

Since those pioneering days, techniques have evolved and have been improved for the successful application of EDTA chelation treatment of the disastrous effects not only of atherosclerosis, but also of circulatory obstructions to the brain in people with some forms of senility. Similar benefits have often been observed amongst those who have experienced cerebral accidents (stroke) or who are suffering from early gangrenous conditions. Relief and marked symptomatic improvement has been gained in countless instances of high blood pressure (essential hypertension) and problems involving peripheral circulation (Reynaud's disease) as well as occlusion of blood flow to the extremities (intermittent claudication).

A description of one of the earliest uses of EDTA in treating chronic cardiovascular disease was given in 1976 by Dr. Norman Clarke, Sr., to the California Medical Association, in testimony before its Advisory Panel on Internal Medicine. He described his introduction to the process by research doctors (Drs. Albert Boyle and Gordon Myers) at Wayne University, Detroit in 1953: They had had preliminary experience in treating two patients at University Hospital, Detroit, who had calcified mitral valves. The patients were almost completely incapacitated . . . the doctors were very pleased with the results [of chelation treatment] because they obtained very satisfactory return of cardiac function.

Dr. Clarke spent many years investigating EDTA's usefulness in treating cardiovascular disease, and in his evidence stated: "In the last 28 years of my experience with EDTA chelation I have given at least 100,000 to 120,000 infusions of EDTA and seen nobody harmed."

He dramatically described the successful treatment of gangrene using EDTA, perfused directly into the site via a drip into the femoral artery, as well as this method's usefulness in cerebrovascular senility: "After all these years, and with all that experience, I am just as certain as can be that EDTA chelation therapy is the best treatment that has ever been brought out for occlusive vascular disease."

Other Benefits from EDTA Infusion

Just as the use of EDTA in treating lead poisoning revealed its ability to remove unwanted calcium, so additional benefits were discovered when circulatory conditions were being treated. Many patients with osteoarthritis and similar problems reported relief of symptoms and an improved range of movement in previously restricted joints.

359

It seems that obstructive calcium deposits in these areas were also being removed during chelation treatment.

Other unexpected benefits which chelation therapy has produced in many patients include a reduction in the amount of insulin which diabetics require to maintain a stable condition, as well as marked improvements in many patients with kidney dysfunction. More surprisingly, perhaps, a great deal of functional improvement in patients with Alzheimer's disease and Parkinson's disease is sometimes seen. Just how chelation could help in these states is not clear, apart from the unpredictable benefits of circulatory enhancement, and it may be that patients who appear to find relief from the symptoms of Alzheimer's and Parkinson's diseases might have had a faulty diagnosis, despite displaying all the classical signs associated with them.

New York studies on hyperactive children, using EDTA, have shown remarkable benefits, thought to relate to the removal of lead which may have accumulated in greater quantities in some of these children, due to their relative deficiency of major protective nutrients such as zinc and vitamin C, not uncommonly observed in such children.

There is also well documented Swiss evidence of chelation therapy offering marked protection against the development of cancer as well as a suggestion that it could be useful in treating some forms of this disease.

Safety

The safety aspect of the use of EDTA in therapy has been phenomenal, with hardly any serious reactions being recorded amongst the host of seriously ill people to whom chelation therapy has been correctly applied.

By 1980 it was estimated by Bruce Halstead, MD, (Halstead 1979) that there had been over 2 million applications of EDTA therapy involving some 100 million infusions, with not a single fatality, in the USA alone. The most effective use of EDTA chelation therapy has, over the 30 years of its successful application, been consistently found to be related to those diseases in which heavy metal or calcium deposits are major factors.

Have there been double blind trials, the yardstick by which so much in medicine is judged? Hardly any, because, as Halstead states: "It is impossible to administer EDTA blindly (i.e., so that neither the doctor nor the patient knows whether real EDTA or a substitute is being used), because it can be readily differentiated from an innocuous placebo by even one unacquainted with the compound."

This is a major obstacle to its acceptance by mainstream medicine, but should not prevent those interested in its claims from examining the objective evidence. It should not require double blind control studies to impress the observer with the possibility that people are actually getting better when severely ill people, with advanced circulatory problems, sometimes involving gangrene, show steady improvement in their functions, better muscular coordination, the disappearance of angina pain, increased ability to walk and work, restoration or improvement of brain function, better skin tone and more powerful arterial pulsations, along with the restoration of normal temperature in the extremities. This is particularly true in many patients who are slated to undergo bypass surgery, and this brings us close to one reason for orthodox medicine's rejection (in the main) of chelation's claims.

It might be that some of the simplistic theories as to how EDTA achieved its results may have prevented some scientists and physicians from taking it seriously or of investigating its potential. The current theories as to how calcium is encouraged to leave atheromatous deposits in blocked arteries have been well investigated by the proponents of chelation therapy and deserve to be seriously considered in view of the vast amount of illness attached to this area of human suffering and the remarkable results demonstrated by chelation physicians.

Bypass surgery and drug treatment of the conditions which chelation so often effectively deals with are very big business indeed. In the USA alone, $4 billion is the current turnover per annum of the bypass industry. A lesser, but nevertheless enormous, sum is involved in medication for conditions which the relatively cheap (and now out of patent) substance EDTA can be shown to help. Such vested interests should not be underestimated when it comes to the lengths to which they will go to try to discredit methods which threaten their stranglehold on the "market." Chelation therapy continues to grow, however, as public awareness and knowledge increases of this safe alternative to surgery and drugs, many of which are of questionable safety and value.

Chapter 38

Dance Therapy

Dance is the most fundamental of the arts, involving direct expression through the body. Thus, it is an intimate and powerful medium for therapy. Based on the assumption that body and mind are interrelated, dance/movement therapy is defined by the American Dance Therapy Association as "the psychotherapeutic use of movement as a process which furthers the emotional, cognitive and physical integration of the individual." Dance/movement therapy effects changes in feelings, cognition, physical functioning, and behavior.

Dance as therapy came into existence in the 1940s, especially through the pioneering efforts of Marian Chace. Psychiatrists in Washington, D.C., found that their patients were deriving benefits from attending Chace's unique dance classes. As a result, Chace was asked to work on the back wards of St. Elizabeth's Hospital with patients who had been considered too disturbed to participate in regular group activities. A non-verbal group approach was needed and dance/movement therapy met that need.

The American Dance Therapy Association (ADTA) was founded in 1966 by 73 charter members in 15 states. Now, the Association has grown to nearly 1200 members in 46 states and 20 foreign countries. ADTA maintains a registry of dance/movement therapists who meet specific educational and clinical practice standards. The title "Dance

---

"Dance/Movement Therapy," an undated document cited January 2002, available online at http://www.ncata.com/dance.html, © National Coalition of Arts Therapies Association (NCATA); reprinted with permission.

Therapist Registered" (DTR) is granted to entry-level dance/movement therapists who have a master's degree which includes 700 hours of supervised clinical internship. The advanced level of registry, Academy of Dance Therapists Registered (ADTR), is awarded only after DTRs have completed 3,640 hours of supervised clinical work in an agency, institution, or special school, with additional supervision from an ADTR. In addition, as part of their written application for review by the credentials committee, applicants for ADTR must document their understanding of theory and practice.

The association has a code of ethics and has established standards for professional practice, education and training. Dance/movement therapy academic programs stress coursework in dance/movement therapy theory and practice, movement observation and analysis, human development, psychopathology, cultural diversity, research skills, and group work. In 1979, ADTA established an approval process for the purpose of evaluating these programs. Research and scholarly writings are published in the *American Journal of Dance Therapy* and in publications funded by the Marian Chace Memorial Fund of the ADTA.

Today, in addition to those with severe emotional disorders, people of all ages and varying conditions receive dance/movement therapy. Examples of these are individuals with eating disorders, adult survivors of violence, sexually and physically abused children, dysfunctional families, the homeless, autistic children, the frail elderly, and substance abusers.

An evolving area of specialization is using dance/movement therapy in disease prevention and health promotion programs and with those who have chronic medical conditions. Many innovative programs provide dance/movement therapy for people with cardiovascular disease, hypertension, chronic pain, or breast cancer.

Research has been undertaken on the effects of dance/movement therapy in special settings (such as prisons and centers for the homeless) and with specific populations including the learning disabled, frail elderly, emotionally disturbed, depressed and suicidal, mentally retarded, substance abusers, visually and hearing impaired, psychotic, and autistic. Those with physical problems (such as amputations, traumatic brain injury, stroke, and chronic pain) and with chronic illnesses (such as anorexia and bulimia, cancer, Alzheimer's disease, cystic fibrosis, heart disease, diabetes, asthma, AIDS, and arthritis) have also been studied.

In institutions, dance/movement therapists may work as administrators as well as clinicians. Dance/movement therapists who are

ADTRs in good standing are also qualified to teach, provide supervision, and engage in private practice.

For further information contact:

The American Dance Therapy Association, Inc.
2000 Century Plaza, Suite 108
Columbia, MD 21044
Tel: 410-997-4040
Fax: 410-997-4048
Internet: http://www.ncata.com
E-Mail: adta@adta.org

Chapter 39

Massage Therapy

Whether seeking relief for a medical condition, searching for a method to help deal with the stresses of daily life or wanting to maintain good health, more and more Americans are turning to therapeutic massage.

Massage doesn't just feel good. Research shows it reduces the heart rate, lowers blood pressure, increases blood circulation and lymph flow, relaxes muscles, improves range of motion, and increases endorphins, the body's natural painkillers. Therapeutic massage may enhance medical treatment and helps people feel less anxious and stressed, relaxed yet more alert.

A writer for the *Chicago Tribune* stated, "Massage is to the human body what a tune-up is to a car." Therapeutic massage can be part of your regular healthcare maintenance.

The consumer demand for massage therapy is fed by the health and fitness movement as well complementary alternative care. Both the demand and the healthcare profession's response are overwhelming:

> Consumers spend $4 billion to $6 billion a year on visits to massage therapists, according to an American Massage Therapy Association (AMTA) analysis of a study by Beth Israel Deaconess Medical Center and Harvard Medical School

"Massage Therapy Enhancing Your Health with Therapeutic Massage," and "Demand for Massage Therapy," used with permission of the American Massage Therapy Association®, © 2001.

published in the *Journal of the American Medical Association* in November 1998.

Current research shows people are getting more massages, and that therapeutic massage has become mainstream, appealing to everyone from young adults to seniors. People are experiencing the therapeutic benefits of massage and report getting massages mostly to relax, relieve aches and pains, and help reduce stress.

A national survey of consumers attitudes about massage, conducted by Opinion Research Corporation International in July 2000, found that, among those people who discussed massage with their primary healthcare provider, 71 percent reported the conversation was favorable and 20 percent found the response from their doctor to be neutral.

The American Massage Therapy Association's membership quadrupled in ten years, to more than 44,000 in 2000.

There also is a growing trend of offering therapeutic massage in the workplace. Your employer may be among those who have learned that massage therapy isn't just a perk, but actually increases employee productivity and morale, and reduces absenteeism.

According to a 1996 survey of employees who regularly receive therapeutic massage onsite at Reebok International Ltd., 98 percent said it helped them reduce work-related stress; 92 percent said it increased alertness, motivation and productivity; 83 percent said it had in some cases sufficiently addressed a problem so medical attention was not necessary; and 66 percent said it had enabled them to stay at work when they would have otherwise gone home sick.

What Is Therapeutic Massage?

Therapeutic massage involves the manipulation of the soft tissue structures of the body to prevent and alleviate pain, discomfort, muscle spasm, and stress; and, to promote health and wellness. AMTA defines massage therapy as a profession in which the practitioner applies manual techniques, and may apply adjunctive therapies, with the intention of positively affecting the health and well-being of the client.

Massage therapy improves functioning of the circulatory, lymphatic, muscular, skeletal, and nervous systems and may improve the rate at which the body recovers from injury and illness. Massage involves holding, causing movement of soft tissue, and/or applying pressure to the body. It comes in many forms, including:

- *Swedish*—a gentle, relaxing massage;
- *Pressure point therapy*—for certain conditions for injuries; and
- *Sports massage*—focuses on muscle groups relevant to the particular sport.

How Can Massage Be Medically Beneficial?

People find that therapeutic massage can help with a wide range of medical conditions, including:

- Allergies
- Anxiety and stress
- Arthritis (osteoarthritis and rheumatoid arthritis)
- Asthma and bronchitis
- Carpal tunnel syndrome
- Chronic and temporary pain
- Circulatory problems
- Depression
- Digestive disorders, including spastic colon, constipation and diarrhea
- Headache, especially when due to muscle tension
- Insomnia
- Myofascial pain (a condition of the tissue connecting the muscles)
- Reduced range of motion
- Sinusitis
- Sports injuries, including pulled or strained muscles and sprained ligaments
- Temporomandibular joint dysfunction (TMJ)

Although massage therapy does not increase muscle strength, it can stimulate weak, inactive muscles and, thus, partially compensate for the lack of exercise and inactivity resulting from illness or injury.

It also can hasten and lead to a more complete recovery from exercise or injury.

Therapeutic massage may not be recommended in some cases, such as in people with:

- inflammation of the veins (phlebitis)
- infectious diseases
- certain forms of cancer
- some skin conditions
- some cardiac problems
- diabetes

If you have one of these or some other diagnosed medical condition, always check with your doctor before seeking a massage.

What Does Research Show about Massage Therapy?

Research on the effects of massage therapy has been ongoing for more than 120 years. A surge in research over the past 20 years has resulted in more than 2,500 published studies.

At the University of Miami School of Medicine's Touch Research Institute, 70 studies on touch—the majority on massage therapy—have been published or are under way. Recent and ongoing research at some of the nation's hospitals, such as Cedars Sinai Medical Center in Los Angeles, is expanding knowledge of the benefits of massage for a variety of injuries and ailments.

Among research findings:

- Massage increases activity level of the body's natural "killer cells," boosting the immune system.
- Office workers massaged regularly were more alert, performed better and were less stressed than those who weren't massaged.
- Massage therapy decreased the effects of anxiety, tension, depression, pain, and itching in burn patients.
- Abdominal surgery patients recovered more quickly after massage.
- Premature infants who were massaged gained more weight and fared better than those who weren't.
- Autistic children showed less erratic behavior after massage therapy.

AMTA, the international 45,000-member professional association for massage therapists, supports research through the AMTA Foundation. AMTA and the AMTA Foundation helped fund research at the Center for Alternative Medicine Research at Boston's Beth Israel Deaconess Medical Center on the use of therapeutic massage for lower back pain. The AMTA Foundation has awarded more than $320,000 since its inception in 1993, to fund massage therapy-related research, community outreach and educational scholarships.

What Is the Cost of Massage Therapy and Will My Insurance Cover It?

While cost depends on the locality, type and length of the massage and the experience of the therapist, fees generally start from $60 an hour.

Responding to consumer demand, many health insurance plans now cover massage provided by a massage therapist or provide "carve out" discount programs for massage. Many Blue Cross and Blue Shield medical plans now offer such discount programs for massage. In a 1998-99 survey of 114 HMOs, by Landmark Healthcare, 11 percent of the HMOs surveyed said they cover therapeutic massage. Some of the largest managed care organizations, including Aetna US Healthcare, Kaiser Permanente and United Healthcare cover massage and other complementary therapies.

The state of Washington requires insurance plans to include every category of regulated healthcare provider in their provider networks, including massage therapists.

Massage therapy is currently regulated in 30 states and the District of Columbia. The remaining states leave any regulation of massage therapy to local municipalities. Statewide regulation of massage therapists may determine if your insurance directly covers massage by a massage therapist. Workers compensation and auto insurance Personal Injury Protection coverage usually cover therapeutic massage.

Check with your healthcare insurance provider. Once massage therapy is prescribed, you or your doctor may need to seek authorization from the insurer if coverage is not clearly spelled out in your policy or plan.

What Can You Expect?

The first appointment generally begins with the massage therapist asking what prompted you to get a massage, your current physical condition, medical history, lifestyle, stress level, and painful areas.

The massage therapist may ask you about your health goals and what you hope the massage will do to help you achieve those goals.

For a full-body massage, you will be asked to remove clothing to your level of comfort. Undressing takes place in private, and a sheet, towel or gown is provided for draping. The therapist will undrape only the part of your body being massaged, ensuring that your modesty is respected at all times. Your massage will take place in a comfortable atmosphere and on a cushioned table. You should expect a peaceful, relaxing experience.

Some massages, such as those onsite at your place of business, are done while you are fully clothed. For this type of massage, often called "seated" massage, you will sit in a specially designed portable chair.

How Can You Find a Qualified Massage Therapist?

Founded in 1943, the American Massage Therapy Association has more than 45,000 members in 30 countries. The Association also offers consumer education materials about the benefits of massage. AMTA has strict membership requirements and also has a Code of Ethics and practice standards that promote the highest quality assurance in the profession.

Physical Benefits of Therapeutic Massage

- Helps relieve stress and aids relaxation
- Helps relieve muscle tension and stiffness
- Fosters faster healing of strained muscles and sprained ligaments; reduces pain and swelling; reduces formation of excessive scar tissue
- Reduces muscle spasms
- Provides greater joint flexibility and range of motion
- Enhances athletic performance
- Promotes deeper and easier breathing
- Improves circulation of blood and movement of lymph fluids
- Reduces blood pressure
- Helps relieve tension-related headaches and the effects of eyestrain
- Enhances the health and nourishment of skin

- Improves posture
- Strengthens the immune system

Massage Therapy and Well-Being: Mental Benefits

- Fosters peace of mind
- Promotes a relaxed state of mental alertness
- Helps relieve mental stress
- Improves ability to monitor stress signals and respond appropriately
- Enhances capacity for calm thinking and creativity
- Satisfies needs for caring—nurturing touch
- Fosters a feeling of well-being
- Reduces levels of anxiety
- Increases awareness of mind-body connection

Public Interest in and Use of Massage Continues to Increase

The cost of healthcare in the United States is estimated to reach $2.2 trillion by 2008 from 1.6 trillion in 1998. Consumers spend between $4 and $6 billion annually on visits to massage therapists—approximately 27% of the $21.2 billion spent on unconventional healthcare in 1997. Consumers visit massage therapists 114 million times each year. About 18% of the 629 million annual visits to alternative healthcare providers. There are numerous indications that massage therapy is gaining acceptance and growing.

Of the types of alternative care explored, people say they would be most likely to use massage therapy (80%), vitamin therapy (80%), herbal therapy (75%), and chiropractic (73%). 54% of primary care physicians and family practitioners say they would encourage their patients to pursue massage therapy as a complement to medical treatment. HMO members using complementary and alternative medicine services rate their satisfaction with HMO-defined acupuncture, naturopathic, and massage benefits as high. 78 of this country's 125 medical schools—including Harvard, Yale, Stanford, Georgetown, and Johns Hopkins—now offer courses in alternative medicine, up from 27 in 1995.

A total of 27% of the adult U.S. population reports having massages in the past 5 years, 15% in the past 12 months. Massage has become increasingly popular among consumers over 45, being used by about a third of this age group versus a quarter of those younger. Massage is also popular among consumers 25 to 34. Those who seek massage therapy from a trained professional average 7 visits per year. Many companies (e.g. G.E., Goldman Sachs, Young & Rubicam, Motorola, and American Airlines) are inviting massage therapists on-site as an employment perk and as a means of reducing stress and absenteeism.

Among organization benefits managers, 8% report that massage is an employee benefit. The number of massage therapists is between 160,000 and 220,000, including students. American Massage Therapy Association's membership increased more than fourfold in the 1990s to over 41,000 members.

Massage Therapy: Massage Has Become Mainstream

American adults are having many more massages than they did even a year ago, pointing to a trend that therapeutic massage is increasingly accepted and appreciated. Consumers visit massage therapists 114 million times each year. Massage is sought out by large numbers of people in all age brackets. Massage is equally popular among men and women in all regions of the country and across most incomes.

Massage is popular among people with some college education (31%) and people with only a high school education (16%), but more popular among college graduates (35%). People earning more than $50,000 are having massages most often (34%). The massage explosion can be attributed partly to the growing population of tired, aging, not-quite-as-limber-as-they-once-were baby boomers, partly to an increased awareness of the effects of stress and of the physiological benefits of "pressing the flesh."

More working-class professionals are using massage therapy to relieve stress and treat sore muscles. Massage therapists that once served only elite professionals or athletes see a wider range of clientele. Doctors are prescribing massage to help patients manage stress and pain. Among emergency room patients, 31% report that they have used massage in the past for painful conditions.

Sports Massage Boosts Athletic Performance

Many athletes are extolling the benefits of massage. More sports teams have begun to hire massage therapists. Many prominent professional athletes rely on massage to help them recover from injuries and muscle soreness.

Massage Therapy: On-Site Massage Offered in the Workplace

The Touch Research Institute at the University of Miami (TRI) has documented the positive effects of massage therapy on job performance and stress reduction. The research indicates that a basic 15-minute chair massage, provided twice weekly, results in decreased job stress and significant increase in productivity. A growing number of businesses and organizations offer massage in the workplace, including the U.S. Department of Justice.

At Boeing and Reebok, headaches, back strain, and fatigue have all fallen since the companies started bringing in massage therapists. More than 80 companies, including many Fortune 500 companies, are using massage therapy to counter such ills as musculoskeletal problems, stress and poor ergonomic design of furniture. By including 15 minutes of free massage therapy once each week, the Calvert Group, an investment firm in Bethesda, MD, reduced its turnover rate to 5% in an industry where the norm is 20%.

Studies show that patients make more visits each year to alternative care practitioners (629 million times per year) than to primary care physicians (386 million), and most of them pay out of their own pockets for the care they receive. More than four in ten adults in the United States (42%) have used some type of alternative healthcare in the past year and many report a likelihood of future usage. Nearly one-half of adults in the United States (45%) say they would be willing to pay more each month to have access to alternative care, and most people (67%) believe the availability of alternative care is an important factor when choosing a health plan.

A survey by the Office of Alternative Medicine found that over half of the conventional physicians in the United States have recommended or tried alternative medicine. Studies show that better-educated, affluent individuals seek out and use alternative medicine more than the less-educated and poor.

Glossary of Terms

Cranio-Sacral is a technique for finding and correcting cerebral and spinal imbalances or blockages that may cause sensory, motor or intellectual dysfunction.

Deep Tissue releases the chronic patterns of tension in the body through slow strokes and deep finger pressure on the contracted areas, either following or going across the grain of muscles, tendons and fascia. It is called deep tissue because it also focuses on the deeper layers of muscle tissue.

Reflexology (zone therapy) is organized around a system of points on the hands and feet that are thought to correspond, or "reflex," to all areas of the body. Though the massage is specific to an area, it is intended to affect the whole body.

Shiatsu and Acupressure are systems of finger-pressure massage, based on Oriental healing concepts, which treat special points along "meridians," the invisible channels of energy flow in the body. Energy blocked along these meridians can cause physical discomfort, so the aim is to release the blockage and re-balance the energy flow. They can be used for the full body or for specific areas of the body.

Sports Massage Therapy is classified into three main categories: maintenance, event and rehabilitation. Maintenance massage is a regular program of massage to help the athlete reach optimal performance through injury-free training. Event massage takes place before, during and/or after competition to supplement an athlete's warm-up, readying the athlete for top performance, and/or to reduce the muscle spasms and metabolic build-up that occurs with vigorous exercise. Such techniques enhance the body's recovery process, improving the athletes return to high-level training and competition, and reducing the risk of injury. Rehabilitation massage techniques are effective in the management of both acute and chronic injuries.

Massage Therapy is a profession in which the practitioner applies manual techniques, and may apply adjunctive therapies, with the intention of positively affecting the health and well-being of the client.

Swedish Massage uses a system of long strokes, kneading, and friction percussive and vibration techniques on the more superficial layers of muscles, combined with active and passive movements of the joints. It is used primarily for full-body sessions and promotes general relaxation, improves blood circulation and range of motion, and relieves muscle tension. Swedish is the most common type of massage.

Trigger Point Therapy (also known as Myotherapy or Neuromuscular Therapy) applies concentrated finger pressure to "trigger points" (painful irritated areas in muscles) to break cycles of spasm and pain.

Chapter 40

Qigong (Ch'i Kung) and T'ai Chi (Taiji)

Qigong (Ch'i Kung)

The history of Qigong (Ch'i Kung) commences beyond the era of written records, in the mists of prehistory. Earliest estimates suggest that self enhancement and empowerment practices date into the time of Chinese shamans, previous to 500 BCE.

While Qigong has strong roots into mystical and philosophical ground, the practical healing and stress management applications are the most popular aspects of the tradition in China today. Both the health and spiritual applications are rapidly gaining in popularity in the Western world as people realize that disease and stress are relieved by peace of mind.

Qigong is one of the four pillars of traditional Chinese medicine: Acupuncture, Massage, Herbal Medicines and Qigong. Of these, Qigong is the one that can be most easily self initiated. Both massage and herbal remedies can also be done as self care, however, Qigong is the mother of Chinese self healing. Patients who use Qigong faithfully need less medication, less acupuncture and heal faster.

"Qigong (Ch'i Kung)," and "Taiji (T'ai Chi)," undated documents by Roger Janke, O.M.D., © Roger Janke, O.M.D. Roger Jahnke is the author of *The Healer Within* (Harper Collins, December 1997) and the soon to be published, *The Healing Promise of Qi* (Contemporary Books, 2002). For more information, go to http://www.healerwithin.com or http://www.qigong-chikung.com or contact The Integral Tai Chi & Qigong Institute, 243 Pebble Beach Santa Barbara, CA 93117, 800-824-4325; cited January 2002; reprinted with permission.

The word Qigong breaks into Qi and Gong: Qi = vitality, energy, life force, Gong = practice, cultivate, refine; Qigong = to cultivate and refine through practice one's vitality or life force. The Chinese believe that the primary mechanism that is triggered by the practice of Qigong is a spontaneous balancing and enhancing of the natural healing resources in the human system. Over thousands of years millions of people have benefited from these practices believing that improving the function of the Qi maintains health and heals disease.

In the paradigm of mechanistic Western science, the practice of Qigong triggers a wide array of physiological mechanisms which have profound healing benefits. It increases the delivery of oxygen to the tissues. It enhances the elimination of waste products as well as the transportation of immune cells through the lymph system. And it shifts the chemistry of the brain and the nervous system.

There are various estimates for the number of varieties of Qigong. There are at least a thousand. Some elaborate and complex, some mysterious and esoteric and some simple and practical. If you adjust to a relaxed, upright posture, take a deep breath and relax your mind—you are already doing Qigong. Try this: sit up, relax your body, take a deep breath, rest your mind for just a moment. Already you are stimulating an automatic self healing response.

On any morning in the parks throughout China you will find literally thousands of people doing Qigong practices. Some practice individually quietly among the trees. Others practice in large groups of hundreds or even thousands. Often, one will see a patient, in hospital pajamas, doing a special form of cancer recovery Qigong-ta form of slow and intentful walking. Or a group might stand in a circle chatting as they do a simple form based on hand movements.

Qigong is one of the most powerful self healing traditions ever developed in human history. It is literally a health wonder of the world.

Taiji (T'ai Chi)

The roots of Taiji (T'ai Chi) go deep into Chinese history. Taiji was originally a martial arts practice called Taijiquan (T'ai Chi Chuan). Quan (Chuan) means fist or boxing. The art has a legendary beginning in the philosophy of Daoism (Taoism). Its origin comes as a part of the history of Zhang, Zhan-feng (Chang San-feng) who was highly enlightened, which allowed him the title of Immortal. Some argue that Zhang was mythic, others that he was historic.

He discovered the Taijiquan in a dream and proved its value by killing a hundred bandits in the Wu Dan Mountains in Hubei Province.

Taijiquan combines the martial skill of Immortal Zhang and his devotion to the deepest principles of Daoism (Taoism). Taiji has evolved in three directions.

Due to its rich heritage in Daoist spirituality, it is a method for spiritual growth. Due to its profound utility as a fighting art it has become the martial art of choice for many serious fighters. In the middle and common to both is Taiji's powerful application as a self-healing tool.

In Chinese tradition there are thousands of methods and practices for self healing generally called Qigong (Ch'i Kung). Taiji is one category of Qigong forms. Taiji consists generally of 108 separate movements that are connected together into a specific order. There are several kinds of Taiji including: Yang Style, Chen Style, Wu Style and others. Most of these forms of Taiji have created a short form, between 20 and 40 movements, that allows for beginners to learn more quickly, elders to have an abbreviated practice and patients who are ill to practice without too much to learn.

The practice triggers health and healing benefits from both the Asian paradigm of energy and the Western paradigm of physiology. The balance and flow of one's internal self healing energies is enhanced by the slow, intentful, meditative movements of Taiji. At the very same time the delivery of oxygen and nutrition from the blood to the tissues is improved. The lymph system's ability to eliminate metabolic by-products and transport immune cells is increased. The biochemical profile of the brain and nervous system is shifted toward recovery and healing.

During the Cultural Revolution in the 1960's, a very dark time in Chinese history, all forms of Qigong that were intellectually or spiritually based became crimes against the "people." Most forms of Taiji were outlawed as well. After this era certain aspects of China's ancient tradition were recovered. For a short period of time Taiji was the only "party certified" system of health enhancement, usually Yang Style Taiji.

As it became clear that many forms of Qigong were beneficial to people's health, the various forms of Taiji re-emerged. Now in China literally millions of citizens practice Taiji every day; some singularly, some in groups numbering into the hundreds, some with swords, some with large red fans.

Because of the widespread popularity of the Taiji concept outside of China, it is typical for people to think of Taiji when thinking of self healing practices from China. However, it is important to remember that there are many self-healing practices from the Chinese tradition.

379

There is a lengthy learning process associated with most forms of Taiji. It may be advisable for some people to explore a number of the more simple Qigong forms, particularly those who are extremely busy, older or dealing with illness.

Chapter 41

Reflexology

What Is Reflexology?

The ancient healing art of reflexology has been known to man for many thousands of years. It was first practiced by the early Indian, Chinese and Egyptian peoples.

In 1913 Dr. William Fitzgerald, an American ear, nose and throat surgeon, introduced this therapy to the West. He noted that pressure on specific parts of the body could have an anaesthetizing effect on a related area. Developing this theory, he divided the body into ten equal and vertical zones, ending in the fingers and toes. He concluded that pressure on one part of a zone could affect everything else within that zone. Thus, reflex areas on the feet and hands are linked to other areas and organs of the body within the same zone.

In the 1930's, Eunice Ingham, a therapist, further developed and refined the zone therapy into what is now known as foot reflexology. She observed that congestion or tension in any part of the foot mirrors congestion or tension in a corresponding part of the body. Thus, when you treat the big toes there is a related effect in the head, and treating the whole foot can have a relaxing and healing effect on the whole body.

How Can Reflexology Help You?

The body has the ability to heal itself. Following illness, stress, injury or disease, it is in a state of "imbalance," and vital energy pathways

"The Healing Art of Reflexology," © 1998 Association of Reflexologists, 27 Old Gloucester Street, London WC1N 3XX, England; reprinted with permission.

are blocked, preventing the body from functioning effectively. Reflexology can be used to restore and maintain the body's natural equilibrium and encourage healing.

A reflexologist uses hands only to apply gentle pressure to the feet. For each person the application and the effect of the therapy is unique. Sensitive, trained hands can detect tiny deposits and imbalances in the feet, and by working on these points the reflexologist can release blockages and restore the free flow of energy to the whole body. Tensions are eased, and circulation and elimination is improved. This gentle therapy encourages the body to heal itself at its own pace, often counteracting a lifetime of misuse.

Who Can Benefit from Reflexology?

Since reflexology treats the whole person, not the symptoms of disease, most people benefit from treatment. The therapy brings relief to a wide range of acute and chronic conditions, and is suitable for all ages. Once your body is in-tune, it is wise to have regular treatments in order to help maintain health and well-being. An increasing number of people are using this safe, natural therapy as a way of relaxing, balancing and harmonizing the body.

What Happens When You Go for Treatment?

On your first visit there is a preliminary talk with the practitioner. The reflexologist then begins to work on your feet, or hands if necessary, noting problem areas. There may be discomfort in some places, but it is fleeting, and is an indication of congestion or imbalance in a corresponding part of the body. For the most part, the sensation is pleasant and soothing. Reflexology will relax you while stimulating the body's own healing mechanisms.

Usually a treatment session lasts for about one hour. A course of treatment varies in length depending on your body's needs. Your reflexologist will discuss this with you at the first session. After the first treatment or two your body may respond in a very definite way: you may have a feeling of well-being and relaxation; or you may feel lethargic, nauseous or tearful, but this is transitory. It is, however, vital information for reflexologists, as it shows how your body is responding to treatment.

Please ensure that your practitioner is professionally qualified and a member of a bona fide organization.

Chapter 42

Reiki

Where does Reiki energy come from?

Reiki energy is a subtle energy. It is different than electricity or chemical energy or other kinds of physical energy. Reiki energy comes from the Higher Power, which exists on a higher dimension than the physical world we are familiar with. When viewed clairvoyantly, Reiki energy appears to come down from above and to enter the top of the practitioners head after which if flows through the body and out the hands. It appears to flow this way because of our perspective. However, the true source of Reiki energy is within ourselves. This does not mean that we use our personal energy when we do Reiki, but that the energy is coming from a transcendental part of ourselves that is connected to an infinite supply of healing energy.

Is Reiki a religion?

Although Reiki energy is spiritual in nature, Reiki is not a religion. Practitioners are not asked to change any religious or spiritual beliefs they may have. They are free to continue believing anything they choose and are encouraged to make their own decisions concerning the nature of their religious practices.

"Reiki, Questions & Answers," © 1999 The International Center for Reiki Training (Southfield, MI); reprinted with permission.

How is a Reiki treatment given?

In a standard treatment Reiki energy flows from the practitioners hands into the client. The client is usually laying on a massage table but treatments can also be given while the client is seated or even standing. The client remains fully clothed. The practitioner places her/his hands on or near the clients body in a series of hand positions. These include positions around the head and shoulders, the stomach, and feet. Other, more specific positions may be used based on the clients needs. Each position is held for three to ten minutes depending on how much Reiki the client needs at each position. The whole treatment usually lasts between 45 and 90 minutes.

What does a Reiki treatment feel like?

What one experiences during a Reiki treatment varies somewhat from person to person. However, feelings of deep relaxation are usually felt by all. In addition, many feel a wonderful glowing radiance that flows through and surrounds the them. As the Reiki energy encourages one to let go of all tension, anxiety, fear or other negative feelings a state of peace and well-being is experienced. Some drift off to sleep or report floating outside their bodies or have visions and other mystical experiences. At the end of the treatment, one feels refreshed with a more positive, balanced outlook.

What can be treated with Reiki?

Reiki has had a positive affect on all forms of illness and negative conditions. This includes minor things like head or stomach aches, bee stings, colds, flu, tension and anxiety as well as serious illness like heart disease, cancer, leukemia, etc. The side effects of regular medical treatments have also been reduced or eliminated. This includes the negative effects of chemotherapy, post operative pain and depression as well as improving the healing rate and reducing the time needed to stay in the hospital. Reiki always helps and in some cases people have experienced complete healings which have been confirmed by medical tests before and after the Reiki treatments. However, while some have experienced miracles, they cannot be guaranteed. Stress reduction with some improvement in ones physical and psychological condition are what most experience.

Does one have to stop seeing a regular doctor or psychologist in order to receive a Reiki treatment?

No. Reiki works in conjunction with regular medical or psychological treatment. If one has a medical or psychological condition, it is recommended that one see a licensed health care professional in addition to receiving Reiki treatments. Reiki energy works in harmony with all other forms of healing, including drugs, surgery, psychological care or any other method of alternative care and will improve the results.

Who can learn to do Reiki?

Reiki is a very simple technique to learn and is not dependent on one having any prior experience with healing, meditation or any other kind of training. It has be successfully learned by over one million people from all walks of life, both young an old. The reason it is so easy to learn that it is not taught in the usual way something is taught. The ability to do Reiki is simply transferred from the teacher to the student through a process called an attunement that takes place during a Reiki class. As soon as one receives an attunement, they have the ability to do Reiki and after that whenever one places their hands on themselves or on another person with the intention of doing Reiki, the healing energy will automatically begin flowing.

How long does it take to learn Reiki?

A beginning Reiki class is taught on a weekend. The class can be one or two days long. I recommend that the minimum time necessary be at least six to seven hours. Along with the attunement, it is necessary that the student be shown how to give treatments and also to practice giving treatments in class.

What is a Reiki attunement?

A Reiki attunement is the process by which a person receives the ability to give Reiki treatments. The attunement is administered by the Reiki Master during the Reiki class. During the attunement, the Reiki Master will touch the students head, shoulders, and hands and use one or more special breathing techniques. The attunement energies will flow through the Reiki Master and into the student. These special energies are guided by the Higher Power and make adjustments in the students energy pathways and connect the student to the source of Reiki. Because the energetic aspect of the attunement is guided by the Higher Power, it adjusts itself to be exactly right for each student. During the attunement, some students feel warmth in the hands, others may see colors or have visions of spiritual beings. However, it is not necessary to have an inner experience for the attunement to have worked. Most simply feel more relaxed.

Can I treat myself?

Yes, once you have received the attunement, you can treat yourself as well as others. This is one of the unique features of Reiki.

I have heard that Reiki can be sent to others at a distance. How does this work?

Yes, in Reiki II, you are given three Reiki symbols. These symbols are empowered by the Reiki II attunement. One of these symbols is for distant healing. By using a picture of the person you would like to send Reiki to or by writing the person's name on a piece of paper or simply by thinking of the person and also activating the distant symbol, you can send Reiki to them no matter where they are. They could be hundreds of miles away, but it makes no difference. The Reiki energy will go to them and treat them. You can also send Reiki to crisis situations or world leaders and the Reiki energy will help them too.

How many levels are there to the Reiki training?

In the Usui/Tibetan system of Reiki taught by the Center, there are four levels. These include one, two, Advanced and Master.

What does it feel like to give a treatment?

When giving a Reiki treatment, the Reiki energy flows through the practitioner before leaving the hands and flowing into the client. Because of this, the practitioner receives a treatment also. As the Reiki energy flows through the practitioner, she/he will feel more relaxed and uplifted. Spiritual experiences sometimes take place. The practitioner sometimes receives insights about what the client needs to know to heal more deeply.

How do I find a Reiki teacher that is right for me?

Reiki teachers or Masters advertise in many magazines and also post notices at health food stores, new age bookstores and other places.

Once you find a Reiki teacher or practitioner you are interested in receiving training or a treatment from, it is a good idea to ask them some important questions. Here are a few that will give you additional information to make a choice.

• How long have you been working with Reiki? What training have you had? How often do you teach? How do you personally use Reiki? What is your lineage?

• What qualifications are required to take Reiki Training?

• What do you cover in your classes? How many hours of class time is included? How much time is instructional, and how much is hands on practice?

• What are the specific things I will be able to do after taking the training?

• What are your fees, and will I get a certificate and a manual?

• Can I take notes and tape record the class?

• How many symbols will I learn?

• Is there a Reiki support group in my area or can you help me establish one?

• Will you openly support me in being a successful Reiki practitioner or Master?

• Do you have a positive respectful attitude toward other Reiki practitioners and Masters regardless of lineage or affiliation?

Be aware of how you feel about their answers and if they are responding in a loving manner that is supportive and empowering. Listen to your heart and you will be guided to the right teacher or practitioner.

Can children learn Reiki?

Yes, Reiki can be taught to anyone. I recommend that a child be old enough to understand what Reiki is and that the child request to receive Reiki.

Is it safe for pregnant woman?

Since Reiki is guided by the Higher Power, the Reiki energy will know the condition of the client or student and adjust appropriately.

Reiki can only do good. Many pregnant women have received treatments with great benefit to them and their unborn child. It has also been used during child birth. Pregnant women have also taken the Reiki training and received the Reiki attunement with beneficial results.

What about babies?

Babies love Reiki. It is very healthy for them. Do not worry about it being too strong. Reiki automatically adjusts to what the baby needs.

Can I treat animals or plants?

Animals love Reiki too. They seem to have a natural understanding of what Reiki is and its benefits. Once a pet has received a Reiki treatment, they will often let you know that they want more. Plants also respond well to Reiki.

Are there any side effects from a Reiki treatment?

Most of the time a person will feel relaxed and uplifted by a Reiki treatment. However, sometimes a person will have what is called a healing crisis. As a person's vibration goes up, toxins that have been stored in the body will be released into the blood stream to be filtered by the liver and kidneys and removed from the system. When this happens, sometimes a person can get a headache or stomach ache or feel weak. If this happens, it is a good idea to drink more water, eat lighter meals and get more rest. The body is cleansing as part of the healing process so this is a good sign.

Can it be used to help groups of people or even global crises?

Yes, this is one of the wonderful benefits of Reiki and is why it is such a wonderful technique for the new millennium. It allows individuals and groups to do something positive about the challenging situations we see on the news involving so many people all over the planet. Reiki can be used to reduce suffering and help people any where in the world. On our Reiki web site at www.reiki.org we list major world events to send Reiki to. As more and more people send Reiki to help the world heal, we will move quickly to a world of peace and harmony.

How much does a treatment usually cost?

A Reiki treatment usually will cost between $25.00 and $100.00 depending on the area of the country. However, some practitioners offer treatments free of charge or for a donation.

Can a person make a living from Reiki?

Yes, if you put your heart into it, you can develop a Reiki practice combined with teaching classes that can bring a regular income. This is a very fulfilling way to earn a living.

Can one become licensed to practice and teach Reiki?

There are no governmental licensing programs at this time. However, the Center does have a licensing program for Reiki teachers.

Does insurance cover Reiki treatments?

Reiki is just starting to be recognized by insurance companies. While not many are covering Reiki treatments, some are. Check with your local insurance company for details.

Can nurses or massage therapists get CEU credit for taking Reiki classes?

Classes taught by our Center Licensed Reiki teachers are approved to give CEU credits to nurses, massage therapists and athletic trainers.

Can you get more than one attunement?

Once you receive a Reiki attunement, it will last your whole life. However, if you get additional attunements for the same level, it will act to refine and strengthen your Reiki energy.

What is lineage?

Reiki is a technique that is passed on from teacher to student over and over. If one has Reiki, than she/he will be part of a secession of teachers leading back to the founder of the system of Reiki one is practicing. In the case of Usui Reiki, the lineage would lead back to Dr. Usui.

Chapter 43

Rolfing

What is Rolfing?

The term "Rolfing" refers to a system of body education and physical manipulation developed by Dr. Ida P. Rolf. It is a method of structural integration that is the product of 50 years of study by Dr. Rolf.

Through guided movements of the client, the Rolfer slowly stretches and repositions the body's fascia, which is the supportive wrapping of the body. This restores normal length and elasticity to the network of deep connective fibers of the fascia and allows these changes in the "wrapping" to occur.

The standard 10-session series may be completed at a rate of one session per week, or spread as long as six months. Sessions can last from 60 minutes to a little over one hour. The results of Rolfing are not only long lasting, they are progressive. Clients report feeling and looking better and better for several months after their last session.

The basic 10-session series does not ever need to be repeated, though people often continue Rolfing later with a three-session series of post 10-week work yearly. This supports an aging process that is more comfortable, more graceful and slower than we have seen previously. We suggest you wait at least six months to a year after your basic 10-series is completed before doing any post 10-week work in

"Questions and Answers," an undated document produced by Alberta Rolfing and Somatic Education Center, available online at http://www.rolfing-ab.com, © Alberta Rolfing and Somatic Education Center; cited January 2002; reprinted with permission.

order to give your body time to make the progressive changes mentioned above.

How old is Rolfing?

Dr. Ida Rolf was a pioneer in the study of the human condition.
She was a Ph.D. in Biochemistry in her early twenties in the 1920's,
when she began her research. She began Rolfing in the 1930's. By the
1950's she was presenting her work to the chiropractic community
throughout North America. In the late fifties and early sixties, she
began teaching "Rolfing" structural integration to pre med. students.
In 1971 the Rolf Institute of Structural Integration was founded. It
is a non-profit organization, focusing on the education and training
of Rolfers, public education of Rolfing and research.

Who benefits from Rolfing?

Athletes, dancers, students of yoga and meditation, musicians,
business people, people riddled with chronic pain and stress, people
from all walks of life and all ages come to Rolfing not only for relief
from their pain and stress, but also for improved performance in their
professions and everyday activities.

Rolfing can also benefit people in psychotherapy by facilitating a
deeper connection to their emotional conflicts, and it can effectively
deepen practices such as meditation, yoga and tai chi.

Who uses Rolfing? How does Rolfing feel?

The area of the body being worked can vary in sensations and feeling depending on the existence of chronic stress, injury and other factors. A new mindset has replaced the old in the Rolfing profession,
making pain a thing of the past. While the work can sometimes be
uncomfortable, it is no longer painful. A pleasure feeling of release
following momentary discomfort is the most common sensation.

Why have I not heard of it before?

The training and selection of Rolfers is a rather selective process
and currently there are approximately 1200 Rolfers in the world. The
international headquarters and educational institute is in Boulder
Colorado, with satellite schools in Munich, Germany and Sau Paulo,
Brazil. Only since the 1950's has Rolfing been researched, refined and
Rolfers trained in structural integration.

How does Rolfing differ from massage or chiropractic care?

In a simplistic manner, massage therapy focuses on working with the musculature. Chiropractic emphasizes manipulation of the bones, particularly the spine. Rolfers focus on manipulation of the "connective tissues" or "fascia" i.e. tendons, ligaments, aponeurosis and fascial sheaths as well as the musculature.

Rolfing also has a very GLOBAL view of the body and is a study of the relationships of all parts moving harmoniously together. Rolfing also considers the profound effect of gravity on human structure.

How are Rolfers trained?

The Rolf Institute of Structural Integration was founded in 1971. Rolfers are trained and certified by the Rolf Institute, headquartered in Bolder, Colorado. The Rolf Institute is the only school accredited to teach Rolfing and is the sole certifying body for Rolfers. It is regulated by the Colorado Department of Higher Education and Private Occupational Schools.

Successful applicants complete a training program that usually requires two years of study and is considered "post graduate" in nature. After initial Certification, Rolfers commit to a program of continuing education for an additional 5 years. The training covers the Biological and Behavioral Sciences, the theory of Rolfing, extensive clinical work under supervision and work with the dynamics of the human structure in motion.

Does insurance cover Rolfing?

Many insurance agencies cover Rolfing in whiplash cases. You'll need to check your individual policy.

Part Six

Alternative Treatments
for Specific Diseases
and Conditions

Chapter 44

Alternative Medicine in Cancer Treatment

Several surveys of CAM use by cancer patients have been conducted with small numbers of patients. One study published in the February 2000 issue of the journal *Cancer* reported that 37 percent of 46 patients with prostate cancer used one or more CAM therapies as part of their cancer treatment. These therapies included herbal remedies, old-time remedies, vitamins, and special diets. A larger study of CAM use in patients with different types of cancer was published in the July 2000 issue of the *Journal of Clinical Oncology*. That study found that 83 percent of 453 cancer patients had used at least one CAM therapy as part of their cancer treatment. The study included CAM therapies such as special diets, psychotherapy, spiritual practices, and vitamin supplements. When psychotherapy and spiritual practices were excluded, 69 percent of patients had used at least one CAM therapy in their cancer treatment.

How are Complementary and Alternative Approaches Evaluated?

It is important that the same scientific evaluation which is used to assess conventional approaches be used to evaluate complementary and alternative therapies. A number of medical centers are evaluating complementary and alternative therapies by developing clinical trials (research studies with people) to test them.

"Questions and Answers about Complementary and Alternative Medicine in Cancer Treatment," Cancer Facts, National Cancer Institute (NCI), reviewed December 2000.

Conventional approaches to cancer treatment have generally been studied for safety and effectiveness through a rigorous scientific process, including clinical trials with large numbers of patients. Often, less is known about the safety and effectiveness of complementary and alternative methods. Some of these complementary and alternative therapies have not undergone rigorous evaluation. Others, once considered unorthodox, are finding a place in cancer treatment—not as cures, but as complementary therapies that may help patients feel better and recover faster. One example is acupuncture. According to a panel of experts at a National Institutes of Health (NIH) Consensus Conference in November 1997, acupuncture has been found to be effective in the management of chemotherapy-associated nausea and vomiting and in controlling pain associated with surgery. Some approaches, such as laetrile, have been studied and found ineffective or potentially harmful.

What Is the Best Case Series Program?

The Best Case Series Program, which was started by the National Cancer Institute (NCI) in 1991, is another way that early data about complementary and alternative approaches are evaluated. The Best Case Series Program is overseen by the NCI's Office of Cancer Complementary and Alternative Medicine (OCCAM). Through the Best Case Series Program, health care professionals who offer CAM services submit their patients' medical records and related materials to OCCAM. The OCCAM conducts a critical review of the materials and presents the approaches that have the most therapeutic potential to the Cancer Advisory Panel for Complementary and Alternative Medicine (CAPCAM) for further review.

CAPCAM was jointly created in 1999 by the NCI and the NIH National Center for Complementary and Alternative Medicine (NCCAM). CAPCAM's membership is drawn from a broad range of experts from the conventional and CAM cancer research and practice communities. CAPCAM evaluates CAM cancer approaches that are submitted through the Best Case Series Program, and makes recommendations to NCCAM on whether and how these approaches should be followed up.

Is NCI Sponsoring Clinical Trials in Complementary and Alternative Medicine?

The NCI is currently sponsoring several clinical trials (research studies with patients) that study complementary and alternative treatments for cancer. Current trials include enzyme therapy with nutritional support for the treatment of inoperable pancreatic cancer, shark cartilage therapy for the treatment of non-small cell lung cancer, and studies of the effects of diet on prostate and breast cancers. Some of these trials compare alternative therapies with conventional treatments, while others study the effects of complementary approaches used in addition to conventional treatments. Patients who are interested in taking part in these or any clinical trials should talk with their doctor.

More information about clinical trials sponsored by the NCI can be obtained from NCCAM, OCCAM, and the NCI's Cancer Information Service (CIS).

What Should Patients Do When Considering Complementary and Alternative Therapies?

Cancer patients considering complementary and alternative therapies should discuss this decision with their doctor or nurse, as they would any therapeutic approach, because some complementary and alternative therapies may interfere with their standard treatment or may be harmful when used with conventional treatment.

When Considering Complementary and Alternative Therapies, What Questions Should Patients Ask Their Health Care Provider?

- What benefits can be expected from this therapy?
- What are the risks associated with this therapy?
- Do the known benefits outweigh the risks?
- What side effects can be expected?
- Will the therapy interfere with conventional treatment?
- Is this therapy part of a clinical trial? If so, who is sponsoring the trial?
- Will the therapy be covered by health insurance?

Chapter 45

Alternative Therapies for Diabetes

Alternative therapies are treatments that are neither widely taught in medical schools nor widely practiced in hospitals. Alternative treatments that have been studied to manage diabetes include acupuncture, biofeedback, guided imagery, and vitamin and mineral supplementation. The success of some alternative treatments can be hard to measure. Many alternative treatments remain either untested or unproven through traditional scientific studies.

Acupuncture

Acupuncture is a procedure in that a practitioner inserts needles into designated points on the skin. Some Western scientists believe that acupuncture triggers the release of the body's natural painkillers. Acupuncture has been shown to offer relief from chronic pain. Acupuncture is sometimes used by people with neuropathy, the painful nerve damage of diabetes.

Biofeedback

Biofeedback is a technique that helps a person become more aware of and learn to deal with the body's response to pain. This alternative therapy emphasizes relaxation and stress-reduction techniques. Guided imagery is a relaxation technique that some professionals who

National Institute of Diabetes and Digestive Diseases (NIDDK), NIH Publication Number 99-4552, 1999.

use biofeedback do. With guided imagery, a person thinks of peaceful mental images, such as ocean waves. A person may also include the images of controlling or curing a chronic disease, such as diabetes. People using this technique believe their condition can be eased with these positive images.

Chromium

The benefit of added chromium for diabetes has been studied and debated for several years. Several studies report that chromium supplementation may improve diabetes control. Chromium is needed to make glucose tolerance factor, which helps insulin improve its action. Because of insufficient information on the use of chromium to treat diabetes, no recommendations for supplementation yet exist.

Magnesium

Although the relationship between magnesium and diabetes has been studied for decades, it is not yet fully understood. Studies suggest that a deficiency in magnesium may worsen the blood sugar control in type 2 diabetes. Scientists believe that a deficiency of magnesium interrupts insulin secretion in the pancreas and increases insulin resistance in the body's tissues. Evidence suggests that a deficiency of magnesium may contribute to certain diabetes complications.

Vanadium

Vanadium is a compound found in tiny amounts in plants and animals. Early studies showed that vanadium normalized blood glucose levels in animals with type 1 and type 2 diabetes. A recent study found that when people with diabetes were given vanadium, they developed a modest increase in insulin sensitivity and were able to decrease their insulin requirements. Currently researchers want to understand how vanadium works in the body, discover potential side effects, and establish safe dosages.

Additional Information on Alternative Therapies for Diabetes

The National Diabetes Information Clearinghouse collects resource information on diabetes for the Combined Health Information Database (CHID). CHID is a database produced by health-related agencies of the Federal Government. This database provides titles, abstracts, and availability information for health information and health education resources.

To provide you with the most up-to-date resources, information specialists at the clearinghouse created an automatic CHID search. To obtain this information, you may view the results of the automatic search on Alternative Therapies for Diabetes.

Chapter 46

Hepatitis C:
Treatment Alternatives

Hepatitis C is a serious communicable (contagious) disease of the liver that is caused by the hepatitis C virus (HCV). Hepatitis C and its implications were identified only recently. There still is much to learn about the disease, the virus that causes it, and treatment options—both conventional and alternative.

Alternative Care

No complementary medicine or alternative medicine therapies have been scientifically proven to cure or even ease symptoms of hepatitis C.

However, some people are turning to herbs for relief. They use herbs either to help with hepatitis itself or to deal with side effects of interferon. These harmful side effects can include: sudden hearing loss; anemia and other forms of low blood cell counts; headaches; heart, eye, liver, or kidney problems; and disorders of the mind, including depression. Among potential herbal therapies (including licorice root, ginseng, ginger, and St. John's wort) for hepatitis C, the most promising alternative treatment seems to be the herb commonly called milk thistle.

Preliminary studies in animals show that milk thistle may help protect the liver from injury by a variety of toxins ("poisons" such as drugs, viruses, alcohol, radiation, and poisonous mushrooms) and limit the damage from them. To date, the most reliable, and also quite preliminary, studies on people show that milk thistle does not cure

Publication Z-04, National Center for Complementary and Alternative Medicine (NCCAM), NCCAM Clearinghouse, May 2000.

liver disease, but that it may improve the way the liver works in patients with cirrhosis. However, there is no current evidence to indicate that milk thistle directly affects HCV.

In Germany, where many herbs are regulated and prescribed like drugs, health authorities have approved milk thistle as a complementary treatment (given in addition to conventional drugs) for cirrhosis, hepatitis, and similar liver conditions. But a great deal of research still is needed before this alternative therapy could be considered a standard treatment option in the United States.

Milk Thistle

Milk thistle originally is from Europe, but now it also is grown in the United States. Its scientific name is *Silybum marianum*. The ingredient that experts believe is responsible for its medicinal qualities is called silymarin. Silymarin is found in the fruits of the milk thistle plant. Studies in animals have shown that this active ingredient promotes the following activities.

- Liver Cell Growth—Silymarin appears to promote the growth of some types of cells in the liver.

- Antioxidation—Silymarin may be an effective "antioxidant," which means it may help fight a destructive chemical process in the body known as "oxidation." In oxidation, harmful substances produced in the body (called free radicals) can damage cells. Some studies suggest that silymarin can prevent these substances from damaging liver cells.

- Antihepatotoxic Activity—Studies suggest that silymarin can block various types of toxins from entering and injuring liver cells.

- Inflammation Inhibition—Silymarin is thought to prevent inflammation (swelling) of the liver; this may be described as displaying anti-inflammatory properties.

Milk thistle is not used to prevent HCV from causing liver disease. Rather, it is used with the hope that it would minimize the damage to the liver that HCV can cause.

Although small, one randomized controlled trial on hepatitis patients suggests that a specific component in silymarin may be beneficial in managing chronic hepatitis. In this study, reported in 1993, 10 patients with chronic hepatitis were assigned to the treatment group and 10 others were assigned to the placebo group. The treatment group received 240 milligrams of silybin, a component of silymarin, two times a day for 1 week. The results of tests that measure how well the liver is functioning showed significant improvement in the treatment group, suggesting that silybin may help treat chronic hepatitis.

Milk thistle in the treatment of liver disease needs to be studied further. Fortunately, negative side effects have not yet been reported, and this herbal therapy may be much less expensive than conventional drug therapies. Yet, it should be mentioned that conventional therapies have been proven to work in a substantial portion of patients.

Because milk thistle does not dissolve well in water, the herb is not effective in the form of a tea. It currently is marketed in the United States as a dietary supplement in the form of capsules containing 200 milligrams of a concentrated extract with 140 milligrams of silymarin.

Other Herbs That May Help

Licorice Root

Herbalists use tea made with licorice root to manage some of the effects hepatitis has on the liver. The scientific name for licorice root is *Glycyrrhiza glabra*, and its active component is called glycyrrhizin. Studies suggest that licorice root displays antiviral and anti-inflammatory properties.

Licorice root does come with a warning, however. If taken regularly (more than 3 grams of licorice root a day for more than 6 weeks, or more than 100 milligrams of glycyrrhizin a day), this herb can cause the following conditions in some people: high blood pressure, sodium and water retention, low potassium levels in the bloodstream, and disturbance of an important electrolyte balancing system in the body. Signs and symptoms of excessive licorice root consumption may include headache, sluggishness, puffiness and swollen ankles, and even heart failure or cardiac arrest (when the heart suddenly stops beating).

Glycyrrhizin has been used in Japan for more than 20 years as a treatment for chronic hepatitis. In a 1998 review 11 of several randomized controlled trials, researchers reported that treatment with glycyrrhizin is effective in easing liver disease in some people. Several of the trials reviewed indicated improvements in liver tissue that had been damaged by hepatitis. Some of them also showed improvements in how well the liver does its job.

A great deal of scientific research still is needed to learn if these alternative therapies are safe and effective in people.

A 1997 experiment suggested that glycyrrhizin also may help prevent the development of liver cancer in patients with chronic hepatitis C. The use of glycyrrhizin as a complementary therapy (in addition to conventional use of interferon drugs) has been studied, but no significant benefit has been found yet.

Ginseng

Tests on animals and on human tissues suggest that ginseng may help the body's disease-fighting and glandular systems. Tests in small animals also suggest that ginseng may help improve the way the liver works and reduce damage to liver tissue caused by hepatitis and similar conditions. However, a search of the current literature shows no studies in people that test ginseng's helpfulness for hepatitis. Only one study, conducted in Italy, shows that ginseng may be helpful for elderly people with liver conditions similar to hepatitis.

There are two true ginsengs—American ginseng (*Panax quinquefolius*) and Asian ginseng (*Panax ginseng*), which includes Chinese, Japanese, and Korean ginseng. Siberian ginseng (*Eleutherococcus senticosus*) is not a true ginseng. It is hard to get authentic ginseng products. Companies that market herbs for sale have poor quality control, so the quality of the different brands varies widely. A 1990 analysis of 54 available ginseng products revealed that 85 percent of them contained little or no ginseng at all. Ginseng most often is taken as a tea.

Herbs That May Ease Interferon's Effects

Ginger

For 2,500 years, the Chinese have used ginger (*Zingiber officinale*) to treat nausea. Some, but not all, research studies confirm that ginger may reduce nausea. This herb may relieve nausea and vomiting caused by interferon drug therapy in some patients with hepatitis C. Ginger generally is recognized as safe and is not known to cause any serious side effects. Ginger is relatively inexpensive and readily available. It most commonly is taken in the form of a tea.

St. John's Wort

Some patients with hepatitis C take the herb St. John's wort (*Hypericum perforatum*) to treat depression caused by interferon drug therapy. Although St. John's wort is not a proven treatment for depression, studies have shown that it does have antidepressive effects over the short term. Although research largely has been done using capsules of this herb, St. John's wort also is taken as a tea. There is no proof yet that St. John's wort is effective and safe over the long term.

St. John's wort does not require a prescription, and it is less expensive and may have fewer side effects than prescription antidepressant drugs. Tests in people reveal it may cause side effects such as fatigue, dry mouth, dizziness, digestive tract symptoms, and increased sensitivity to sunlight.

Chapter 47

Alternative Treatments for Headaches

The successful treatment of conditions ranging from the common cold to many cancers remains beyond the reach of modern medicine, despite its tremendous advances. It is not surprising, then, that patients seek a variety of alternative or complimentary therapies. Complementary techniques are those that lack definitive proof of efficacy and are not accepted by the medical mainstream. While many treatments widely used in modern medicine also lack scientific proof, they are not considered complementary or alternative because of their wide acceptance by the medical establishment.

Headaches and Alternatives

While the experience of an occasional headache may be universal and usually is tolerable, chronic headache is an important cause of distress and disability. The vast majority of people who suffer from headaches have either tension-type or migraine headaches. Headache only recently began to receive attention from the pharmaceutical industry and organized medicine. Selective serotonin-agonist drugs like sumatriptan have revolutionized treatment of migraines and dramatically changed the lives of millions of people. However, even these "designer" drugs do not work for at least 30% of patients. Unpleasant side effects may occur, and a very small proportion of patients can suffer serious side effects. These concerns encourage many patients who have tried conventional therapy for migraines to explore complementary therapies. Most headache sufferers, however, have never seen a physician for their headaches and may turn directly to complementary treatments, which seem cheaper, safer (though this may not always be the case), and more holistic.

In numerous double-blind treatment trials, a large proportion (30-40%) of headache patients respond favorably to placebo. This "placebo effect" can account for completely useless therapies being effective in some patients. If a particular therapy appears to be clearly ineffective, but at the same time is harmless and inexpensive, I would not discourage an interested patient from trying such an approach, in hopes of a favorable placebo response.

Types of Complementary Therapies

Acupuncture

This ancient method has recently received a boost in popularity because of the consensus statement by a panel convened by the National Institutes of Health. This statement strongly suggests that acupuncture is a legitimate therapy proven to be effective for some conditions and deserving additional studies for others. The panel concluded that nausea and acute dental pain clearly respond to acupuncture, while many painful conditions, including headaches, may respond to acupuncture but require additional studies.

Acupuncture treatment is done using very thin disposable needles, which cause very little discomfort or pain. In patients with chronic headaches treatment involves ten or more weekly 20-minute sessions. Electrical stimulation of the needles is frequently used instead of the traditional twirling of the needles.

Double-blind study of acupuncture is very difficult because blinding for insertion of a needle is impossible, and inserting needles into non-acupuncture points has been shown to relieve pain. A large number of animal studies indicate that different mechanisms of action (involving different chemical substances) may be involved in pain relief from acupuncture. Only about 70% of humans and animals respond to acupuncture. Patients with chronic headaches who did not respond to acupuncture were shown to have low endorphin levels.

Despite the lack of definitive proof of its efficacy, acupuncture has a significant potential to help some patients with headaches. Issues of cost, convenience and patient preferences should be taken into the account when deciding on this treatment.

412

Mind-Body Techniques

Biofeedback is another therapy where definitive proof will be hard to obtain. Most specialty headache clinics offer biofeedback, which strongly suggests that a large number of patients benefit from it (but does not prove its efficacy).

Biofeedback is only one of many relaxation and stress management techniques which can be equally effective if strictly adhered to. This is a big "if." Biofeedback is a preferred technique because it gives the patient a structure and a therapist, who acts as a coach.

The essence of biofeedback, which is often combined with behavior modification, is to teach a patient how to encounter stress without adverse physiological effects. A typical course of biofeedback consists of 8-10 weekly 30-45 minute sessions. Learning to control body functions such as temperature can be achieved only by first learning to relax the skeletal muscles. This is achieved through progressive relaxation, visualization and breathing techniques. Most important though is the daily practice of these techniques. The practice sessions can be only a few seconds or minutes long, but have to be very frequent. A conscious effort is required in the first few weeks of training, but gradually self-monitoring and very brief relaxation techniques become a subconscious habit. This appears to allow many patients to lower tension throughout the day and this results in fewer headaches. Children are especially adept at biofeedback. They can often learn not only how to prevent their headaches in 4 to 5 sessions, but at times can learn how to stop their headache once it begins.

Nutritional Therapies

Dietary approaches to the treatment of migraines are widely advocated, but have very little scientific basis, which places them in the category of complementary methods. Dietary avoidance is a widely-advocated strategy. Migraine can be triggered in susceptible individuals by tyramine-containing foods, some food additives and sugar substitutes, as well as by skipping meals. Some patients report that their headaches get better with elimination of wheat, sugar, or milk products from their diets. While we do not have scientific proof, it is possible to speculate on why these dietary changes may work. If the patient is so inclined there is no reason to discourage her from trying these dietary changes, which are usually safe and inexpensive. Strict vegetarian and other unusual diets, on the other hand, can lead to vitamin B12 and other deficiencies, which can make headaches worse and cause other health problems.

Magnesium is a vital element which plays an important role in the pathogenesis of migraines. Many studies have found low magnesium levels in the serum and tissues of migraine patients. In one study, an intravenous infusion of 1 gram of magnesium sulfate was given to 40 consecutive patients with acute migraine. Twenty-one (53%) had very good and sustained relief of their headache. Of the responders, 86% had low serum ionized magnesium levels, while of the non-responders only 16% had low values. A study of intravenous magnesium in the treatment of cluster headaches suggests a possible 40% success rate in this difficult-to-treat disorder. Oral magnesium supplementation was attempted as preventive therapy of migraines in three double-blind trials. Two of the three trials were positive, while one was negative. The negative study might have used a more poorly absorbed salt of magnesium. The absorption of various salts of magnesium has not been studied, so it is difficult to recommend a specific product to patients interested in trying magnesium for their headaches. Magnesium oxide, magnesium diglycinate and slow-release magnesium chloride seem to work for some patients when used in 400-600 mg daily dose.

Wider availability of serum ionized magnesium testing may enable us to identify patients who have low ionized magnesium levels and who are most likely to benefit from magnesium supplementation. In order to remove magnesium from the list of complementary therapies and move it into the mainstream we need large trials unequivocally proving its efficacy.

Riboflavin or vitamin B2 has been reported to relieve migraine headaches better than placebo. The maximum effect was achieved after three months of daily intake of 400 mg of riboflavin. The study involved only 55 patients, but the treatment is very benign and potentially very effective, which makes riboflavin a good candidate for further extensive trials.

Herbal Remedies

Feverfew is the only herbal remedy studied in double-blind fashion. In a trial of 24 patients, a daily dose of feverfew was found to be better than placebo as prophylactic therapy for migraines, though the difference was not dramatic. Because feverfew is fairly safe and may help some patients, this is the herb to recommend to patients interested in herbal remedies.

Guarana is a relatively recent import from Brazil, which is being used for headache relief. It may very well have some analgesic properties because of its high caffeine content. However, daily caffeine consumption is one of the leading causes of rebound headaches. Guarana and all other caffeine-containing foods, drinks and medications should be avoided in patients with frequent headaches. Anecdotal reports suggest that ingestion of ginger, gingko or valerian root, all of which are well tolerated, may help some patients with headaches.

Aromatherapy

Aromatherapy may not appear as far fetched if we consider how much of our brain is devoted to olfaction and that strong odors can almost instantly induce a migraine. A double-blind study of healthy volunteers showed that an external application of peppermint extract raises pain threshold and has strong relaxing effects, while eucalyptus has calming and relaxing effects and improves cognitive performance without analgesic effect. Another study which used peppermint oil for tension headaches showed positive results. This gives some scientific support to a variety of topical products being promoted for the treatment of headaches.

Homeopathy

Homeopathy is based on an unproved concept of using extremely small amounts of substances (usually herbal), which in large amounts can induce a symptoms which are being treated. Since the treatment is extremely benign and relatively inexpensive it can be tried by patients who believe that it may help.

Physical Approaches

Regular and frequent aerobic exercise as a treatment for headaches is impossible to study in a double-blind trial and would require a very large comparative trial to confirm efficacy. However, there is little doubt that it offers effective relief for many stress-provoked conditions, including headaches. Other unsubstantiated but anecdotally effective modalities include application of heat and cold, massage and many other similar techniques. As long as they are safe and affordable, patients should not be discouraged from trying them.

Chiropractic manipulation has several potential benefits, which must be weighed against possible complications. Controlled trials in tension headache have yielded mixed results, while small trials looking at migraine prevention have been encouraging. More than 100 cases of serious complications of this approach have been reported. The number of unreported complications must be certainly much larger. Most of the complications involve neck manipulation resulting in a stroke. Because there is no proof that this treatment works, and in view of the potential for very serious complications it seems prudent to strongly discourage headache patients from trying chiropractic treatment.

Chapter 48

Alternative Medicine for Menopause

For many women, menopause brings relief from monthly periods, freedom from worry about unplanned pregnancy, and excitement about entering a new phase of life. For many others, menopause brings physical and emotional upheaval linked to changes occurring as the female body makes its transition out of the child-bearing years.

Whether you're among the former or the latter or somewhere in between, chances are that you will at some point seek relief from the symptoms of menopause, which include insomnia, depression, stiff joints, bloating, vaginal dryness, sore breasts, and hot flashes. Hot flashes, which are characterized by a sudden increase in heart rate, peripheral blood flow, and sweating, are for many women the most uncomfortable aspect of menopause. Research suggests that about 75 percent of menopausal women are affected at one time or another by hot flashes, 15 percent of them seriously so. These figures suggest that four to five million U.S. women currently are severely affected by hot flashes.

Modern science has linked hot flashes to a decline in estrogen levels, which in menopausal women are only about 10 percent of their former levels. For the past several decades, conventional medicine has treated hot flashes and other menopausal discomforts with estrogen replacement therapy (ERT). Because ERT is contraindicated for women with a history of cancer, hormone replacement therapy (HRT),

"Menopause: Herbs That Can Ease the Transition," an undated document, © Herbs for Health Magazine; reprinted with permission from *Herbs for Health Magazine*, Real Health Media, Loveland, CO; cited January 2002.

which combines estrogen with a synthetic progesterone, is often used instead. But many women don't want to take the potential increased risk of cancer associated with ERT, or they dislike the cyclical bleeding often caused by HRT, or they don't want to take pills. Some women can't tolerate the side effects associated with these treatments. Despite the high interest of women in alternatives to ERT and HRT, however, little scientific investigation of alternatives has been done.

Traditional herbal medicine has for years offered a variety of treatments to ease hot flashes. Few of them have been sufficiently researched, but black cohosh (*Cimicifuga racemosa*) and vitex (*Vitex agnus-castus*), or chaste tree—both of which contain estrogen-like compounds—have shown promise in relieving menopausal complaints. Further work is needed to determine how effective these herbal remedies are as actual substitutes for ERT. Dong quai (*Angelica sinensis*), an herb commonly used in traditional Chinese medicine, has been shown to relieve menopause symptoms in many women; how it works is not clearly understood.

Black Cohosh

North American Indians and eclectic physicians of the nineteenth century alike used black cohosh in decoctions to treat gynecological problems. Today's herbalists and homeopaths also value it for this purpose; herbalists also prescribe it as a hormone regulator and as a diuretic to relieve water retention.

Studies carried out in Europe have verified black cohosh's effectiveness in reducing the secretion of LH, which has been implicated in causing hot flashes. Experiments with rats in the 1980s showed that a methanol extract of black cohosh contains substances that bind to estrogen receptors, causing a selective reduction in luteinizing hormone (LH), which has been implicated in causing hot flashes. Experiments with rats in the 1980s showed that a methoanol extract of black cohosh causing a selective reduction of LH. In 1991, researchers at the University of Göttingen in Germany performed a study of a commercial ethanol extract of black cohosh called Remifemin. The study involved 110 menopausal women between the ages of 50 and 54 who had received no estrogen replacement therapy for at least six months and complained of menopausal symptoms. The researchers found that the product reduced LH, and they isolated three active, as yet unidentified compounds in black cohosh that work together to suppress the hormone.

Today in Germany, black cohosh is a main ingredient of three commercial drugs used for menopausal discomforts. Germany's Commission E, a governmental panel that studies and makes recommendations about medicinal herbs, has found black cohosh to be a safe and reasonably effective treatment of nervous conditions associated with menopause. However, the U.S. Food and Drug Administration in 1986 found no pharmacologic evidence of therapeutic value in black cohosh and cautioned against its overuse.

Vitex

Hippocrates recommended vitex in the fourth century B.C. to treat injuries, inflammations, and swelling of the spleen. Its common name, chaste tree, is derived from the belief that it would suppress libido; European Catholics placed blossoms of the plant at the clothing of novice monks. Like black cohosh, contemporary herbalists value vitex for its hormone-regulating action and often prescribe it to treat not only hot flashes, but depression and vaginal dryness as well.

Vitex is believed to act on the hypothalamus and pituitary, regulating progesterone levels. Most of the clinical studies of vitex have been done in Europe and were noncontrolled. Two surveys of gynecological practices in Germany investigated the effect of vitex on 1,542 women aged thirteen to sixty-two with gynecological complaints. The women took forty drops of a commercial vitex product for an average length of 166 days. Physicians and patients agreed that the vitex product relieved fluid retention, bloating, breast tenderness, headache, and fatigue. Two percent of the patients reported side effects that included nausea, other gastric complaints, and diarrhea. Symptoms improved after an average of 25.3 days of taking the vitex drops. Additional anecdotal clinical reports indicate that vitex may help manage hot flashes, although further investigation is needed.

In Europe, vitex has been used for about forty years in a commercial alcohol-based tincture of the fruits known as Agnolyt; 100 mg of the solution is standardized to contain 9 g of the fruit. Recommended dosage is forty drops with liquid in the morning for several months to offset fluid retention and other discomforts. A solid extract equivalent of the tincture has been developed for those who are sensitive to alcohol.

Side effects from using vitex are rare, and there are no known interactions with other drugs. Commission E has supported the use of chaste-tree berries to treat menstrual disorders and mastodynia (painful breasts).

Dong Quai

Known as a blood-purifying tonic in traditional Chinese medicine, dong quai is one of the best-selling Chinese herbal products in North America. Western herbalists view dong quai as having tonic and regulatory effects on the female reproductive system, and it is often used to treat menopausal symptoms. Scientific investigations have confirmed dong quai's pain-relieving, antispasmodic, and anti-inflammatory activity. It is generally believed to lower blood pressure and to soothe discomforts associated with menopause.

Herbalists view dong quai as the "female ginseng," referring to its ability to revitalize and renourish the female body by correcting hormonal imbalances; they call upon this Chinese relative of the herb angelica to regulate and normalize hormonal production.

In traditional Chinese medicine, dong quai is often used in conjunction with other herbs. In a clinical study in China, Si Wu Tang, a well-known formula that contains dong quai, was used in conjunction with herbs that tonify the spleen to treat forty-three menopausal women. Seventy percent of the women reported that the combination relieved hot flashes, dizziness, blurred vision, stomachaches, and constipation. Dong quai root is small and ivory in color; it can be purchased sliced and pressed, or in powder, tincture, or extract forms.

Be Informed

Women who have uncomfortable menopause symptoms or are preparing for menopause should become as knowledgeable as possible about the choices that are open to them. Talk to health-care providers and read more about menopause, its effects, and treatment options. Learning about various herbs' physiological actions, including side effects and contraindications, can help a woman decide whether herbal remedies are right—and safe—for her.

Estrogen's Role

Menopause, the cessation of menstruation, marks the end of a woman's childbearing years, but hormonal changes leading up to this milestone have begun several years earlier. Each month for some thirty-five or forty years, follicle-stimulating hormone (FSH) from the pituitary gland stimulates the ripening of an egg in the ovary and an increase in the ovarian hormone estrogen. The increase in estrogen signals the uterine lining (endometrium) to thicken in preparation for receiving a fertilized egg and also stimulates the production of luteinizing hormone (LH) in the pituitary. LH triggers ovulation and production of a second ovarian hormone, progesterone, which continues preparing the endometrium for implantation of the egg. If the egg is not fertilized, however, the production of progesterone declines, and the endometrium is shed as menstrual fluid.

During these years, a feedback system involving the hypothalamus and pituitary (both in the brain) and the ovaries keeps production of the various hormones in balance. At some point, however, usually in a woman's mid forties, the amount of estrogen and progesterone secreted by the ovaries declines. Ovulation and menstrual periods become irregular. When ovulation ceases completely, progesterone no longer is produced, but some estrogen is, so the endometrium continues to build up as usual. Without progesterone to regulate the cycle, however, it grows and grows until it breaks down, causing spotting. Not until estrogen levels become too low to stimulate endometrial growth does menstruation stop once and for all.

What Are Hot Flashes?

Hot flashes usually affect women who are in the transition to menopause or in menopause, either naturally or because of medical intervention. They often occur during the first two years of menopause and decrease over time; for some women, hot flashes begin during menstruation.

The frequency and intensity of hot flashes vary from woman to woman. A "typical" hot flash lasts three to six minutes; it can last thirty. Hot flashes can occur over six months to two years—or up to forty years. They occur spontaneously and without warning signs, although some women link them to psychological stress, a hot environment, and caffeine or alcohol consumption.

The mechanism that causes hot flashes is unclear, although they have been linked to declining estrogen levels. Many women have found that they can deal with them nonmedically. By observing the conditions surrounding you at the time of a hot flash, you may be able to exert some control.

You may wish to keep a record of the time and severity of a hot flash to see whether there is a pattern. Dressing (and undressing) in layers can help you tolerate overheated offices and meeting rooms: at least one study has confirmed that the frequency and intensity of hot flashes decline dramatically when women are in a cool environment.

Recent research suggests that exercise and healthy eating habits may be just as effective in reducing hot flashes as estrogen and hormone replacement therapy. Smoking also plays a role; it has been shown to reduce estrogen levels, so quitting may help decrease the incidence of hot flashes along with decreasing the incidence of cancer, heart disease, and stroke.

Self-Esteem and Depression

A recent study performed at the University of Pennsylvania's Department of Anthropology found that menopausal depression may be linked to cultural attitudes. The study included fifteen sociocultural groups in different parts of the world. It found that in non-Western cultures where older women gain enhanced status, political power, and decision-making authority, the depression associated with menopause in Western societies is often nonexistent. The study concluded that Western "negative stressors," such as the views that menopause is a time of loss and that aging women have lost their societal value, may work in conjunction with fluctuating hormone levels to exacerbate feelings of low self-esteem.

An Herbal Approach

Here's a formula developed by herbalist and author Kathi Keville that contains tinctures of black cohosh, vitex, and dong quai, as well as tinctures of other herbs traditionally used to relieve menopausal symptoms:

- Asian ginseng (*Panax ginseng*) is among the most important herbs in traditional Chinese medicine. It is the exception to many herbs in that nearly 3,000 studies have explored a wide range of its medicinal benefits. Herbalists prescribe it as a tonic used to treat the nervous and hormonal systems and fatigue. It is not known to cause adverse reactions.

- Chinese medicine values licorice (*Glycyrrhiza glabra*) for its ability to replenish vital energy; people with high blood pressure or edema should use it sparingly.

- Herbalists often prescribe motherwort (*Leonurus cardiaca*) to treat anxiety and vaginal dryness, among other conditions. It is considered a gentle sedative that corrects over-rapid heart beats. Pregnant women shouldn't use it.

- Herbalists use the roots and leaves of dandelion (*Taraxacum officinale*) to treat a variety of ailments, including mood swings. Insufficient research has been done to support either side of this argument. In rare cases, the therapeutic use of dandelion has produced a skin rash.

- St. John's-wort (*Hypericum perforatum*) has traditionally been used to treat mild depression and anxiety. When taking therapeutic doses of its extract, it's best to avoid sunlight as the herb has caused photodermatitis in animals.

Menopause Tincture

1 teaspoon black cohosh root tincture

1 teaspoon vitex berry tincture

1/2 teaspoon ginseng root tincture

1/2 teaspoon licorice root tincture

1/2 teaspoon dong quai root tincture

1/2 teaspoon motherwort tincture

You may prepare the tinctures of the individual herbs yourself or purchase them. Take 1 teaspoon of the Menopause Tincture three times a day, mixed in a small amount of warm water.

Alternatively, dried herbs can be combined in the same proportions. To use, pour a cup of boiling water over 1 to 2 teaspoons of the mixture and let it steep; strain. Drink a cup of this tea three times a day. To relieve water retention, add 1 teaspoon dandelion root tincture. For depression or nervousness, add 1 teaspoon tincture of St. John's-wort flowering tops. If making an infusion, use fresh St. John's-wort, not dried.

Chapter 49

Alternative Medicine for Pain Management

Responding to a Public Need

"Pain is a widespread public health problem," says Christine Goertz, D.C., Ph.D., a program officer for the Division. "We're looking at alternative medicine because there is so much consumer interest in it, and managing pain is of primary importance to the public."

Take chronic back pain, for example. "Acupuncture, chiropractic, and massage all are being sought by people with chronic back pain because conventional medicine often provides no long-term solution," says Dr. Nahin. Drugs have not been effective in treating back pain, or they have side effects that some people cannot tolerate.

In addition, a growing number of conventional practitioners (physicians, registered nurses, physical therapists, etc.) are interested in alternative treatments for pain, "because their patients need and demand them," says Dr. Nahin. "Practitioners and their patients are more willing to try different types of treatments."

Responding to these critical needs, the NCCAM funds several randomized clinical trials of CAM treatments for managing pain. For example, NCCAM-funded trials in Boston, MA, and Seattle, WA, are comparing CAM treatments with standard medical therapy for back pain.

Other pain management research projects funded by the NCCAM include studies of acupuncture for osteoarthritis, fibromyalgia, dental

"Studying Pain Management: CAM Research Challenges," National Center for Complementary and Alternative Medicine, *NCCAM Newsletter*, Summer 2000.

pain, and carpal tunnel syndrome; chiropractic for chronic pelvic pain in women; and relaxation, guided imagery, and chamomile tea for abdominal pain in children.

Dr. Goertz points out that both CAM and conventional medicine practitioners are interested in this research. "They're excited by opportunities to access NIH funding for the first time" to begin clinical research on CAM treatments. However, the research has its challenges.

Producing a Placebo

"Alternative medicine does not always fit in a box," says Dr. Goertz, referring to chiropractic, acupuncture, massage, and other CAM therapies that require physical intervention. A randomized, controlled trial requires that one group of patients receives a placebo (a presumably pharmaceutically inactive or "fake" treatment), and it is difficult to devise a hands-on treatment that mimics acupuncture, for example.

For chiropractic and osteopathic manipulation, "there's a lot of discussion about sham manipulation," according to Dr. Goertz, a chiropractor herself. "Some chiropractic researchers have tried massage or thrust [manual force] that they believe is not strong enough to produce an effect," says Dr. Goertz.

In a research setting, attempts have been made to include patients who have never had real treatment by a chiropractic or acupuncturist so they do not know the difference between real and sham chiropractic or acupuncture procedures, and that poses another challenge. "It's more and more difficult to find patients who are naive to alternative therapies," says Dr. Goertz. "The subject pool gets smaller as time goes on."

When used, sham treatment provides some other information as well. For example, "the amount of attention from a CAM practitioner you get as a patient usually exceeds the attention you would get from a conventional doctor," says Marguerite Evans, M.S., R.D., another program officer for the Division. Even patients in the control group (the comparison or placebo group) receive a comparable amount of the practitioner's time as well as physical contact, which may have an effect on the patient.

Standardizing Holistic Treatments

Another challenge to research is the individualized, holistic nature of CAM treatment itself. To yield good, consistent data, studies must ensure that all treatment is the same (standardized). "One thing to be mindful of is the extent to which standardizing a protocol takes away some therapeutic benefit," says Dr. Goertz.

Ms. Evans points out how this concern multiplies with larger, multicenter trials. "You have to train a number of people to do the CAM intervention the same way to all patients at all centers, and train several people to collect the data in a standard fashion. This is common to any trial," she notes.

Measuring Outcomes

Yet another challenge lies in measuring the results of studies to ease pain. Although a number of reliable tools to measure pain have been validated by research, such as patient questionnaires, "it is hard to measure pain, and you rely mostly on patient perceptions," says Dr. Goertz.

From a research point of view, "you want to see a double-blind, placebo-controlled trial with a physiologic mechanism or other outcome measure," she says. Studies of pain so far cannot show the kind of concrete outcome data as, for example, studies that can demonstrate how insulin reduces high blood sugar levels in diabetics.

Facilitating Research

Chiropractic and acupuncture have been used in the United States for many years, so it is not surprising that a significant proportion of NCCAM-funded studies, especially those for pain, focus on chiropractic, acupuncture, or both. CAM practitioners have been interested in conducting research for some time, but funding has been limited.

According to Dr. Goertz, the availability of NCCAM research funds will not only enable CAM practitioners to undertake large, well-designed, rigorously controlled trials, but it also will encourage researchers from more mainstream fields to take part in such studies. "This, along with consumer interest, will cause a boom in CAM research," Dr. Goertz predicts.

Part Seven

Controversial Cancer Treatments

Chapter 50

Questionable Cancer Therapies

The American Cancer Society (ACS) has defined questionable methods as lifestyle practices, clinical tests, or therapeutic modalities that are promoted for general use for the prevention, diagnosis, or treatment of cancer and which are, on the basis of careful review by scientists and/or clinicians, deemed to have no real evidence of value. Under the rules of science (and federal law), proponents who make health claims bear the burden of proof. It is their responsibility to conduct suitable studies and report them in sufficient detail to permit evaluation and confirmation by others.

The ACS evaluates cancer methods by asking three questions:

- Has the method been objectively demonstrated in the peer-reviewed scientific literature to be effective?

- Has the method shown potential for benefit that clearly exceeds the potential for harm?

- Have objective studies been correctly conducted under appropriate peer review to answer these questions?

Typical Misrepresentations

Proponents of questionable methods typically claim that marketplace demand and testimonials from satisfied customers are proof that their remedies work. However, proponents almost never keep score or reveal what percentage of their cases end in failure. Cancer cures attributed to questionable methods usually fall into one or more of five categories: (1) the patient never had cancer; (2) a cancer was cured or put into remission by proven therapy, but questionable therapy was also used and erroneously credited for the beneficial result; (3) the cancer is progressing but is erroneously represented as slowed or cured; (4) the patient has died as a result of the cancer (or is lost to follow-up) but is represented as cured; or (5) the patient had a spontaneous remission (very rare) or slow-growing cancer that is publicized as a cure.

Promoters of questionable methods often misrepresent their methods as "alternatives." Genuine alternatives are comparable methods that have met the criteria for safety and effectiveness. Experimental alternatives are unproven but have a plausible rationale and are undergoing responsible investigation. Questionable "alternatives" are unproven and lack a scientifically plausible rationale. When referring to the latter, we use quotation marks because they are not true alternatives. Some promoters of "alternative" methods are physicians or other highly educated scientists who have strayed from scientific thought. The factors that motivate them can include delusional thinking, misinterpretation of personal experience, financial considerations, and pleasure derived from notoriety and/or patient adulation.

Misinformation about questionable cancer therapies is spread through books, articles, audiotapes, videotapes, talk shows, news reports, lectures, health expositions, "alternative" practitioners, information and referral services, and word of mouth. Promoters typically explain their approach in commonsense terms and appear to offer patients an active role in their care: (a) cancer is a symptom, not a disease; (b) symptoms are caused by diet, stress, or environment; (c) proper fitness, nutrition, and mental attitude allow biologic and mental defense against cancer; and (d) conventional therapy weakens the body's reserves, treats the symptoms rather than the disease. Questionable therapies are portrayed as natural and nontoxic, while standard (responsible) therapies are portrayed as highly dangerous.

During the past few years, the news media have publicized "alternative" methods in ways that are causing great public confusion. Most of these reports have contained no critical evaluation and have featured the views of proponents and their satisfied clients. Many have exaggerated the significance of the National Institutes of Health

(NIH)'s Office of Alternative Medicine (OAM)—now called the Center for Research in Alternative and Complementary Medicine—whose creation was spearheaded by promoters of questionable cancer therapies who wanted more attention paid to their methods. Most of the its advisory panel members have been promoters of "alternative" therapies. In 1994, the OAM's first director resigned, charging that political interference had hampered his ability to carry out OAM's mission in a scientific manner. The OAM has funded several dozen studies related to "alternative" methods, including a few related to cancer treatment. However, it remains to be seen whether such research will yield useful results. Even if it does, the benefit is unlikely to outweigh the publicity bonanza given to questionable methods. Some of today's "alternative" methods are described below in alphabetical order.

Antineoplastons

Stanislaw R. Burzynski, M.D., has given the name "antineoplastons" to substances he claims can "normalize" cancer cells that are constantly being produced within the body. He has published many papers stating that antineoplastons extracted from urine or synthesized in his laboratory have proven effective against cancer in laboratory experiments. He also claims to have helped many people with cancer get well. A 1992 analysis concluded that none of Burzynski's "antineoplastons" has been proven to normalize tumor cells.

Cancell

Cancell—originally called Entelev and recently renamed Cantron—is a liquid claimed to cure cancer by "lowering the voltage of the cell structure by about 20%," causing cancer cells to "digest" and be replaced with normal cells. Accompanying directions have warned that bottles of Cancell should not be allowed to touch each other or be placed near any electrical appliance or outlet.

Cancell has also been promoted for the treatment of AIDS, amyotrophic lateral sclerosis, multiple sclerosis, Alzheimer's disease, "extreme cases of emphysema and diabetes," and several other diseases. In 1989, the FDA reported that Cancell contained inositol, nitric acid, sodium sulfite, potassium hydroxide, sulfuric acid, and catechol. Subsequently, its promoters claimed to be modifying the formulation to make it more effective. They have also claimed that Cancell can't be analyzed because it varies with atmospheric vibrations and keeps changing its energy. Laboratory tests conducted between 1978 and 1991 by the NCI found no evidence that Cancell was effective against cancer. The FDA has obtained an injunction forbidding its distribution to patients.

Cell Specific Cancer Therapy

According to information that was on the promoter's web site during 1997, Cell Specific Cancer Therapy (CSCT) is applied with a device that is four inches thick, shaped like a donut, and exposes the patient to a magnetic field that is much weaker than that of magnetic resonance imaging. It is available at a clinic in the Dominican Republic. The advertised fee is $20,000, payable in advance, but the fee may be reduced or waived for people unable to pay. CSCT is claimed not to cure cancer but to "destroy active cancerous cells in a body and to do so without causing any damage to healthy cells." Its objective is to destroy enough cancerous cells that the body's immune system is "once again able to take over and do its normal job." The device is claimed to "detect cancerous cells with a sensitivity much greater than that of either conventional magnetic resonance imaging (MRI) or CAT scans" and to destroy cancer cells without harming adjacent normal cells." The promoter claims that cancerous cells have an "atypical metabolic mechanism that makes them "susceptible to polarizing electromagnetic fields." There is no scientific evidence that magnetic energy can selectively destroy cancer cells. Similar treatment is offered at the Davidson Cancer Clinic in Mexico, whose proprietor is facing criminal charges for fraud.

Clark's "Cure for All Cancers"

Hulda Clark, Ph.D., N.D., claims that (a) all cancers and many other diseases are caused by "parasites, toxins, and pollutants;" (b) cancers can be detected with a blood test for ortho-phospho-tyrosine and a device that identifies diseased organs and toxic substances; (c) cancers can be cured by killing the parasites and ridding the body of environmental chemicals; (d) black walnut hulls, wormwood, and common cloves can rid the body of over 100 types of parasites; (d) the amino acids ornithine and arginine improve this recipe. Her book *Cure for All Cancers*, contains 103 case histories of her supposed cancer cures. However, judging from her descriptions (a) most did not have cancer, and (b) of those that did, most had received standard medical treatment or their tumors were in early stages.

Devices

Many types of devices are used with unfounded claims that they are effective against cancer. These include devices that pass low-voltage electrical current through tumors or the body, "electroacupuncture" devices purported to measure the electrical resistance of "acupuncture points," electrical devices claimed to "charge" blood samples taken from patients and later reinjected, negative ion generators claimed to have an effect against tumors, radionics devices claimed to diagnose and cure cancer by analyzing and emitting radio waves at the correct frequencies, magnets claimed capable of curing cancers by "improving circulation" or by intracellular effects, and projectors of colored light claimed to exert healing effects.

Essiac

Essiac is an herbal remedy that was prescribed and promoted for about 50 years by Rene M. Caisse, a Canadian nurse who died in 1978. Shortly before her death, she turned over the formula and manufacturing rights to the Resperin Corporation, a Canadian company that has provided it to patients under a special agreement with Canadian health officials. Several reports state that the formula contains burdock, Indian rhubarb, sorrel, and slippery elm, but there may be additional ingredients. Essiac tea claimed to be Caisse's original formulation is also marketed in the United States. Several animal tests using samples of Essiac have shown no antitumor activity. Nor did a review of data on 86 patients performed by the Canadian federal health department during the early 1980s.

Fresh Cell Therapy

Fresh cell therapy, also called live cell therapy or cellular therapy, involves injections of fresh embryonic animal cells taken from the organ or tissue that corresponds to the unhealthy organ or tissue in the patient. Proponents claim that the recipient's body automatically transports the injected cells to the target organ where they repair and rejuvenate the ailing cells. The American Cancer Society states that fresh cell therapy has no proven benefit and has caused serious side effects (infections and immunologic reactions to the injected protein) and death. In 1984, The FDA issued an Import Alert asking the U.S. Customs and Postal Services to block the importation of all "cell therapy" powders and extracts intended for injection.

435

Gerson Method

Proponents of the Gerson diet claim that cancer can be cured only if toxins are eliminated from the body. They recommend "detoxification" with frequent coffee enemas and a low-sodium diet that includes more than a gallon a day of juices made from fruits, vegetables, and raw calf's liver. This method was developed by Max Gerson, a German-born physician who emigrated to the United States in 1936 and practiced in New York City until his death in 1959. Gerson therapy is still available at Hospital Meridien in Tijuana, Mexico and, since February 1997, at the Gerson Healing Center in Sedona, Arizona.

Gerson therapy is still actively promoted by his daughter, Charlotte Gerson, through lectures, talk show appearances, and publications of the Gerson Institute in Bonita, California. Gerson protocols have included liver extract injections, ozone enemas, "live cell therapy," thyroid tablets, royal jelly capsules, linseed oil, castor oil enemas, clay packs, laetrile, and vaccines made from influenza virus and killed Staphylococcus aureus bacteria.

In 1947, the NCI reviewed ten cases selected by Dr. Gerson and found his report unconvincing. That same year, a committee appointed by the New York County Medical Society reviewed records of 86 patients, examined ten patients, and found no evidence that the Gerson method had value in treating cancer. An NCI analysis of Dr. Gerson's book *A Cancer Therapy: Results of Fifty Cases* concluded in 1959 that most of the cases failed to meet the criteria (such as histologic verification of cancer) for proper evaluation of a cancer case. A recent review of the Gerson treatment rationale concluded: (a) the "poisons" Gerson claimed to be present in processed foods have never been identified, (b) frequent coffee enemas have never been shown to mobilize and remove poisons from the liver and intestines of cancer patients, (c) there is no evidence that any such poisons are related to the onset of cancer, (d) there is no evidence that a "healing" inflammatory reaction exists that can seek out and kill cancer cells.

Greek Cancer Cure

The principal proponent of the Greek Cancer Cure was microbiologist Dr. Hariton-Tzannis Alivizatos, of Athens, Greece, who died in 1991. He claimed to have a blood test that could determine the type, location, and severity of any cancer. He also asserted that his "serum" enabled the patient's immune system to destroy cancer cells, and helped the body rejuvenate parts destroyed by cancer. Knowledgeable observers believe that the principal ingredient of the so-called Greek Cancer Cure was niacin. The American Cancer Society and the NCI asked Alivizatos several times for detailed information on his methods, but he never replied.

Hoxsey Treatment

Naturopath Harry Hoxsey promoted an herbal treatment consisting of an externally used paste or powder and a tonic taken orally. The external preparations contained corrosive agents such as arsenic sulfide. The internal medicine, said to be adjusted on a case-by-case basis, contained potassium iodide and such things as red clover, licorice, burdock root, Stillingia root, Berberis root, pokeroot, cascara, prickly ash bark, and buckthorn bark. Hoxsey said that the formulas were developed in 1840 by his great grandfather and passed to him by his father while the latter was dying of cancer.

Hoxsey's treatment was offered at clinics in the United States from 1924 until repeated clashes with the FDA led him to close his main clinic in Dallas in the late 1950s. In 1963, Hoxsey's former chief nurse Mildred Nelson began offering it at a clinic in Tijuana, Mexico. Hoxsey himself contracted prostate cancer in 1967 and underwent surgery after treating himself unsuccessfully with his tonic. Most of the herbs in the tonic have been tested for antitumor activity in cancer, with negligible results for a few and no results for the others. Some of these herbs, most notably pokeroot, have toxic side effects. The NCI evaluated case reports submitted by Hoxsey and concluded that no assessment was possible because the records did not contain adequate information. Hoxsey died in 1974. Nelson died in January 1999.

Hydrazine Sulfate

In the mid-1970s, hydrazine sulfate was proposed for treating the progressive weight loss and debilitation characteristic of advanced cancer. Based on animal data and preliminary human studies, it has also been claimed to cause tumor regression and subjective improvement in patients. However, three recent trials sponsored by the National Cancer Institute demonstrated no benefit attributable to hydrazine sulfate.

"Hyperoxygenation" Therapies

"Hyperoxygenation" therapy—also called "bio-oxidative therapy" and "oxidative therapy"—is based on the erroneous concept that cancer is caused by oxygen deficiency and can be cured by exposing cancer cells to more oxygen than they can tolerate. The most touted agents are hydrogen peroxide, germanium sesquioxide, and ozone. Although these compounds have been the subject of legitimate research, there is little or no evidence that they are effective for the treatment of any serious disease, and each has demonstrated potential for harm. Germanium products have caused irreversible kidney damage and death. The FDA has banned their importation and seized products from several U.S. manufacturers.

Immuno-Augmentative Therapy

Immuno-augmentative therapy (IAT) was developed by Lawrence Burton, Ph.D., a zoologist who claimed he could stimulate the immune system's natural ability to detect and destroy cancer cells. He claimed to accomplish this by injecting protein extracts isolated with processes he had patented. However: (a) the immune system does not detect and destroy cancer cells as Burton postulated, and (b) the substances he claimed to use cannot be produced by the procedures described in his patent applications and have not been demonstrated to exist in the human body.

Iscador

Iscador is an extract of mistletoe first proposed for the treatment of cancer in 1920 by Rudolph Steiner, a Swiss physician who espoused occult beliefs. Steiner founded the Society for Cancer Research to promote mistletoe extracts and occult-based practices he called anthroposophical medicine. A 1962 report by the society claimed that the time of picking the plants was important because they react to the influences of the sun, moon, and planets. Various mistletoe juice preparations have been studied with the hope of finding an effective anticancer agent. However, in 1984, the expert working group of the Swiss Society for Oncology concluded that there was no evidence that Iscador was effective against human cancers.

Kelley/Gonzalez Metabolic Therapy

In the 1960s, William Donald Kelley, D.D.S., developed a program for cancer patients that involved dietary measures, vitamin and enzyme supplements, and computerized "metabolic typing." Kelley classified people as "sympathetic dominant," "parasympathetic dominant," or metabolically "balanced" and made dietary recommendations for each type. He claimed that his "Protein Metabolism Evaluation Index" could diagnose cancer before it was clinically apparent and that his Kelley Malignancy Index could detect "the presence or absence of cancer, the growth rate of the tumor, the location of the tumor mass, prognosis of the treatment, age of the tumor and the regulation of medication for treatment."

In 1970, Kelley was convicted of practicing medicine without a license after witnesses testified that he had diagnosed lung cancer on the basis of blood from a patient's finger and prescribed dietary supplements, enzymes, and a diet as treatment.

Laetrile

Laetrile, which achieved great notoriety during the 1970s and early 1980s, is the trade name for a synthetic relative of amygdalin, a chemical in the kernels of apricot pits, apple seeds, bitter almonds, and some other stone fruits and nuts. Many laetrile promoters have called it "vitamin B17" and falsely claimed that cancer is a vitamin deficiency disease that laetrile can cure. Claims for laetrile's efficacy have varied considerably. First it was claimed to prevent and cure cancer. Then it was claimed not to cure, but to "control" cancer while giving patients an increased feeling of well being. More recently, laetrile has been claimed to be effective, not by itself, but as one component of "metabolic therapy."

Laetrile was first used to treat cancer patients in California in the 1950s. According to proponents, it kills tumor cells selectively while leaving normal cells alone. Although laetrile has been promoted as safe and effective, clinical evidence indicates that it is neither. When subjected to enzymatic breakdown in the body, it forms glucose, benzaldehyde, and hydrogen cyanide. Some cancer patients treated with laetrile have suffered nausea, vomiting, headache and dizziness, and a few have died from cyanide poisoning. Laetrile has been tested in at least 20 animal tumor models and found to have no benefit either alone or together with other substances. Several case reviews have found no benefit for the treatment of cancer in humans.

Livingston-Wheeler Regimen

Virginia C. Livingston, M.D., who died in 1990, postulated that cancer is caused by a bacterium she called Progenitor cryptocides, which invades the body when "immunity is stressed or weakened."

439

She claimed to combat this by strengthening the body's immune system with vaccines (including one made from the patient's urine); "detoxification" with enemas; digestive enzymes; a vegetarian diet that avoided chicken, eggs, and sugar; vitamin and mineral supplements; visualization; and stress reduction. She claimed to have a very high recovery rate but published no clinical data to support this. Scientists who attempted to isolate the organism she postulated found that it was a common skin bacterium. Researchers at the University of Pennsylvania Cancer Center compared 78 of its patients with similar patients treated at the Livingston-Wheeler Clinic. All had advanced cancers for which no proven treatment was known. As expected, the study found no difference in average survival time of the two groups. However, Livingston-Wheeler patients reported more appetite difficulties and pain.

Macrobiotics

Macrobiotics is a quasireligious philosophical system that advocates a semivegetarian diet. ("Macrobiotic" means "way of long life.") Macrobiotic diets have been promoted for maintaining general health and for preventing and "relieving" cancer and other diseases. The optimal diet is said to balance "yin" and "yang" foods. It is composed of whole grains (50 to 60% of each meal), vegetables (25 to 30% of each meal), whole beans or soybean-based products (5 to 10% of daily food), nuts and seeds (small amounts as snacks), miso soup, herbal teas, and small amounts of white meat or seafood once or twice weekly. Some macrobiotic diets contain adequate amounts of nutrients, but others do not.

Macrobiotic practitioners may base their recommendations on "pulse diagnosis" and other unscientific procedures related to Chinese medicine. Pulse diagnosis supposedly involves six pulses at each wrist that correspond to twelve internal spheres of bodily function. Other diagnostic methods include "ancestral diagnosis," "astrological diagnosis," "aura and vibrational diagnosis," "environmental diagnosis" (including consideration of celestial influences" and tidal motions), and "spiritual diagnosis" (an evaluation of "atmospheric vibrational conditions" to identify spiritual influences, including "visions of the future").

The diet itself can cause cancer patients to undergo serious weight loss. In July 2001, Kushi's wife and colleague Aveline died of cervical cancer. According to an *Associated Press* obituary, she underwent standard radiation treatment when the cancer was discovered. When the cancer spread to her bones and she was told that no standard treatment was available, relied on acupuncture and "Eastern" methods.

Metabolic Therapy

Proponents of "metabolic therapy" claim to diagnose abnormalities at the cellular level and correct them by normalizing the patient's metabolism. They regard cancer, arthritis, multiple sclerosis, and other "degenerative" diseases as the result of metabolic imbalance caused by a buildup of "toxic substances" in the body. They claim that scientific practitioners merely treat the symptoms of the disease while they treat the cause by removing "toxins" and strengthening the immune system so the body can heal itself. The "toxins" are neither defined nor objectively measurable. "Metabolic" treatment regimens vary from practitioner to practitioner and may include a "natural food" diet, coffee enemas, vitamins, minerals, glandulars, enzymes, laetrile, and various other nostrums that are not legally marketable in the United States. No scientific study has ever shown that "metabolic therapy" or any of its components is effective against cancer or any other serious disease.

Pau D'arco

Pau d'arco tea, sold through health food stores and by mail, is also called taheebo, lapacho, lapacho morado, ipe roxo, or ipes. The tea is claimed to be an ancient Inca Indian remedy prepared from the inner bark of various species of Tabebuia, an evergreen tree native to the West Indies and Central and South America. However, stories about its origins contain geographic and botanical errors. Proponents claim that pau d'arco tea is effective against cancer and many other ailments. Tabebuia woods contains lapachol, which has been demonstrated to have antitumor activity in a few animal tumor models. However, no published study has shown a significant effect on cancer in humans. Studies during the early 1970s found that lapachol is not as readily absorbed by humans as by rats, and that plasma levels high enough to influence tumors would be accompanied by anticoagulant effects. Even low doses can cause nausea and vomiting and can interfere with blood clotting. Some researchers believe that lapachol should be studied further using vitamin K to inhibit its anticoagulant activity.

Psychic Surgery

Psychic surgery is claimed to remove tumors without leaving a skin wound. Actually, its practitioners use sleight-of-hand to create the illusion that surgery is being performed. A false finger or thumb may be used to store a red dye that appears as "blood" when the skin is "cut." Animal parts or cotton wads soaked in the dye are palmed and then exhibited as "diseased organs" supposedly removed from the patient's body. (However, one Philippine "healer" has been reported to use human blood, which raises the possibility that HIV or hepatitis B could be transmitted.) The American Cancer Society has concluded that "all demonstrations to date of psychic surgery have been done by various forms of trickery." Most "psychic surgeons" practice in the Philippines or Brazil, but some have made tours within the United States. A few have been prosecuted for theft and/or practicing medicine without a license.

Psychologic Methods

Various psychologic methods are being promoted to cancer patients as cures or adjuncts to other treatment. The techniques include imagery, visualization, meditation, progressive muscle relaxation, and various forms of psychotherapy. These techniques may reduce stress, alleviate depression, help control pain, and enhance patients' feelings of mastery and control. Individual and group support can have a positive impact on quality of life and overall attitude. A positive attitude may increase a patient's chance of surviving cancer by increasing compliance with proven treatment. However, it has not been demonstrated that emotions directly influence the course of the disease.

Revici Cancer Control

Revici Cancer Control (also called lipid therapy and "biologically guided chemotherapy") is based on the notion that cancer is caused by an imbalance between constructive ("anabolic") and destructive ("catabolic") body processes. Its main proponent, Emanuel Revici, M.D., prescribed lipid alcohols, zinc, iron, and caffeine, which he classified as anabolic, and fatty acids, sulfur, selenium, and magnesium, which he classified as catabolic. His formulations were based on his interpretation of the specific gravity, pH (acidity), and surface tension of single samples of the patient's urine. Scientists who have offered to evaluate Revici's methods were unable to reach an agreement with him on procedures to ensure a valid test. However, his method of urinary interpretation is obviously not valid. The specific gravity of urine reflects the concentration of dissolved substances and depends largely on the amount of fluid a person consumes. The acidity depends mainly on diet, but varies considerably throughout the day. Thus, even when these values are useful for a metabolic determination, information from a single urine sample would be meaningless. The surface tension of urine has no medically recognized diagnostic value. In 1993, following a lengthy struggle with New York State licensing authorities, Revici's medical license was permanently revoked. He died in January 1998 at the age of 101. His treatment is still available at the Revici Life Sciences Center, which reportedly is overseen by Keith Korins, M.D., and Revici's niece.

714-X

714-X is a chemical solution produced in Quebec by Gaston Naessens, who also operates the International Academy of Somatidian Orthobiology. He claims that 714-X can "fluidify the lymph" and "direct nitrogen into the cancerous cells in order to stop their toxic secretions which block the organism's defense system." 714-X has been analyzed by the Canadian Health Protection Branch and found to contain a mixture of camphor, ammonium chloride and nitrate, sodium chloride, ethyl alcohol, and water. The Health Protection Branch has received no scientific data to support claims that 714-X can cure cancer or AIDS. Its Expert Advisory Committee has deplored its use for these purposes and warned that there could be adverse side effects.

In 1956, in connection with alleged cancer remedy called GN-24, Naessens was convicted of illegal medical practice and ordered by a French court to pay the maximum applicable fine. He was prosecuted again in 1964 after another alleged cancer remedy he administered in Corsica was proven not to work.

Shark Cartilage

Powdered shark cartilage is purported to contain a protein that inhibits the growth of new blood vessels needed for the spread of cancer. Although a modest anti-angiogenic effect has been observed in laboratory experiments, it has not been demonstrated that feeding shark cartilage to humans significantly inhibits angiogenesis in patients with cancer. Even if direct applications were effective, oral administration would not work because the protein would be digested rather than absorbed intact into the body. (If the proteins could enter the body, they would cause an immune response that would make the individual allergic to them and could trigger disastrous allergic responses with further exposure to the protein.)

443

Vitamin C

The claim that vitamin C is useful in the treatment of cancer is largely attributable to Linus Pauling, Ph.D. During the mid-1970s, Pauling began claiming that high doses of vitamin C are effective in preventing and curing cancer. In 1976 and 1978, he and a Scottish surgeon, Ewan Cameron, reported that a group of 100 terminal cancer patients treated with 10,000 mg of vitamin C daily had survived three to four times longer than historically matched patients who did not receive vitamin C supplements. However, Dr. William DeWys, chief of clinical investigations at the NCI, found that the patient groups were not comparable. The vitamin C patients were Cameron's, while the other patients were managed by other physicians. Cameron's patients were started on vitamin C when he labeled them "untreatable" by other methods, and their subsequent survival was compared to the survival of the "control" patients after they were labeled untreatable by their doctors. DeWys found that Cameron's patients were labeled untreatable much earlier in the course of their disease—which meant that they entered the hospital before they were as sick as the other doctors' patients and would naturally be expected to live longer. Nevertheless, to test whether Pauling might be correct, the Mayo Clinic conducted three double-blind studies involving a total of 367 patients with advanced cancer. All three studies found that patients given 10 g of vitamin C daily did no better than those given a placebo. Despite many years of taking huge daily amounts of vitamin C, both Pauling and his wife Ava died of cancer—she in 1981 and he in 1994.

Chapter 51

714-X

714-X was developed over 30 years ago in a privately funded laboratory in Quebec, Canada, where it continues to be produced. The primary component of 714-X is naturally-derived camphor that has been chemically altered by the addition of an extra nitrogen atom and then combined with ammonium salts, sodium chloride, and ethanol.

The laboratory currently makes 714-X available through physicians in Canada (where it is available on compassionate grounds only, but not approved for general therapeutic use), Mexico, and some western European countries. Since the production of 714-X is not regulated, there is no guarantee that rigorous quality control procedures are followed to assure manufacturing consistency and product safety. The Food and Drug Administration (FDA) has not approved 714-X for use in the United States.

Before researchers can conduct clinical drug research in the United States, they must file an Investigational New Drug (IND) application with the FDA. The IND application process is highly confidential, and IND information can be disclosed only by the applicants. To date, no investigators have announced that they have applied for an IND to study 714-X as a treatment for cancer.

714-X is usually administered by injection into lymph nodes in the groin, but it can be administered nasally, using a nebulizer, for patients with lung or oral cancers. The producers of 714-X do not recommend intravenous or oral administration. A usual treatment cycle

CancerNet, National Cancer Institute (NCI), 2000; available online at http://www.cancer.gov.

consists of daily injection for 21 days followed by a 3-day rest period. Between three and 12 treatment cycles are recommended, depending on the stage of the cancer. It has been suggested that 714-X is more effective if administered early in the disease process and before chemotherapy or radiation therapy, but that it can also be used in conjunction with conventional treatments. It has been recommended that vitamin B12 supplements, vitamin E supplements, and alcohol be avoided during 714-X therapy.

History

Little documentation exists regarding the development of 714-X and its mechanism of action. It appears to have been developed in the 1960s on the basis of earlier studies that used a high-magnification, dark-field microscope called a somatoscope. With the somatoscope, researchers were able to examine living cells in fresh blood and tissue samples taken from healthy individuals and individuals with serious diseases, including cancer. The study of living cells (as opposed to the dead cells examined with a conventional light microscope or an electron microscope) led to the theory that microorganisms distinct from bacteria, viruses, and fungi exist normally in the blood and play a role in cancer development. These microorganisms, which were called "somatids," are said to exist in multiple forms, some of which appear only in individuals affected by degenerative diseases or cancer. The forms associated with disease reportedly secrete toxic substances and growth hormones that disrupt normal cellular metabolism and damage the immune system. In this compromised environment, cells that have become cancerous are allowed to proliferate. It was also suggested that cancer cells trap nitrogen, thereby depriving the rest of the body of the nitrogen needed for normal cellular metabolism. In addition, it was proposed that cancer cells secrete a toxic substance (co-cancerogenic K factor) that further inhibits the immune system. The producers of 714-X state that cancer can be diagnosed, and its development and spread can be predicted, by studying blood samples with the somatoscope. No evidence has been published in peer-reviewed, scientific journals to support these proposals, and the somatid theory of cancer development is not widely accepted.

It has been proposed that 714-X works by protecting, stabilizing, and reactivating the patient's immune system, so the body can defend itself against tumor growth and metastasis. The camphor component of 714-X is purportedly attracted to cancer cells, where the added nitrogen is released, thus preventing tumor cells from depleting the nitrogen required by normal cells, including immune system cells, for proper metabolism and function.

Laboratory/Animal/Preclinical Studies

There have been no laboratory or animal studies published in peer-reviewed, scientific journals in which the safety or the efficacy of 714-X was evaluated. Results of studies using tumor models in rats, dogs, and cows were presented at a scientific conference in 1982, and no benefit of 714-X could be demonstrated.

A few laboratory and animal studies have suggested that camphor (a component of 714-X) may be able to enhance the immune response observed after vaccine administration and increase the sensitivity of tumor cells to radiation therapy. In one series of studies, investigators used camphor vapors as a "conditioned stimulus" to promote an immune response. These studies demonstrated that mice exposed to camphor vapors at the same time they received an antitumor vaccine showed decreased growth of transplanted lymphoma cells and increased survival when they were re-exposed to camphor vapors plus the vaccine or to camphor vapors alone, in comparison with mice re-exposed to only the vaccine. These investigators also demonstrated that exposure to camphor vapors led to an increase in natural killer cells and in tumor-specific cytotoxic T cells. Another study reported that breast adenocarcinoma cells transplanted under the skin of mice responded better to local radiation therapy when small doses of camphor were given by intraperitoneal injection before irradiation. Finally, researchers examined nine compounds, including a camphor-containing compound, for their ability to inhibit the activity of estrone sulfatase, an enzyme involved in the production of estrone, which is a precursor of the various forms of estrogen. Estrogens are thought to promote the growth of hormone-dependent breast cancer cells. The camphor-containing compound showed only modest inhibition of estrone sulfatase activity in human breast cancer cells grown in the laboratory.

Human/Clinical Studies

No clinical trials, clinical series, or case reports have been published in peer-reviewed, scientific journals to support the safety or the efficacy of 714-X. A number of anecdotal reports and testimonials have been published in newspapers and other non-medical literature. The producers of 714-X state that they have tried to document the long-term experience of patients treated with 714-X, but they have encountered difficulty in obtaining information from patients and their health-care providers.

Adverse Effects

714-X is reported to be nontoxic, with the only side effects of treatment being local redness, tenderness, and swelling at injection sites.

Levels of Evidence for Human Studies of Cancer Complementary and Alternative Medicine

To assist readers in evaluating the results of human studies of CAM treatments for cancer, the strength of the evidence (i.e., the "levels of evidence") associated with each type of treatment is provided whenever possible. To qualify for a levels of evidence analysis, a study must 1) be published in a peer-reviewed, scientific journal; 2) report on a therapeutic outcome(s), such as tumor response, improvement in survival, or measured improvement in quality of life; and 3) describe clinical findings in sufficient detail that a meaningful evaluation can be made. No levels of evidence analysis could be performed for 714-X because no study of its use in humans has been published in a peer-reviewed, scientific journal.

Chapter 52

Antineoplastons

Antineoplastons are a group of synthetic compounds that were originally isolated from human blood and urine by Stanislaw Burzynski, M.D., Ph.D., in Houston, Texas. Dr. Burzynski has used antineoplastons to treat patients with a variety of cancers. In 1991, the National Cancer Institute (NCI) conducted a review to evaluate the clinical responses in a group of patients treated with antineoplastons at the Burzynski Research Institute in Houston.

The medical records of seven brain tumor patients who were thought to have benefited from treatment with antineoplastons were reviewed by NCI. This did not constitute a clinical trial but, rather, was a retrospective review of medical records, called a "best case series." The reviewers of this series found evidence of antitumor activity, and NCI proposed that formal clinical trials be conducted to further evaluate the response rate and toxicity of antineoplastons in adults with advanced brain tumors.

Investigators at several cancer centers developed protocols for two phase II clinical trials with review and input from NCI and Dr. Burzynski. These NCI-sponsored studies began in 1993 at the Memorial Sloan-Kettering Cancer Center, the Mayo Clinic, and the Warren Grant Magnussen Clinical Center at the National Institutes of Health. Patient enrollment in these studies was slow, and by August 1995 only nine patients had entered the trials. Attempts to reach a

"National Cancer Institute-Sponsored Clinical Trials of Antineoplastons," Cancer Facts, National Cancer Institute (NCI), February 1999.

449

consensus on proposed changes to increase accrual could not be reached by Dr. Burzynski, NCI staff, and investigators, and on August 18, 1995, the studies were closed prior to completion. A paper describing this research, "Phase II Study of Antineoplastons A10 (NSC 648539) and AS2-1 (NSC 620261) in Patients with Recurrent Glioma," appears in *Mayo Clinic Proceedings* 1999, 74:137-145. Because of the small number of patients in these trials, no definitive conclusions can be drawn about the effectiveness of treatment with antineoplastons.

Chapter 53

Cancell

Cancell is also known as Entelev, Sheridan's Formula, Jim's Juice, Crocinic Acid, JS-114, JS-101, 126-F, and Cantron. It has been promoted as a therapy for cancer and a wide range of other diseases. The U.S. Food and Drug Administration has listed the components of Cancell as inositol, nitric acid, sodium sulfite, potassium hydroxide, sulfuric acid, and catechol. Cancell can be administered orally or rectally. It can also be applied to the skin of the wrist or the ball of the foot.

Cancell was developed by James V. Sheridan, a former researcher at the Michigan Cancer Center, in the 1930s. Mr. Sheridan and his associate, Edward J. Sopcak, offered the mixture free of charge to any seriously ill patient who requested it.

The principal manufacturers of Cancell state that they have performed numerous animal experiments with the mixture, and that it has been used by many cancer patients. However, these findings have not been published in peer-reviewed, scientific journals, and no clinical trials (research studies with patients) of Cancell have been conducted. The National Cancer Institute (NCI) has evaluated Cancell in the laboratory and in animal studies and found that it had no effect on cancer cells.

Because studies of Cancell have not shown it to be effective in treating cancer, it has not been approved by the U.S. Food and Drug Administration (FDA). In 1989, the FDA obtained a permanent injunction

Cancer Facts, National Cancer Institute (NCI), November 2000.

against the manufacturers of Cancell. The injunction prohibited the manufacture or distribution of the product. The Cancell mixture is reportedly being sold under various names as a dietary supplement in health food stores.

More detailed information about Cancell can be found in the National Cancer Institute's PDQ database for cancer information. This information is available from the NCI's Cancer Information Service (CIS) at 1-800-4-CANCER (1-800-422-6237), or on the CancerNet Web site at http://cancernet.nci.nih.gov/cam/cancell.htm on the Internet.

Cancer patients considering complementary and alternative medicine should discuss this decision with their doctor or nurse, as they would any therapeutic approach, because some complementary and alternative therapies may interfere with their standard treatment or may be harmful when used with conventional treatment. Here are some questions patients may want to ask their health care provider:

- What benefits can be expected from this therapy?
- What are the risks associated with this therapy?
- Do the known benefits outweigh the risks?
- What side effects can be expected?
- Will the therapy interfere with conventional treatment?
- Will the therapy be covered by health insurance?

Chapter 54

Cartilage (Bovine and Shark)

General Information

Bovine cartilage and shark cartilage have been investigated as treatments for cancer, psoriasis, arthritis, and a number of other medical conditions for more than 30 years. At least some of the interest in cartilage as a treatment for cancer arose from the mistaken belief that sharks, whose skeletons are made primarily of cartilage, are not affected by this disease. Although reports of malignant tumors in sharks are rare, a variety of cancers have been detected in these animals. Nonetheless, several substances that have antitumor activity have been identified in cartilage. More than a dozen clinical studies of cartilage as a treatment for cancer have already been conducted, and additional clinical studies are now under way.

The absence of blood vessels in cartilage led to the hypothesis that cartilage cells (also known as chondrocytes) produce one or more substances that inhibit blood vessel formation. The formation of new blood vessels, or angiogenesis, is necessary for tumors to grow larger than a few millimeters in diameter (i.e., larger than approximately 100,000 to 1,000,000 cells) because tumors, like normal tissues, must obtain most of their oxygen and nutrients from blood. A developing tumor, therefore, cannot continue to grow unless it establishes connections to the circulatory system of its host. It has been reported that tumors can initiate the process of angiogenesis when they contain as few as 100 cells. Inhibition of angiogenesis at this early stage may, in some

CancerNet, National Cancer Institute (NCI), 2000.

instances, lead to complete tumor regression. The possibility that cartilage could be a source of one or more types of angiogenesis inhibitors for the treatment of cancer has prompted much research.

The major structural components of cartilage include several types of the protein collagen and several types of glycosaminoglycans, which are polysaccharides. Chondroitin sulfate is the major glycosaminoglycan in cartilage. Although there is no evidence that the collagens in cartilage, or their breakdown products, can inhibit angiogenesis, there is evidence that shark cartilage contains at least one angiogenesis inhibitor that has a glycosaminoglycan component. Other data indicate that most of the antiangiogenic activity in cartilage is not associated with the major structural components.

Some glycosaminoglycans in cartilage reportedly have anti-inflammatory and immune system-stimulating properties, and it has been suggested that either they or some of their breakdown products are toxic to tumor cells. Thus, the antitumor potential of cartilage may involve more than one mechanism of action.

Cartilage products are sold commercially in the United States as dietary supplements. More than 40 different brand names of shark cartilage alone are available to consumers. In the United States, dietary supplements are regulated as foods, not drugs. Therefore, premarket evaluation and approval by the Food and Drug Administration (FDA) are not required unless specific disease prevention or treatment claims are made. Because manufacturers of cartilage products are not required to show evidence of anticancer or other biologic effects, it is unclear whether any of these products has therapeutic potential. In addition, individual products may vary considerably from lot to lot because standard manufacturing processes do not exist and binding agents and fillers may be added during production.

To conduct clinical drug research in the United States, researchers must file an Investigational New Drug (IND) application with the FDA. To date, IND status has been granted to at least four groups of investigators to study cartilage as a treatment for cancer. Because the IND application process is confidential and because the existence of an IND can be disclosed only by the applicants, it is not known whether other applications have been made.

In animal studies, cartilage products have been administered in a variety of ways. In some studies, oral administration of either liquid or powdered forms has been used. In other studies, cartilage products have been given by injection (intravenous or intraperitoneal), applied topically, or placed in slow-release, plastic pellets that were surgically implanted. Most of the latter studies investigated the effects of cartilage products on the development of blood vessels in the chorioallantoic membrane of chicken embryos, the cornea of rabbits, or the conjunctiva of mice.

In human studies, cartilage products have been administered topically or orally, or they have been given by enema or subcutaneous injection. For oral administration, liquid, powdered, and pill forms have been used. The dose and duration of cartilage treatment have varied in human studies, in part because different types of products have been tested.

History

The therapeutic potential of cartilage has been investigated for more than 30 years. As noted previously, cartilage products have been tested as treatments for cancer, psoriasis, and arthritis. Cartilage products have also been studied as enhancers of wound repair and as treatments for osteoporosis, ulcerative colitis, regional enteritis, acne, scleroderma, hemorrhoids, severe anal itching, and the dermatitis caused by poison oak and poison ivy.

Early studies of cartilage's therapeutic potential used extracts of bovine cartilage. The ability of these extracts to suppress inflammation was first described in the early 1960s. The first report that bovine cartilage contains at least one angiogenesis inhibitor was published in the mid-1970s. The use of bovine cartilage extracts to treat patients with cancer and the ability of these extracts to kill cancer cells directly and to stimulate animal immune systems were first described in the mid- to late-1980s.

In contrast, the first report that shark cartilage contains at least one angiogenesis inhibitor was published in the early 1980s, and the only published report to date of a clinical trial of shark cartilage as a treatment for cancer appeared in the late 1990s. The more recent interest in shark cartilage is due, in part, to the greater abundance of cartilage in this animal and its apparently higher level of antiangiogenic activity. It has been estimated that 6% of the body weight of a shark is composed of cartilage, compared with less than 1% of the body weight of a cow. In addition, it has been estimated that, on a weight-for-weight basis, shark cartilage contains 1,000 times more antiangiogenic activity than bovine cartilage.

As indicated previously, at least three different mechanisms of action have been proposed to explain the anticancer potential of cartilage: 1) it is toxic to cancer cells; 2) it stimulates the immune system; and 3) it inhibits angiogenesis. There is only limited evidence to support the first two mechanisms of action; however, the evidence in favor of the third mechanism is more substantial.

The process of angiogenesis requires at least four coordinated steps, each of which may be a target for inhibition. First, tumors must communicate with the endothelial cells that line the inside of nearby blood vessels. This communication takes place, in part, through the secretion of angiogenesis factors, such as vascular endothelial growth factor (VEGF). Second, the "activated" endothelial cells must divide to produce new endothelial cells, which will be used to make the new blood vessels. Third, the dividing endothelial cells must migrate toward the tumor. To accomplish this, they must produce enzymes called matrix metalloproteinases, which will help them carve a pathway through the tissue elements that separate them from the tumor. Fourth, the new endothelial cells must form the hollow tubes that will become the new blood vessels. It is conceivable that some angiogenesis inhibitors may be able to block more than one step in this process.

It is important to note that cartilage is relatively resistant to invasion by tumor cells and that tumor cells use matrix metalloproteinases when they migrate during the process of metastasis. Therefore, if the angiogenesis inhibitors in cartilage are also inhibitors of matrix metalloproteinases, then the same molecules may be able to block both angiogenesis and metastasis. It should also be noted that shark tissues other than cartilage have been reported to produce antitumor substances.

Laboratory/Animal/Preclinical Studies

The antitumor potential of cartilage has been investigated extensively in laboratory and animal studies. Some of these studies have focused on the toxicity of cartilage products toward cancer cells in vitro.

In one study, cells from 22 freshly isolated human tumors (nine ovary, three lung, two brain, two breast, and one each of sarcoma, melanoma, colon, pancreas, cervix, and testis) and three human cultured cell lines (breast cancer, colon cancer, and myeloma) were treated with Catrix, which is a commercially available powdered preparation of bovine cartilage. In the study, the growth of all three cultured cell lines and of cells from approximately 70% of the tumor specimens was inhibited by 50% or more when Catrix was used at high concentrations (1 to 5 milligrams per milliliter of culture fluid). It is unclear, however, whether the inhibitory effect of Catrix in this study was specific to the growth of cancer cells because its effect on the growth of normal cells was not tested. In addition, the "toxic" component of Catrix has not been identified, and it has not been shown that equivalent inhibitory concentrations of this component can be achieved in the bloodstream of patients who may be treated with either injected or oral formulations of this product.

A liquid (i.e., aqueous) extract of shark cartilage, called AE-941/ Neovastat, has also been reported to inhibit the growth of a variety of cancer cell types in vitro. However, these results have not been published in a peer-reviewed, scientific journal.

In contrast, a commercially available preparation of powdered shark cartilage (no brand name given) was reported to have no effect on the growth of human astrocytoma cells in vitro. In this published study, the shark cartilage product was tested at only one concentration (0.75 milligrams per milliliter).

The immune system-stimulating potential of cartilage has also been investigated in laboratory and animal studies, but just one study has been published in the peer-reviewed, scientific literature. In that study, Catrix was shown to stimulate the production of antibodies by mouse B cells (B lymphocytes) both in vitro and in vivo. However, increased antibody production in vivo was observed only when Catrix was given by intraperitoneal or intravenous injection. It was not observed when oral formulations of Catrix were used. It is important to note that, in most experiments, the proliferation of mouse B cells (i.e., normal, nonmalignant cells) in vitro was increasingly inhibited as the concentration of Catrix was increased (tested concentration range: 1 to 20 milligrams per milliliter). Catrix has also been reported to stimulate the activity of mouse macrophages in vivo, but results demonstrating this effect have not been published in a peer-reviewed, scientific journal. To date, no studies of the immune system-stimulating potential of shark cartilage have been reported.

A large number of laboratory and animal studies have been published concerning the antiangiogenic potential of cartilage. Overall, these studies have revealed the presence of at least three angiogenesis inhibitors in bovine cartilage and, in shark cartilage, of at least two.

Three angiogenesis inhibitors in bovine cartilage have been very well characterized. They are relatively small proteins with molecular masses that range from 23,000 to 28,000. These proteins, called cartilage-derived inhibitor (CDI), cartilage-derived antitumor factor (CATF), and cartilage-derived collagenase inhibitor (CDCI) by the researchers who purified them, have been shown to block endothelial cell proliferation in vitro and new blood vessel formation in the chorio-allantoic membrane of chicken embryos. Two of the proteins (CDI and CDCI) have been shown to inhibit matrix metalloproteinase activity in vitro, and one (CDI) has been shown to inhibit endothelial cell migration in vitro. These proteins do not block the proliferation of normal cells or of tumor cells in vitro. When the amino acid sequences of CDI, CATF, and CDCI were determined, it was discovered that they were the same as those of proteins known otherwise as TIMP-1 (tissue inhibitor of matrix metalloproteinases 1), ChMI (chondromodulin I), and TIMP-2 (tissue inhibitor of matrix metalloproteinases 2), respectively.

A possible fourth angiogenesis inhibitor in bovine cartilage has been purified not from cartilage but from the culture fluid of bovine chondrocytes grown in the laboratory. This inhibitor, which has been named chondrocyte-derived inhibitor (ChDI), is a protein that has a molecular mass of approximately 36,000. It has been reported that ChDI and CDI/TIMP-1 have similar antiangiogenic activities, but the relationship between these proteins is unclear because amino acid sequence information for ChDI is not available. Thus, whether CDI/TIMP-1 is a breakdown product of ChDI or whether ChDI is truly the fourth angiogenesis inhibitor identified in bovine cartilage is unknown.

As indicated previously, shark cartilage, like bovine cartilage, contains more than one type of angiogenesis inhibitor. One shark cartilage inhibitor, named U-995, reportedly contains two small proteins, one with a molecular mass of approximately 14,000 and the other with a molecular mass of approximately 10,000. Both proteins have shown antiangiogenic activity when tested individually. The exact relationship between these two proteins, as well as their relationship to the larger bovine angiogenesis inhibitors, is not known because amino acid sequence information for U-995 is not available. U-995 has been reported to inhibit endothelial cell proliferation, endothelial cell migration, and matrix metalloproteinase activity in vitro and the formation of new blood vessels in the chorioallantoic membrane of chicken embryos. It does not appear to inhibit the proliferation of other types of normal cells or of cancer cells in vitro. Intraperitoneal, but not oral, administration of U-995 has been shown to inhibit the growth of mouse sarcoma-180 tumors implanted subcutaneously on the backs of mice and the formation of lung metastases of mouse B16-F10 melanoma cells injected into the tail veins of mice.

The second angiogenesis inhibitor identified in shark cartilage appears to have been studied independently by three groups of investigators. This inhibitor, which was named SCF2 by one of the groups, is a proteoglycan that has a molecular mass of less than 10,000. Proteoglycans are combinations of glycosaminoglycans and protein. The principal glycosaminoglycan in SCF2 is keratan sulfate. SCF2 has been shown to block endothelial cell proliferation in vitro, the formation of new blood vessels in the chorioallantoic membrane of chicken embryos, and tumor-induced angiogenesis in the cornea of rabbits.

Other studies have indicated that AE-941/Neovastat, the previously mentioned aqueous extract of shark cartilage, has antiangiogenic activity, but the molecular basis for this activity has not been defined. Therefore, whether AE-941/Neovastat contains U-995 and/ or SCF2 or some other angiogenesis inhibitor is not known. It has been reported that AE-941/Neovastat inhibits endothelial cell proliferation and matrix metalloproteinase activity in vitro and the formation of new blood vessels in the chorioallantoic membrane of chicken embryos. It may also inhibit the action of vascular endothelial growth factor (VEGF), thus interfering with the communication between tumor cells and nearby blood vessels. AE-941/Neovastat has also been reported to inhibit the growth of DA3 mammary adenocarcinoma cells and the metastasis of Lewis lung carcinoma cells in vivo in mice. In the Lewis lung carcinoma experiments, AE-941/Neovastat reportedly enhanced the antimetastatic effect of the chemotherapy drug cisplatin. It is important to note, however, that most of the results obtained with AE-941/Neovastat have not been published in peer-reviewed, scientific journals.

Additional in vivo studies of the antitumor potential of shark cartilage have been published in the peer-reviewed, scientific literature. In one study, oral administration of powdered shark cartilage (no brand name given) was shown to inhibit chemically induced angiogenesis in the mesenteric membrane of rats. In another study, oral administration of powdered shark cartilage (no brand name given) was shown to reduce the growth of GS-9L gliosarcomas in rats. In contrast, it was reported in a third study that oral administration of two powdered shark cartilage products, Sharkilage and MIA Shark Powder, did not inhibit the growth or the metastasis of SCCVII squamous cell carcinomas in mice.

Human/Clinical Studies

More than a dozen clinical studies of cartilage as a treatment for cancer have been conducted since the early 1970s. However, results from only three studies have been published in peer-reviewed, scientific journals. Although additional clinical studies are now under way, the cumulative evidence to date is inconclusive regarding the effectiveness of cartilage as a cancer treatment in humans.

Two of the three published clinical studies evaluated the use of Catrix, the previously mentioned powdered preparation of bovine cartilage, as a treatment for various solid tumors. One of these studies was a case series that included 31 patients; the other was a phase II clinical trial that included nine patients.

In the case series, all patients were treated with subcutaneously injected and/or oral Catrix; however, three patients (one with squamous cell carcinoma of the skin and two with basal cell carcinoma of the skin) were treated with topical preparations as well. The individual dose, the total dose, and the duration of Catrix treatment in this series varied from patient to patient; however, the minimum treatment duration was 7 months, and the maximum duration was more than 10 years.

Eighteen patients had been treated with conventional therapy (surgery, chemotherapy, radiation therapy, hormone therapy) within 1 year of the start of Catrix treatment; nine patients received conventional therapy concurrently (at the same time) with Catrix treatment; and seven patients received conventional therapy both prior to and during Catrix treatment. It was reported that 19 patients had a complete response, 10 patients had a partial response, and one patient had stable disease following Catrix treatment. The remaining patient did not respond to cartilage therapy. Eight of the patients with a complete response received no prior or concurrent conventional therapy. Approximately half of the patients with a complete response eventually experienced recurrent cancer.

This clinical study had several weaknesses that could have affected its outcome, including the absence of a control group and the receipt of prior and/or concurrent conventional therapy by the majority of patients.

In the phase II trial, Catrix was administered by subcutaneous injection only. All patients in this trial had progressive disease following radiation therapy and/or chemotherapy. Identical individual doses of Catrix were given to each patient, but the duration of treatment and the total delivered dose varied because of disease progression or death. The minimum duration of Catrix treatment in this study was 4 weeks. It was reported that one patient (with metastatic renal cell carcinoma) had a complete response that lasted more than 39 weeks. The remaining eight patients did not respond to Catrix treatment. The researchers in this trial also investigated whether Catrix had an effect on immune system function in these patients. No consistent trend or change in the numbers, percentages, or ratios of white blood cells (i.e., total lymphocyte counts, total T cell counts, total B cell counts, percentage of T cells, percentage of B cells, ratio of helper T cells to cytotoxic T cells) was observed, although increased numbers of T cells were found in three patients.

Partial results of a third clinical study of Catrix are described in an abstract submitted for presentation at a scientific conference, but complete results of this study have not been published in a peer-reviewed, scientific journal. In the study, 35 patients with metastatic renal cell carcinoma were divided into four groups, and the individuals in each group were treated with identical doses of subcutaneously injected and/or oral Catrix. Three partial responses and no complete responses were observed among 22 evaluable patients who were treated with Catrix for more than 3 months. Two of the 22 evaluable patients were reported to have stable disease and 17 were reported to have progressive disease following Catrix therapy. No relationship could be established between Catrix dose and tumor response in this study.

The third published study of cartilage as a treatment for cancer was a phase I/II trial that tested the safety and the efficacy of orally administered Cartilade, a commercially available powdered preparation of shark cartilage, in 60 patients with various types of advanced solid tumors. All but one patient in this trial had been treated previously with conventional therapy. According to the design of the study, no additional anticancer treatment could be given concurrently with Cartilade therapy. No complete responses or partial responses were observed among 50 evaluable patients who were treated with Cartilade for at least 6 weeks. However, stable disease that lasted 12 weeks or more was reported for 10 of the 50 patients. All 10 of these patients eventually experienced progressive disease.

Partial results of three other clinical studies of powdered shark cartilage are described in two abstracts submitted for presentation at scientific conferences, but complete results of these studies have not been published in peer-reviewed, scientific journals. All three studies were phase II clinical trials that involved patients with advanced disease; two of the studies were conducted by the same group of investigators. These three studies enrolled 20 patients with breast cancer, 12 patients with prostate cancer, and 12 patients with primary brain tumors. All patients had been treated previously with conventional therapy. No other anticancer treatment was allowed concurrently with cartilage therapy. In two of the studies, the name of the cartilage product was not identified; however, in the third study, the commercially available product BeneFin was used. Ten patients in each study completed at least 8 weeks of treatment and were, therefore, considered evaluable for response. No complete responses or partial responses were observed in any of the studies. Two patients in each study were reported to have stable disease that lasted 8 weeks or more.

The safety and the efficacy of AE-941/Neovastat, the previously mentioned aqueous extract of shark cartilage, have also been examined in clinical studies. However, results of these studies have been described only in abstracts presented at scientific conferences and in press releases by the manufacturer and not in peer-reviewed, scientific journals.

The exact number of clinical studies of AE-941/Neovastat is difficult to determine because of inconsistencies in the information that is available. It appears that at least two clinical studies have been conducted: 1) a phase I/II trial of oral AE-941/Neovastat as a single agent in 80 patients with advanced lung cancer and 72 patients with advanced prostate cancer, and 2) a study of oral AE-941/Neovastat plus chemotherapy and/or radiation therapy in 126 patients with various types of solid tumors. The phase I/II trial has been variously described as a single phase I/II study, two phase I studies, two phase II studies, a study that involved only patients with advanced lung cancer, and a study that involved both patients with advanced lung cancer and patients with advanced prostate cancer.

It has been reported that AE-941/Neovastat has little toxicity, and there are indications from a retrospective analysis of data from the phase I/II trial that it may have anticancer activity in humans. In addition, there is evidence from a randomized clinical trial that examined the effect of AE-941/Neovastat on the angiogenesis associated with surgical wound repair that this extract contains at least one antiangiogenic component that is orally bioavailable.

On the basis of laboratory, animal, and human data provided by the manufacturer, two randomized phase III trials of AE-941/Neovastat in patients with advanced cancer have been approved by the FDA. In one trial, treatment with oral AE-941/Neovastat plus chemotherapy and radiation therapy is being compared to treatment with placebo plus the same chemotherapy and radiation therapy in patients with stage III non-small cell lung cancer. In the other trial, treatment with oral AE-941/Neovastat is being compared to treatment with placebo in patients with metastatic renal cell carcinoma. Both trials are currently enrolling patients.

Adverse Effects

The side effects associated with cartilage therapy are generally described as mild-to-moderate in severity. Inflammation at injection sites, dysgeusia, fatigue, nausea, dyspepsia, fever, dizziness, and edema of the scrotum have been reported after treatment with the bovine cartilage product Catrix. Nausea, vomiting, abdominal cramping and/or bloating, constipation, hypotension, hyperglycemia, generalized weakness, and hypercalcemia have been associated with the use of powdered shark cartilage. The high level of calcium in shark cartilage may contribute to the development of hypercalcemia. In addition, one case of hepatitis has been associated with the use of powdered shark cartilage. Nausea and vomiting are the most commonly reported side effects following treatment with AE-941/ Neovastat, the aqueous extract of shark cartilage.

Chapter 55

Coenzyme Q10

General Information

Coenzyme Q10 (also known as Co Q10, Q10, vitamin Q10, ubiqui-
none, or ubidecarenone) is a benzoquinone compound synthesized
naturally by the human body. The "Q" and the "10" in the name refer
to the quinone chemical group and the 10 isoprenyl chemical subunits,
respectively, that are part of this compound's structure. The term "coenzyme" denotes it as an organic (contains carbon atoms), nonprotein
molecule necessary for the proper functioning of its protein partner
(an enzyme or an enzyme complex). Coenzyme Q10 is used by cells of
the body in a process known variously as aerobic respiration, aerobic
metabolism, oxidative metabolism, or cell respiration.

Through this process, energy for cell growth and maintenance is
created inside cells in compartments called mitochondria. Coenzyme
Q10 is also used by the body as an endogenous antioxidant. An antioxidant is a substance that protects cells from free radicals, which are
highly reactive chemicals, often containing oxygen atoms, capable of
damaging important cellular components such as DNA and lipids. In
addition, the plasma level of coenzyme Q10 has been used, in studies, as a measure of oxidative stress (a situation in which normal
antioxidant levels are reduced).

Coenzyme Q10 is present in most tissues, but the highest concentrations are found in the heart, the liver, the kidneys, and the pancreas. The lowest concentration is found in the lungs. Tissue levels

CancerNet, National Cancer Institute (NCI), December 2000.

of this compound decrease as people age, due to increased requirements, decreased production, or insufficient intake of the chemical precursors needed for synthesis. In humans, normal blood levels of coenzyme Q10 have been defined variably, with reported values ranging from 0.30 to 3.84 micrograms per milliliter.

Given the importance of coenzyme Q10 to optimal cellular energy production, use of this compound as a treatment for diseases other than cancer has been explored. Most of these investigations have focused on coenzyme Q10 as a treatment for cardiovascular disease. In patients with cancer, coenzyme Q10 has been shown to protect the heart from anthracycline-induced cardiotoxicity (anthracyclines are a family of chemotherapy drugs, including doxorubicin, that have the potential to damage the heart) and to stimulate the immune system. Stimulation of the immune system by this compound has also been observed in animal studies and in humans without cancer. In part because of its immunostimulatory potential, coenzyme Q10 has been used as an adjuvant therapy in patients with various types of cancer.

While coenzyme Q10 may show indirect anticancer activity through its effect(s) on the immune system, there is evidence to suggest that analogs of this compound can suppress cancer growth directly. Analogs of coenzyme Q10 have been shown to inhibit the proliferation of cancer cells in vitro and the growth of cancer cells transplanted into rats and mice. In view of these findings, it has been proposed that analogs of coenzyme Q10 may function as antimetabolites to disrupt normal biochemical reactions that are required for cell growth and/or survival and, thus, that they may be useful for short periods of time as chemotherapeutic agents.

Several companies distribute coenzyme Q10 as a dietary supplement. In the United States, dietary supplements are regulated as foods not drugs. Therefore, premarket evaluation and approval by the Food and Drug Administration (FDA) are not required unless specific disease prevention or treatment claims are made. Because dietary supplements are not formally reviewed for manufacturing consistency, there may be considerable variation from lot to lot.

To conduct clinical drug research in the United States, researchers must file an Investigational New Drug (IND) application with the FDA. The IND application process is highly confidential, and IND information can be disclosed only by the applicants. To date, no investigators have announced that they have applied for an IND to study coenzyme Q10 as a treatment for cancer.

In animal studies, coenzyme Q10 has been administered by injection (intravenous, intraperitoneal, intramuscular, or subcutaneous).

In humans, it is usually taken orally as a pill (tablet or capsule), but intravenous infusions have been given. Coenzyme Q10 is absorbed best with fat; therefore, lipid preparations are better absorbed than the purified compound. In human studies, supplementation doses and administration schedules have varied, but usually have been in the range of 90 to 390 milligrams per day.

History

Coenzyme Q10 was first isolated in 1957, and its chemical structure (benzoquinone compound) was determined in 1958. Interest in coenzyme Q10 as a therapeutic agent in cancer began in 1961, when a deficiency was noted in the blood of both Swedish and American cancer patients, especially in the blood of patients with breast cancer. A subsequent study showed a statistically significant relationship between the level of plasma coenzyme Q10 deficiency and breast cancer prognosis. Low blood levels of this compound have been reported in patients with malignancies other than breast cancer, including myeloma, lymphoma, and cancers of the lung, prostate, pancreas, colon, kidney, and head and neck. Furthermore, decreased levels of coenzyme Q10 have been detected in malignant human tissue, but increased levels have been reported as well.

A large amount of laboratory and animal data on coenzyme Q10 has accumulated since 1962. Research into cellular energy producing mechanisms that involve this compound was awarded the Nobel Prize in chemistry in 1978. Some of the accumulated data show that coenzyme Q10 stimulates animal immune systems, leading to higher antibody levels, greater numbers and/or activities of macrophages and T cells (T lymphocytes), and increased resistance to infection. Coenzyme Q10 has also been reported to increase IgG (immunoglobulin G) antibody levels and to increase the CD4 to CD8 T-cell ratio in humans. CD4 and CD8 are proteins found on the surface of T cells, with CD4 and CD8 identifying "helper" T cells and "cytotoxic" T cells, respectively; decreased CD4 to CD8 T-cell ratios have been reported for cancer patients. Research subsequently delineated the antioxidant properties of coenzyme Q10.

Proposed mechanisms of action for coenzyme Q10 that are relevant to cancer include its essential function in cellular energy production and its stimulation of the immune system (the two of which may be related), as well as its role as an antioxidant. Coenzyme Q10 is essential to aerobic energy production, and it has been suggested that increased cellular energy may lead to increased antibody synthesis in B cells

(B lymphocytes). As noted previously, coenzyme Q10 can also behave as an antioxidant. In this capacity, coenzyme Q10 is thought to stabilize cell membranes (lipid-containing structures essential to maintaining cell integrity) and to prevent free radical damage to other important cellular components. Free radical damage to DNA (and possibly to other cellular molecules) may be a factor in cancer development.

Laboratory/Animal/Preclinical Studies

Laboratory work on coenzyme Q10 has focused primarily on its structure and its function in cell respiration. Studies in animals have demonstrated that coenzyme Q10 is capable of stimulating the immune system, with treated animals showing increased resistance to protozoal infections and to viral and chemically induced neoplasia. Early studies of coenzyme Q10 showed increased hematopoiesis (the formation of new blood cells) in monkeys, rabbits, and poultry. Coenzyme Q10 demonstrated a protective effect on the heart muscle of mice, rats, and rabbits given the anthracycline anticancer drug doxorubicin. Although another study confirmed this protective effect with intraperitoneal administration of doxorubicin in mice, it failed to demonstrate a protective effect when the anthracycline was given intravenously, which is the route of administration in humans. Researchers in one study sounded a cautionary note when they found that coadministration of coenzyme Q10 and radiation therapy decreased the effectiveness of the radiotherapy. In this study, mice inoculated with human small cell lung cancer cells (a xenograft study), and then given coenzyme Q10 and single-dose radiation therapy, showed substantially less inhibition of tumor growth than mice in the control group that were treated with radiation therapy alone. Since radiation leads to the production of free radicals, and since antioxidants protect against free radical damage, the effect in this study might be explained by coenzyme Q10 acting as an antioxidant. As noted previously, there is some evidence from laboratory and animal studies that analogs of coenzyme Q10 may exhibit direct anticancer activity.

Human/Clinical Studies

The use of coenzyme Q10 as a treatment for cancer in humans has been investigated in only a limited manner. With the exception of a single randomized trial, which involved 20 patients and tested the ability of coenzyme Q10 to reduce the cardiotoxicity caused by anthracycline drugs, the studies that have been published consist of anecdotal reports, case reports, case series, and uncontrolled clinical studies.

In view of the promising results from animal studies, coenzyme Q10 was tested as a protective agent against the cardiac toxicity observed in cancer patients treated with the anthracycline drug doxorubicin. It has been postulated that doxorubicin interferes with energy generating biochemical reactions that involve coenzyme Q10 in heart muscle mitochondria and that this interference can be overcome by coenzyme Q10 supplementation. Studies with adults and children, including the aforementioned randomized trial, have confirmed the decrease in cardiac toxicity observed in animal studies.

The potential of coenzyme Q10 as an adjuvant therapy for cancer has also been explored. In view of observations that blood levels of coenzyme Q10 are frequently reduced in cancer patients, supplementation with this compound has been tested in patients undergoing conventional treatment. An open-label (nonblinded), uncontrolled clinical study in Denmark followed 32 breast cancer patients for 18 months. The disease in these patients had spread to the axillary lymph nodes, and an unreported number had distant metastases. The patients received antioxidant supplementation (vitamin C, vitamin E, and beta-carotene), other vitamins and trace minerals, essential fatty acids, and coenzyme Q10 (at a dose of 90 milligrams per day), in addition to standard therapy (surgery, radiation therapy, and chemotherapy, with or without tamoxifen). The patients were seen every 3 months to monitor disease status (progressive disease or recurrence), and, if there was a suspicion of recurrence, mammography, bone scan, x-ray, or biopsy was performed. The survival rate for the study period was one hundred percent (four deaths were expected). Six patients were reported to show some evidence of remission; however, incomplete clinical data were provided, and information suggestive of remission was presented for only three of the six patients. None of the six patients had evidence of further metastases.

For all 32 patients, decreased use of painkillers, improved quality of life, and an absence of weight loss were reported. Whether painkiller use and quality of life were measured objectively (e.g., from pharmacy records and validated questionnaires, respectively) or subjectively (from patient self-reports) was not specified.

In a follow-up study, one of the six patients with a reported remission and a new patient were treated for several months with higher doses of coenzyme Q10 (390 and 300 milligrams per day, respectively). Surgical removal of the primary breast tumor in both patients had been incomplete. After 3 to 4 months of high-level coenzyme Q10 supplementation, both patients appeared to experience complete regression of their residual breast tumors (assessed by clinical examination and mammography). It should be noted that a different patient identifier was used in the follow-up study for the patient who had participated in the original study. Therefore, it is impossible to determine which of the six patients with a reported remission took part in the follow-up study. In the follow-up study report, the researchers noted that all 32 patients from the original study remained alive at 24 months of observation, whereas six deaths had been expected.

In another report by the same investigators, three breast cancer patients were followed for a total of 3 to 5 years on high-dose coenzyme Q10 (390 milligrams per day). One patient had complete remission of liver metastases (determined by clinical examination and ultrasonography), another had remission of a tumor that had spread to the chest wall (determined by clinical examination and chest X-ray), and the third patient had no microscopic evidence of remaining tumor after a mastectomy (determined by biopsy of the tumor bed).

All three of the above-mentioned human studies had important design flaws that could have influenced their outcome. Study weaknesses include the absence of a control group (i.e., all patients received coenzyme Q10), possible selection bias in the follow-up investigations, and multiple confounding variables (i.e., the patients received a variety of supplements in addition to coenzyme Q10, and they received standard therapy either during or immediately before supplementation with coenzyme Q10). Thus, it is impossible to determine whether any of the beneficial results was directly related to coenzyme Q10 therapy.

Anecdotal reports of coenzyme Q10 lengthening the survival of patients with pancreatic, lung, rectal, laryngeal, colon, and prostate cancers also exist in the peer-reviewed, scientific literature. The patients described in these reports also received therapies other than coenzyme Q10, including chemotherapy, radiation therapy, and surgery.

Adverse Effects

No serious toxicity associated with the use of coenzyme Q10 has been reported. Doses of 100 milligrams per day or higher have caused mild insomnia in some individuals. Liver enzyme elevation has been detected in patients taking doses of 300 milligrams per day for extended periods of time, but no liver toxicity has been reported. Researchers in one cardiovascular study reported that coenzyme Q10 caused rashes, nausea, and epigastric (upper abdominal) pain that required withdrawal of a small number of patients from the study. Other reported side effects have included dizziness, photophobia (abnormal visual sensitivity to light), irritability, headache, heartburn, and fatigue.

Certain lipid-lowering drugs, such as the "statins" (lovastatin, pravastatin, and simvastatin) and gemfibrozil, as well as oral agents that lower blood sugar, such as glyburide and tolazamide, cause a decrease in serum levels of coenzyme Q10 and reduce the effects of coenzyme Q10 supplementation. Beta-blockers (drugs that slow the heart rate and lower blood pressure) can inhibit coenzyme Q10-dependent enzyme reactions. The contractile force of the heart in patients with high blood pressure can be increased by coenzyme Q10 administration. Coenzyme Q10 can reduce the body's response to the anticoagulant drug warfarin. Finally, coenzyme Q10 can decrease insulin requirements in individuals with diabetes.

Chapter 56

Hydrazine Sulfate

General Information

Hydrazine sulfate has been investigated as a treatment for cancer for more than 30 years. It has been studied, in combination with established treatments, as a first-line agent in cancer chemotherapy. It has also been investigated as a treatment for cancer-related anorexia (loss of appetite) and cachexia (loss of muscle mass and body weight). Similar to other hydrazine compounds, it has a core chemical structure consisting of two nitrogen atoms and four hydrogen atoms.

Several companies distribute hydrazine sulfate as a dietary supplement. In the United States, dietary supplements are regulated as foods not drugs. Therefore, premarket evaluation and approval by the Food and Drug Administration (FDA) are not required unless specific disease prevention or treatment claims are made. Because dietary supplements are not formally reviewed for manufacturing consistency, there may be considerable variation from lot to lot.

To conduct clinical drug research in the United States, researchers must file an Investigational New Drug (IND) application with the FDA. To date, the FDA has granted IND status to at least three groups of investigators to study hydrazine sulfate as a treatment for cancer.

In animal studies, hydrazine sulfate has been added to the drinking water or the food supply, or it has been given by injection. In clinical trials involving patients with cancer, hydrazine sulfate has been

CancerNet, National Cancer Institute (NCI), January 2001.

administered in pills or capsules. In the clinical trials conducted thus far, the dose and the duration of hydrazine sulfate administration have varied.

History

During the past 90 years, hydrazine compounds have been studied in animal cells grown in the laboratory, in live animals, and in humans. More than 400 hydrazine analogs (related compounds) have been screened for their ability to kill tumors. In 1996, a retrospective review of scientific studies in which the anticancer activity of hydrazine analogs was investigated found that 65 of 82 evaluated compounds showed some anticancer activity in xenograft models (tumor cells of one species transplanted to another species). Seven of the 82 tested compounds showed activity against human tumor cells and were, therefore, selected for further testing in pilot studies and phase I clinical trials. Among these seven compounds, only procarbazine (a methylhydrazine derivative; also called ibenzmethyzin or natulan) completed preliminary testing in humans. Procarbazine exhibited anticancer activity in patients with Hodgkin's disease, melanoma, and lung carcinoma, and it was ultimately used in several first-line treatment regimens in the 1960s. In view of the initial success with procarbazine, hydrazine sulfate, which is similar in chemical composition, was investigated for anticancer activity beginning in the 1970s. During this period, investigation of hydrazine sulfate as a treatment for cancer-related cachexia was also initiated. Research on hydrazine sulfate both as a single agent and in combination with standard chemotherapy regimens continued through the mid-1990s.

Although it was proposed in the early 1900s that hydrazine compounds are toxic to animals and to humans, they have been administered as antidepressant (e.g., iproniazid), chemotherapy (e.g., procarbazine), and antituberculosis (e.g., isoniazid) drugs. In addition to medicinal uses, hydrazine compounds have been used in industry and agriculture as components of rocket fuel, as herbicides, and as antioxidants in boiler and cooling-tower water. Many scientists consider hydrazine sulfate and other hydrazine analogs to be cancer-causing agents, and they have expressed concern about the safety of these compounds. In the Ninth Report on Carcinogens 2000, hydrazine and hydrazine sulfate are listed by the U.S. Department of Health and Human Services' National Toxicology Program as "reasonably anticipated to be human carcinogens." When the antituberculosis drug isoniazid and hydrazine antidepressants are combined with purified

DNA in the laboratory, they produce hydrogen peroxide and free radicals that can damage the DNA. Hydrazine compounds have been reported to cause mutations and chromosome damage in bacteria and in plant and animal cells.

Two mechanisms of action have been proposed for hydrazine sulfate to explain its potential antitumor and anticachexia properties. Both mechanisms involve the utilization of glucose (sugar), which tumors require as a main source of energy for growth. In one proposed mechanism, hydrazine sulfate blocks gluconeogenesis through inhibition of the enzyme phosphoenolpyruvate carboxykinase. Gluconeogenesis is a process by which extra glucose (in addition to that obtained from the diet) can be formed in the liver and the kidneys from the breakdown products of sugars, lipids (fats), and proteins. It has been suggested that cachexia occurs because the body must use increasing amounts of energy and other resources, including its own protein, to meet the demand for glucose by tumors. Blocking gluconeogenesis, and interfering with the supply of nutrients to tumors, has been proposed as one way to inhibit tumor growth and to prevent cachexia.

In the second proposed mechanism, hydrazine sulfate inhibits tumor necrosis factor-alfa (TNF-alfa) activity. TNF-alfa, which is also known as cachectin, is one of a number of substances normally produced by white blood cells of the body in response to infection by microorganisms and in response to other stimuli, such as tissue damage. Higher than normal TNF-alfa production has been observed in white blood cells obtained from cancer patients. It has been suggested that higher than normal levels of TNF-alfa can cause the anorexia, the increased energy expenditure, and the increased muscle protein breakdown seen in cancer patients. Some of the muscle protein breakdown products would become available for gluconeogenesis. Inhibition of TNF-alfa activity might, therefore, inhibit tumor growth and prevent cachexia.

Laboratory/Animal/Preclinical Studies

Hydrazine compounds have been studied both as potential anticancer drugs and as cancer-causing agents. Early studies of hydrazines, including hydrazine sulfate, were conducted to determine whether these compounds could cause cancer in healthy laboratory animals. Substantial increases in tumor incidence were observed in most studies that used rats, mice, or hamsters. Hydrazine administration was associated with increases in lung, liver, and breast tumors in rats, increases in lung and liver tumors in mice, and increases in liver tumors in hamsters. In one study, hydrazine sulfate increased the incidence of lung tumors in both males and females of the mouse strain C3H, but reduced the incidence of breast adenocarcinomas in C3H females.

Animal studies of hydrazine sulfate as a treatment for cancer have investigated this compound as a single agent and in combination with established chemotherapy drugs. In studies conducted in one laboratory, hydrazine sulfate alone was found to cause dose-dependent inhibition of tumor growth in rats bearing Walker 256 carcinosarcoma or Murphy-Sturm lymphosarcoma tumors and in mice bearing B-16 melanoma tumors. Hydrazine sulfate alone had no effect on solid tumors formed from L-1210 leukemia cells in mice. In work performed in another laboratory, hydrazine sulfate alone inhibited the growth of FBCa bladder cancer tumors in one of two experiments in rats, but it had no effect on the growth of 13762NF mammary adenocarcinomas in rats. Findings from a third laboratory demonstrated that hydrazine sulfate alone had no effect on the growth of Dunning prostate cancer tumors in rats. It is important to note that the best tumor responses to hydrazine sulfate as a single agent (i.e., tumor reductions of approximately 50% or more) were accompanied by substantial losses in animal body weight. This finding appears to be inconsistent with the proposed use of hydrazine sulfate as an anticachexia agent.

In other experiments, hydrazine sulfate was combined with individual chemotherapy drugs (cyclophosphamide, mitomycin C, methotrexate, bleomycin, 5-fluorouracil, carmustine (BCNU), or neocarcinostatin) to treat Walker 256 carcinosarcoma tumors in rats and solid L-1210 leukemia tumors in mice. For both tumor types, enhanced anticancer effects were observed. In the experiments with L-1210 tumors, cyclophosphamide and mitomycin C were more effective when combined with hydrazine sulfate than they were when used alone. As indicated previously, hydrazine sulfate alone had no effect against solid L-1210 tumors.

Addition of the drug clofibrate to the hydrazine sulfate plus chemotherapy drug combinations was reported to produce even greater antitumor effects. Clofibrate lowers blood lipid levels and has the potential to inhibit gluconeogenesis by limiting the availability of lipid breakdown products for the synthesis of glucose. This three-drug treatment regimen, however, was tested against only one type of tumor (Walker 256 carcinosarcomas in rats).

Hydrazine sulfate has also been tested in combination with drugs that affect the uptake of glucose by cells. The combination of hydrazine sulfate and phloretin, a drug that blocks glucose uptake, showed greater activity against FBCa bladder cancer tumors in rats than was found with hydrazine sulfate alone; however, this combination did not exhibit enhanced antitumor activity against 13762NF mammary adenocarcinomas in rats. When hydrazine sulfate was combined with the drug phlorizden, which is similar to phloretin, using the same two tumor models, no increase in anticancer activity was observed. When hydrazine sulfate was combined with the drug phenformin, which increases glucose uptake by cells (and lowers blood glucose levels), enhanced antitumor activity against Walker 256 carcinosarcomas in rats was observed.

In the 1980s, the National Cancer Institute (NCI) conducted preclinical studies of hydrazine sulfate as a single agent, using many of the animal tumor models described above. With the exception of borderline activity against Walker 256 carcinosarcomas in rats, no evidence of antitumor activity was found. In view of these results, NCI recommended against further evaluation of hydrazine sulfate as an anticancer agent. However, clinical investigation of this compound continued, largely because of its potential as a treatment for cancer-related anorexia and cachexia.

Human/Clinical Studies

Hydrazine sulfate has been studied extensively in patients with advanced cancer. These studies have evaluated the following: a) tumor response and/or survival among patients with various types of cancer, b) changes in body weight, c) carefully measured quality of life, and d) changes in nutritional or metabolic status. Clinical studies of hydrazine sulfate have been funded by a pharmaceutical company, the Russian government, and grants from the NCI. They have also been sponsored by the North Central Cancer Treatment Group (NCCTG) and the Cancer and Leukemia Group B (CALGB).

The first clinical tests of hydrazine sulfate as a treatment for cancer were conducted in the mid-1970s by a pharmaceutical company. In an uncontrolled study of 158 patients with advanced disease, it was found that 45 of 84 evaluable patients had subjective improvements (i.e., the patients reported an increase in appetite, a decrease in weight loss, an increase in strength, or a decrease in pain) and that 14 had objective improvements (i.e., there was measurable tumor regression, stable disease, or improvement in a cancer-related disorder) in response to treatment with hydrazine sulfate. Among the patients with objective responses, two had long-term (17 and 18 months) stabilization of their disease and seven had measurable tumor regression, although the extent and duration of these regressions were not specified. Major weaknesses of this study included the absence of a control (i.e., comparison) group and the fact that 74 of the 158 initially recruited patients could not be evaluated because of poor prognosis, missing documentation, insufficient duration of treatment, and/or concurrent therapy (i.e., therapy given at the same time) with other anticancer drugs.

In 1976, Russian investigators reported findings from 95 patients with advanced cancer who had been treated with hydrazine sulfate after all previous therapy (surgery, chemotherapy, and/or radiation therapy) had failed. Three partial responses (i.e., reductions in tumor size of greater than 50% observed for a period of 4 weeks or more) and no complete responses were noted after 1 to 5 months of treatment. Tumor regressions of 50% or less and stable disease (i.e., cessation of tumor growth for a period of 1.5 to 2.0 months or more) were reported for 16 and 20 patients, respectively.

In 1981, the same investigators published findings from 225 patients with advanced disease who had been treated with hydrazine sulfate after all previous therapy had failed. It appears that the 225 patients described in this second report included the 95 patients described in the first report. Partial responses and stable disease were reported for four and 95 patients, respectively, after 1 to 6 months of treatment. No patient experienced a complete response. Subjective improvements in appetite, weight stabilization or gain, pain, fever, breathing, and/or mental outlook were reported by 147 patients.

In 1995, the same Russian investigators published findings from 740 patients with advanced cancer. Once again, it appears that 225 of these 740 patients were described in the earlier reports. Partial responses and stable disease were reported for 25 and 263 patients, respectively. Complete responses were noted for six patients. Subjective improvements in cancer-related symptoms were reported by 344 patients.

In 1994, the same investigators reported findings from a clinical series involving 46 patients with malignant brain tumors (38 with glioblastomas, four with astrocytomas, and four with meningiomas) and six patients with benign brain tumors. These patients were not described in the other reports. All patients in this series appear to have been treated with surgery in addition to hydrazine sulfate therapy, and at least some of the patients were also treated with radiation therapy. Complete or partial regression of neurologic symptoms (e.g., seizures, headaches, sensory and motor disorders, and hallucinations) was reported for 73% of the patients. In addition, longer than average survival was reported for most patients. Among the patients with glioblastomas, the increase in average survival time was from 6 months to more than 13 months.

Evaluation of the findings from these Russian clinical series is made difficult by the limited information provided about the patients and their treatment histories. In addition, insufficient information was given about study design and methodology. The absence of control groups; the receipt of prior or concurrent surgery, chemotherapy, and/or radiation therapy by all patients; and the reliance on subjective measures of quality of life are major study weaknesses. Therefore, it is difficult to ascribe any of the positive findings to treatment with hydrazine sulfate.

In contrast with the previously described clinical series, three NCI-funded clinical series found no complete responses or partial responses among a total of 79 patients treated with hydrazine sulfate. In addition, only temporary, minor improvements in appetite, pain, and weight stabilization or gain were reported by the patients in these series. A weakness in these three clinical series was the absence of control groups.

Findings from four placebo-controlled, randomized clinical trials, however, also fail to support the effectiveness of hydrazine sulfate as a cancer treatment in humans. In these trials, survival, objective tumor response, and carefully measured quality of life were major endpoints.

One of the trials involved 65 patients with advanced non-small cell lung cancer and examined the effects of hydrazine sulfate on survival and nutritional status. In this trial, patients received either hydrazine sulfate or placebo in addition to a multiple-drug chemotherapy regimen. When all patients were evaluated, no improvement in survival was found with hydrazine sulfate therapy. In addition, no differences were noted in objective tumor response between the hydrazine sulfate group and the placebo group. However, on the basis of caloric intake and the maintenance of serum albumin levels, the nutritional status of the patients in the hydrazine sulfate group was judged better than that of the patients in the placebo group. However, the moderate increases in body weight associated with hydrazine sulfate use did not achieve statistical significance.

A CALGB-sponsored trial also evaluated the use of hydrazine sulfate as a treatment for patients with advanced non-small cell lung cancer. In this trial, 266 patients received either hydrazine sulfate or placebo in addition to a multiple-drug chemotherapy regimen. No differences in survival, objective tumor response, anorexia, weight gain or loss, or nutritional status were observed between the hydrazine sulfate group and the placebo group. However, the quality of life of the patients who received hydrazine sulfate was found to be statistically significantly worse than that of the patients who received placebo.

The use of hydrazine sulfate as a treatment for patients with non-small cell lung cancer was also evaluated in an NCCTG-sponsored trial. In this trial, 243 patients were randomly assigned to receive either hydrazine sulfate or placebo in addition to a multiple-drug chemotherapy regimen. No statistically significant differences were found between the hydrazine sulfate group and the placebo group with respect to either survival or quality of life.

Another NCCTG-sponsored trial tested hydrazine sulfate alone versus placebo in the treatment of 127 patients with metastatic colorectal cancer. In this trial, the patients who received hydrazine sulfate had, on average, shorter survival than the patients who received placebo, a finding that was statistically significant. There were no statistically significant differences between the hydrazine sulfate group and the placebo group with respect to weight gain or loss, anorexia, or quality of life.

Four other clinical trials did find some objective evidence of benefit with hydrazine sulfate therapy. These trials had either nutritional status or metabolic status as the primary endpoint. In a placebo-controlled, randomized trial involving 38 patients with advanced disease, hydrazine sulfate was found to improve the abnormal glucose metabolism seen in cancer patients. In another placebo-controlled, randomized trial that involved 101 patients with advanced cancer and weight loss, the use of hydrazine sulfate was associated with statistically significant improvements in appetite and either weight increase or weight maintenance. However, the higher average caloric intake observed in this study for patients treated with hydrazine sulfate compared with patients treated with placebo was not statistically significant. Two other clinical studies involving a total of 34 patients with either lung cancer or colon cancer found that hydrazine sulfate was able to reduce the body protein breakdown associated with cancer cachexia. In view of the totality of evidence, the overall importance of the findings from these four clinical trials is not clear.

Finally, a search of the PDQ clinical trials database indicates that no clinical trials of hydrazine sulfate as a therapy for cancer are being conducted at this time.

Adverse Effects

The side effects associated with hydrazine sulfate use have been mainly neurologic and gastrointestinal. Nausea and/or vomiting, dizziness, and sensory and motor neuropathies have been reported. The sensory and motor neuropathies have included paresthesias (abnormal touch sensations, such as burning or prickling, in the absence of external stimuli) of the upper and lower extremities (i.e., the arms and the legs, including the hands and the feet), polyneuritis (simultaneous inflammation of several peripheral nerves), and impaired fine motor function (e.g., an impaired ability to write). Other side effects have included dry skin and/or itching, insomnia, and hypoglycemia. One case of fatal liver and kidney failure and one case of severe encephalopathy (an injury to the brain) have been associated with the use of hydrazine sulfate. In general, the side effects of hydrazine sulfate treatment have been described as mild to moderate in severity, and their incidence appears to have been low. Most side effects are reported to resolve when treatment is stopped.

Hydrazine sulfate is said to be incompatible with certain types of tranquilizers, barbiturates, alcohol, and foods high in tyramine content (e.g., aged cheeses and fermented products). Use of these products reportedly decreases the effectiveness of hydrazine sulfate treatment and increases its side effects.

481

Chapter 57

Laetrile/Amygdalin

General Information

The term "laetrile" is an acronym (laevorotatory and mandelo-nitrile) used to describe a purified form of the chemical amygdalin, a cyanogenic glucoside (a plant compound that contains sugar and produces cyanide) found in the pits of many fruits and raw nuts and in other plants, such as lima beans, clover, and sorghum. In the 1970s, laetrile gained popularity as an anticancer agent. By 1978, more than 70,000 individuals in the United States were reported to have been treated with it. Laetrile has been used for cancer treatment both as a single agent and in combination with a metabolic therapy program that consists of a specialized diet, high-dose vitamin supplements, and pancreatic enzymes.

In the United States, researchers must file an Investigational New Drug (IND) application with the Food and Drug Administration (FDA) to conduct clinical drug research in human subjects. In 1970, an application for an IND to study laetrile was filed by the McNaughton Foundation (San Ysidro, California). This request was initially approved, but later rejected because preclinical evidence in animals showed that laetrile was not likely to be effective as an anticancer agent and because there were questions about how the proposed study was to be conducted. Laetrile supporters viewed this reversal as an attempt by the U.S. government to block access to new and promising cancer therapies, and pressure mounted to make laetrile available to

CancerNet, National Cancer Institute (NCI), December 2000.

the public. Court cases in Oklahoma, Massachusetts, New Jersey, and California challenged the FDA's role in determining which drugs should be available to cancer patients. Consequently, laetrile was legalized in more than 20 states during the 1970s. In 1980, the U.S. Supreme Court overturned decisions by the lower courts, thereby reaffirming the FDA's position that drugs must be proven to be both safe and effective before widespread public use. As a result, the use of laetrile as a cancer therapy is not approved in the United States, but it continues to be manufactured and administered as an anticancer treatment, primarily in Mexico.

Although the names laetrile, Laetrile, and amygdalin are often used interchangeably, they are not the same product. The chemical composition of U.S. patented Laetrile (mandelonitrile-beta-glucuronide), a semi-synthetic derivative of amygdalin, is different from the laetrile/amygdalin produced in Mexico (mandelonitrile beta-D-gentiobioside), which is made from crushed apricot pits. Mandelonitrile, which contains cyanide, is a structural component of both products. It has been proposed that cyanide is the active cancer-killing ingredient in laetrile, but two other breakdown products of amygdalin, prunasin (which is similar in structure to Laetrile) and benzaldehyde, may also be cancer cell inhibitors. The studies discussed in this summary used either Mexican laetrile/amygdalin or the patented form. In most instances, the generic term "laetrile" will be used here; however, a distinction will be made between the products when necessary.

Laetrile can be administered orally as a pill, or it can be given by injection (intravenous or intramuscular). It is commonly given intravenously over a period of time followed by oral maintenance therapy. The incidence of cyanide poisoning is much higher when laetrile is taken orally because intestinal bacteria and some commonly eaten plants contain enzymes (beta-glucosidases) that activate the release of cyanide after laetrile has been ingested. Relatively little breakdown to yield cyanide occurs when laetrile is injected. Administration schedules and the length of treatment in animal models and humans vary widely.

Human/Clinical Studies

Laetrile has been used as an anticancer treatment in humans worldwide. Although many anecdotal reports and case reports are available, findings from only two clinical trials have been published. No controlled clinical trial (a trial including a comparison group that receives no additional treatment, a placebo, or another treatment) of laetrile has ever been conducted.

Case reports and reports of case series have provided little evidence to support laetrile as an anticancer treatment. The absence of a uniform documentation of cancer diagnosis, the use of conventional therapies in combination with laetrile, and variations in the dose and duration of laetrile therapy complicate evaluation of the data. In a case series published in 1962, findings from ten patients with various types of metastatic cancer were reported. These patients had been treated with a wide range of doses of intravenous Laetrile (total dose range, 9 to 133 grams). Pain relief (reduction or elimination) was the primary benefit reported. Some objective responses (responses that are measured rather than based on opinion), such as decreased adenopathy (swollen lymph nodes) and decreased tumor size, were noted. Information on prior or concurrent therapy was provided; however, patients were not followed long-term to determine whether the benefits continued after treatment was stopped. Another case series that was published in 1953 included 44 cancer patients and found no evidence of objective response that could be attributed to laetrile. Most patients with reported cancer regression in this series received recent or concurrent radiation therapy or chemotherapy. Thus, it is impossible to determine which treatment produced the positive results.

Benzaldehyde, which is one of laetrile's breakdown products, has also been tested for anticancer activity in humans. Two clinical series reported a number of responses to benzaldehyde in patients with advanced cancer for whom standard therapy had failed. In one series, 19 complete responses and 10 partial responses were reported among 57 patients who had received either oral or rectal beta-cyclodextrin benzaldehyde; however, precise response durations were specified for only two of the patients. Another series by the same investigators used 4,6-benzylidene-alpha-D-glucose, which is an intravenous formulation of benzaldehyde. In this series, seven complete responses and 29 partial responses were reported among 65 patients, with response durations ranging from 1.5 to 27 months. No toxicity was associated with either preparation of benzaldehyde, and it was reported that the responses persisted as long as treatment was continued. Almost all of the patients in these two series had been treated previously with chemotherapy or radiation therapy, but the elapsed time before the initiation of benzaldehyde treatment was not disclosed.

In 1978, the NCI requested case reports from practitioners who believed their patients had benefited from laetrile treatment. Ninety-three cases were submitted, and 67 were considered evaluable for response. An expert panel concluded that two of the 67 patients had complete responses and that four others had partial responses while using laetrile. On the basis of these six responses, the NCI agreed to sponsor phase I and phase II clinical trials.

The phase I study was designed to test the doses, routes of administration, and the schedule of administration judged representative of those used by laetrile practitioners. The study involved six cancer patients. The investigators found that intravenous and oral amygdalin showed minimal toxicity under the conditions evaluated; however, two patients who ate raw almonds while undergoing oral treatment developed symptoms of cyanide poisoning.

The phase II study was conducted in 1982 and was designed to test the types of cancer that might benefit from laetrile treatment. The majority of patients had breast, colon, or lung cancer. To be eligible for the trial, patients had to be in good general condition (not totally disabled or near death), and they must not have received any other cancer therapy for at least one month before treatment with amygdalin. Amygdalin, evaluated for potency and purity by the NCI, was administered intravenously for 21 days, followed by oral maintenance therapy, utilizing doses and procedures similar to those evaluated in the phase I study. Vitamins and pancreatic enzymes were also administered as part of a metabolic therapy program that included dietary changes to restrict the use of caffeine, sugar, meats, dairy products, eggs, and alcohol. A small subset of patients received higher-dose amygdalin therapy and higher doses of some vitamins as part of the trial.

Patients were followed until there was definite evidence of cancer progression, elevated blood cyanide levels, or severe clinical deterioration. Among 175 evaluable patients, only one patient met the criteria for response. This patient, who had gastric carcinoma with cervical lymph node metastasis, experienced a partial response that was maintained for 10 weeks while on amygdalin therapy. Fifty-four percent of patients had measurable disease progression at the end of the intravenous course of treatment, and all patients had progression seven months after completing intravenous therapy. Seven percent of patients reported an improvement in performance status (ability to work or to perform routine daily activities) at some time during therapy, and 20 percent claimed symptomatic relief. In most patients, these benefits did not persist. Blood cyanide levels were not elevated after intravenous amygdalin treatment; however, they were elevated after oral therapy.

On the basis of this phase II study, NCI concluded that no further investigation of laetrile was warranted. However, several concerns have been expressed about the way the study was conducted.

Variations in commercial preparations of laetrile from Mexico, the primary supplier, have been documented. Incorrect product labels have been found, and samples contaminated with bacteria and other substances have been identified. When a comparison was made of products manufactured in the United States and Canada, differences in chemical composition were noted, and neither product was effective in killing cultured human cancer cells.

Adverse Effects

The side effects associated with laetrile treatment mirror the symptoms of cyanide poisoning. Cyanide is a neurotoxin that can cause nausea and vomiting, headache, dizziness, cyanosis (bluish discoloration of the skin due to oxygen-deprived hemoglobin in the blood), liver damage, hypotension (abnormally low blood pressure), ptosis (droopy upper eyelid), ataxic neuropathies (difficulty walking due to damaged nerves), fever, mental confusion, coma, and death. Oral laetrile causes more severe side effects than injected laetrile. These side effects can be potentiated (increased) by the concurrent administration of raw almonds or crushed fruit pits, eating fruits and vegetables that contain beta-glucosidase (e.g., celery, peaches, bean sprouts, carrots), or taking high doses of vitamin C.

Chapter 58

Mistletoe

General Information

Mistletoe, a parasitic plant, holds interest as a possible anticancer agent because extracts derived from it have been shown to kill cancer cells in vitro and to stimulate immune system cells both in vitro and in vivo. Several components of mistletoe, namely alkaloids, viscotoxins, and lectins, may be responsible for these effects. Alkaloids comprise a large group of nitrogen-containing chemicals produced by plants, and some alkaloids, from other types of plants, are widely used as cancer chemotherapy agents. Limited experimental evidence indicates that mistletoe alkaloids may also have anticancer activity. Viscotoxins are small proteins that exhibit cell-killing activity and possible immune system stimulating activity. Lectins are complex molecules that contain both protein and sugars and are capable of binding to the outside of cells (e.g., immune system cells) and inducing biochemical changes in them. In view of mistletoe's ability to stimulate the immune system, it has been classified as a type of biological response modifier. Biological response modifiers constitute a complex group of biologic substances that have been used individually, or in combination with other agents, to treat cancer or to lessen the adverse effects of anticancer drugs.

"Mistletoe (PDQ)," and undated fact sheet produced by the National Cancer Institute (NCI); available online at http://www.cancer.gov; cited December 2001.

Mistletoe is used mainly in Europe and Asia, where commercially available products are marketed under the brand names Iscador, Eurixor, Helixor, Isorel, Vysorel, and ABNOBAviscum. These products are not sold commercially in the United States. Mistletoe products have not been tested and found by the U.S. Food and Drug Administration (FDA) to be safe and effective in treating cancer in humans. Before researchers can conduct clinical drug research in the United States, they must file an Investigational New Drug (IND) application with the FDA. To date, no investigators have announced that they have applied for an IND to study mistletoe as a treatment for cancer.

Mistletoe grows on various trees such as apple, oak, maple, elm, pine, and birch. Each mistletoe species (e.g., *Viscum album Loranthacea* [*Viscum album L.* or "European mistletoe"] and *Viscum album coloratum* ["Korean mistletoe"]) is capable of growing on a variety of trees. The chemical composition of commercial mistletoe products varies greatly depending on the species of the host tree, the time of year harvested, the species of mistletoe, how it is prepared for use, and the commercial producer. This summary discusses research using primarily *Viscum album L.*

Mistletoe extracts are prepared as aqueous solutions or solutions of water and alcohol, and they can be fermented or unfermented. For example, Iscador is an aqueous extract of *Viscum album L.* that is available in both fermented and unfermented forms. In addition, Iscador products can be subdivided according to the species of host tree. IscadorM is obtained from apple trees, IscadorP comes from pine trees, IscadorQ comes from oak trees, and IscadorU comes from elm trees. Helixor is an unfermented aqueous extract of *Viscum album L.*, with HelixorA from spruce trees, HelixorM from apple trees, and HelixorP from pine trees. Helixor is reported to be standardized by its biologic effect on human leukemia cells grown in the laboratory. Eurixor is an unfermented aqueous extract of *Viscum album L.* obtained from poplar trees. As indicated previously, there are several potentially active components in mistletoe, and some researchers contend the formulation of mistletoe extracts should vary according to the type of tumor, patient gender, and the method of administration. In this chapter, the exact type of mistletoe extract or mistletoe product used in individual studies will be specified wherever possible.

In modern studies, mistletoe extracts have been administered by intramuscular injection, subcutaneous injection (sometimes in the vicinity of a tumor), or intravenous infusion.

Human/Clinical Studies

Mistletoe has been used for centuries to treat a number of ailments in humans, but scientific data from controlled or uncontrolled studies of cancer are limited and often of poor quality. To a great extent, research in this area has concentrated on immune system effects. Relatively few studies have used tumor response or survival as study endpoints, and conflicting results have been obtained. Furthermore, the use of different mistletoe products, or combinations of mistletoe products, from one study to the next makes comparison of the findings difficult, and, in some studies, patients have required different doses of the same product to achieve comparable effects on immune system function. Although there is substantial evidence of mistletoe's ability to modulate the human immune system, there is no evidence that this enhanced immunity leads to improved cancer cell destruction.

It has been suggested that mistletoe may fail to inhibit tumor growth in humans because 1) antibodies can be produced against the active component(s), 2) plasma proteins may break down or interfere with the active component(s), or 3) the plant lectins in mistletoe extracts may not be able to bind to certain types of human cells.

Several studies involving patients with breast cancer have demonstrated that extracts of *Viscum album L.*, or the lectin ML-I purified from them, can stimulate increases in a variety of white blood cell types and may be able to induce cells to repair damaged DNA. A limited study of eight patients with cancer (type not specified) found higher serum levels of the cytokines interleukin-6 and tumor necrosis factor-alfa after a single intravenous infusion of the mistletoe lectin ML-I. In addition, 25 of 36 patients with advanced breast cancer showed higher white blood cell counts and higher production of the cytokines interleukin-1-alfa, interleukin-2, interferon-gamma, and tumor necrosis factor-alfa (all of which are immune system enhancers) when the mistletoe product Eurixor (given by subcutaneous injection) was added to their treatment regimen. Higher production of the neuropeptide beta-endorphin and higher quality of life (determined by use of a standardized questionnaire) were also reported for these 25 patients. A prospective, randomized study of 47 patients with advanced breast cancer found that subcutaneous treatment with Eurixor produced increases in serum beta-endorphin levels and immune system function that were statistically significantly correlated. The authors of this latter study concluded that their data showed the existence of a link between the immune system and the neuroendocrine system.

Another randomized study involving 38 patients with glioma demonstrated that subcutaneous injections of Eurixor could enhance immune system function and improve the quality of life (determined by use of a standardized questionnaire) in individuals treated with tumor destructive therapy (i.e., surgery, perioperative dexamethasone treatment, and local radiation therapy). However, an analysis that included all 38 patients in this study showed that Eurixor treatment did not improve disease-free survival or overall survival.

In a case series involving 168 patients with malignant pleural effusions, injection of *Viscum album L.* extracts into the effusions led to a decline in the number of tumor cells and an increase in the number of white blood cells in this fluid in some patients (the number of patients with responses was not specified). Another case series involving 23 patients with various types of cancer showed no partial remissions or complete remissions, or any effect on tumor markers, after treatment with the mistletoe lectin ML-I.

A phase I/II trial involving 16 patients with stage III or stage IV pancreatic cancer showed no partial remissions or complete remissions following subcutaneous treatment with Eurixor, although it was reported that quality of life (measured by use of a standardized questionnaire) was stabilized for approximately half of the patients. A phase II trial involving 14 patients with stage IV kidney cancer found no measurable response to therapy or improvement in survival after subcutaneous treatment with copper ion-supplemented extracts of *Viscum album L.* (males were treated with IscadorQ and females were treated with IscadorM).

In 1994, a review article on mistletoe use in human cancer evaluated 11 controlled clinical trials. The primary reports of these trials were published in German, and none of the trials is included in the discussion above. The authors of the review article initially identified 13 trials, but two trials were excluded because they failed to meet eligibility criteria for inclusion in the analysis. Only preliminary results were available from one of the excluded trials, and detailed information on the design and conduct of this trial was lacking. The method of selecting the control group in the second excluded trial left open the possibility that the control group and the group treated with mistletoe were not equivalent. Most of the 11 evaluated trials recruited patients with a single type of cancer, including lung, colorectal, gastric, breast, and female genital cancers. Survival duration was the principle endpoint measured in these trials. Ten trials reported beneficial effects with mistletoe use, but, according to the reviewers, these positive trials all had serious shortcomings (flaws in study design, incomplete data reporting, etc.), which make it difficult to draw meaningful conclusions from the data. The trial judged to have the best design showed no difference in lung cancer survival between patients given IscadorQ and IscadorU and patients given either a multivitamin preparation as a placebo or Polyerga, a substance previously shown in laboratory studies to have immune system stimulating effects. The number of patients enrolled in each of the 11 trials was not presented in the review.

Finally, a protocol for a randomized, phase III trial of adjuvant therapy with IscadorM versus interferon-alfa versus interferon-gamma versus no further treatment following potentially curative surgery for high-risk stage I or stage IIB melanoma was found in the closed section of the PDQ clinical trials database.[http://cancernet. nci.nih.gov] This trial, which had a goal of recruiting more than 800 patients over a 4-year period, was sponsored by a European clinical trials organization. Preliminary findings from this trial have been reported in abstract form, with no benefit in disease-free survival or overall survival shown for either interferon or Iscador.

Adverse Effects

Although numerous formulations of mistletoe have been used in human studies, the associated side effects have been minimal and non-life threatening. Common side effects found with mistletoe-product injection include soreness and inflammation at the injection site, headache, fever, and chills. Seizures, slowing of the heart rate, abnormally high blood pressure, abnormally low blood pressure, vomiting, and death have been reported after ingestion of mistletoe plants and berries. The severity of the toxic effects associated with mistletoe ingestion may depend on the amount consumed and the type of mistletoe plant.

Levels of Evidence for Human Studies of Cancer Complementary and Alternative Medicine

To assist readers in evaluating the results of human studies of CAM treatments for cancer, the strength of the evidence (i.e., the "levels of evidence") associated with each type of treatment is provided whenever possible. To qualify for a levels of evidence analysis, a study must 1) be published in a peer-reviewed, scientific journal; 2) report on a therapeutic outcome(s), such as tumor response, improvement in survival, or measured improvement in quality of life; and 3) describe clinical findings in sufficient detail that a meaningful evaluation can be made. Separate levels of evidence scores are assigned to qualifying human studies on the basis of statistical strength of the study design and scientific strength of the treatment outcomes (i.e., endpoints) measured. The resulting two scores are then combined to produce an overall score.

Part Eight

Skeptical Points of View

Chapter 59

Magnet Therapy: Questions about Its Efficacy

During the past few years, magnetic devices have been claimed to relieve pain and to have therapeutic value against a large number of diseases and conditions. The way to evaluate such claims is to ask whether scientific studies have been published. Pulsed electromagnetic fields—which induce measurable electric fields—have been demonstrated effective for treating slow-healing fractures and have shown promise for a few other conditions. However, few studies have been published on the effect on pain of small, static magnets marketed to consumers.[1] Explanations that magnetic fields "increase circulation," "reduce inflammation," or "speed recovery from injuries" are simplistic and are not supported by the weight of experimental evidence.[2]

The main basis for the claims is a double-blind test study, conducted at Baylor College of Medicine in Houston, which compared the effects of magnets and sham magnets on knee pain. The study involved 50 adult patients with pain related to having been infected with the polio virus when they were children. A static magnetic device or a placebo device was applied to the patient's skin for 45 minutes. The patients were asked to rate how much pain they experienced when a "trigger point was touched." The researchers reported that the 29 patients exposed to the magnetic device achieved lower pain scores than did the 21 who were exposed to the placebo device.[3] Although this study is cited by nearly everyone selling magnets, it provides no legitimate basis for concluding that magnets offer any health-related benefit:

- Although the groups were said to be selected randomly, the ratio of women to men in the experimental group was twice that of the control group. If women happen to be more responsive to placebos than men, a surplus of women in the "treatment" group would tend to improve that group's score.

- The age of the placebo group was four years higher than that of the control group. If advanced age makes a person more difficult to treat, the "treatment" group would again have a scoring advantage.

- The investigators did not measure the exact pressure exerted by the blunt object at the trigger point before and after the study.

- Even if the above considerations have no significance, the study should not be extrapolated to suggest that other types of pain can be relieved by magnets.

- There was just one brief exposure and no systematic follow-up of patients. Thus there was no way to tell whether any improvement would be more than temporary.

- The authors themselves acknowledge that the study was a "pilot study." Pilot studies are done to determine whether it makes sense to invest in a larger more definitive study. They never provide a legitimate basis for marketing any product as effective against any symptom or health problem.

Two better-designed, longer-lasting pain studies have been negative:

- Researchers at the New York College of Podiatric Medicine have reported negative results in a study of patients with heel pain. Over a 4-week period, 19 patients wore a molded insole containing a magnetic foil, while 15 patients wore the same type of insole with no magnetic foil. In both g roups, 60% reported improvement, which suggests that the magnetic foil conveyed no benefit.[4]

- More recently, researchers at the VA Medical Center in Prescott, Arizona conducted a randomized, double-blind, placebo-controlled, crossover study involving 20 patients with chronic back pain, of the use of magnets to treat back pain. Each patient was exposed to real and sham bipolar permanent magnets during alternate weeks, for 6 hours per day, 3 days per week for a week, with a 1-week period between the treatment weeks. No difference in pain or mobility was found between the treatment and sham-treatment periods.[5]

Legal and Regulatory Actions

In 1998, Magnetherapy, Inc., of West Palm Beach, Florida, signed an Assurance of Voluntary Compliance with the State of Texas to pay a $30,000 penalty and to stop claiming that wearing its magnetic device near areas of pain and inflammation will relieve pain due to arthritis, migraine headaches, sciatica or heel spurs. The agreement also requires Magnetherapy to stop making claims that its magnets can cure, treat, or mitigate any disease or can affect any change in the human body, unless its devices are FDA-approved for those purposes.[6] Ads for the company's Tectonic Magnets had featured testimonials from athletes, including golfers from the senior pro tours. Various ads had claimed that Tectonic Magnets would provide symptomatic relief from certain painful conditions and could restore range of motion to muscles and joints. The company had provided retailers with display packages that included health claims, written testimonials, and posters of sports stars. Texas Attorney General Dan Morales stated that some claims were false or unsubstantiated and others had rendered the product unapproved medical devices under Texas law. In 1997, the FDA had warned Magnetherapy to stop claiming that its products would relieve arthritis; tennis elbow; low back pain; sciatica; migraine headache; muscle soreness; neck, knee, ankle, and shoulder pain; heel spurs; bunions; arthritic fingers and toes; and could reduce pain and inflammation in the affected areas by increasing blood and oxygen flow.[7]

In 1999, the FTC obtained a consent agreement barring two companies from making unsubstantiated claims about their magnetic products. Magnetic Therapeutic Technologies, of Irving, Texas, is barred from claiming that its magnetic sleep pads or other products: (a) are effective against cancers, diabetic ulcers, arthritis, degenerative joint conditions, or high blood pressure; (b) could stabilize or increase the T-cell count of HIV patients; (c) could reduce muscle spasms in persons with multiple sclerosis; (d) could reduce nerve spasms associated with diabetic neuropathy; (e) could increase bone density, immunity, or circulation; or (f) are comparable or superior to prescription pain medicine. Pain Stops Here! Inc., of Baiting Hollow, N.Y., may no longer claim that its "magnetized water" or other products are useful against cancer, diseases of the liver or other internal organs, gallstones, kidney stones, urinary infection, gastric ulcers, dysentery, diarrhea, skin ulcers, bed sores, arthritis, bursitis, tendonitis, sprains, strains, sciatica, heart disease, circulatory disease, arthritis, autoimmune illness, neuro-degenerative disease, and allergies, and could stimulate the growth of plants.

On August 8, 2000, the Consumer Justice Center, of Laguna Niguel, California filed suit in Orange County Superior Court charging that Florsheim and a local shoe store (Shoe Emporium) made false and fraudulent claims that their MagneForce shoes (a) correct "magnetic deficiency," (b) "generate a deep-penetrating magnetic field which increases blood circulation; reduces leg and back fatigue; and provides natural pain relief and improved energy level."; and (c) their claims are established and proven by scientific studies.[8] A few days after this suit was filed, Florsheim removed the disputed ad from its Web site.

The Bottom Line

There is no scientific basis to conclude that small, static magnets can relieve pain or influence the course of any disease. In fact, many of today's products produce no significant magnetic field at or beneath the skin's surface.

References

1. Livingston JD. Magnetic therapy: Plausible attraction. *Skeptical Inquirer* 25-30, 58, 1998.

2. Ramey DW. Magnetic and electromagnetic therapy. *Scientific Review of Alternative Medicine* 2(1):13-19, 1998.

3. Vallbona C, Hazelwood CF, Jurida G. Response of pain to static magnetic fields in postpolio patients: A double-blind pilot study. *Archives of Physical and Rehabilitative Medicine* 78:1200-1203, 1997.

4. Caselli MA and others. Evaluation of magnetic foil and PPT Insoles in the treatment of heel pain. *Journal of the American Podiatric Medical Association* 87:11-16, 1997.

5. Collacott EA and others. Bipolar permanent magnets for the treatment of chronic low back pain. *JAMA* 283:1322-1325, 2000.

6. Morales halts unproven claims for magnet therapy. News release, April 9, 1998.

7. Gill LJ. Letter to William L. Roper, Feb 3, 1997.

8. Jeff Wynton and the Consumer Justice Center v. Florsheim Group, Inc., Shoe Emporium. Superior Court of California, Orange County, Case #00CC09419, filed Aug 8, 2000.

Chapter 60

Therapeutic Touch:
An Opposing Point of View

Therapeutic touch (TT) method in which the hands are used to "direct human energies to help or heal someone who is ill." Proponents claim that the patient's "energy field" can be detected and intentionally manipulated by the therapist. They theorize that healing results from a transfer of "excess energy" from healer to patient. Their reports claim that TT is effective against scores of diseases and conditions.

Therapeutic Touch was conceived in the early 1970s by Dolores Krieger, Ph.D., R.N., a faculty member at New York University's Division of Nursing. The "human energy field" TT theorists postulate resembles the "magnetic fluid" or "magnetic force" hypothesized during the 18th century by Anton Mesmer and his followers. Mesmerism held that illnesses are caused by obstacles to the free flow of this fluid and that skilled healers ("sensitives") could remove these obstacles by making passes with their hands. Some aspects of mesmerism were revived in the nineteenth century by Theosophy, an occult religion that incorporated Eastern metaphysical concepts and underlies many current "New Age" ideas. Dora Kunz, who is considered TT's co-developer, was president of the Theosophical Society of America from 1975 to 1987. She collaborated with Krieger on the early TT studies and claims to be a fifth-generation "sensitive" and a "gifted healer."

"Therapeutic Touch," by Stephen Barrett, M.D. © 2000 Quackwatch, and "Further Notes on Therapeutic Touch," by Kevin Courcey, R.N., an undated document produced by Quackwatch, available online at http://www.quackwatch. com/01QuackeryRelatedTopics/tt2.html, cited January 2002, © Quackwatch; reprinted with permission.

Today's proponents state that more than 100,000 people worldwide have been trained in TT technique, including at least 43,000 health care professionals, and that about half of those trained actually practice it. TT generally involves four steps: (1) "centering," a meditative process said to align the healer with the patent's energy level, (2) "assessment," said to be performed by using one's hands to detect forces emanating from the patient, (3) "unruffling the field," said to involve sweeping "stagnant energy" downward to prepare for energy transfer, and (4) transfer of "energy" from practitioner to patient. "Noncontact therapeutic touch" is done the same way, except that the "healer's" hands are held a few inches away from the body. TT is sometimes used together with massage.

There is no scientific evidence that the "energy transfer" postulated by proponents actually occurs. It is safe to assume that any reactions to the procedure are psychological responses to the "laying on of hands."

In 1996, Linda Rosa, R.N., published a critique of all of the studies related to TT she could locate in nursing journals and elsewhere. She concluded: "The more rigorous the research design, the more detailed the statistical analysis, the less evidence that there is any observed—or observable—phenomenon."

During the past two years, Rosa's daughter Emily has tested 21 TT practitioners to determine whether they could detect one of her hands near theirs. Each subject was tested ten or twenty times. During the tests, the practitioners rested their forearms and hands, palms up, on a flat surface, approximately 10 to 12 inches apart. Emily then hovered her hand, palm down, a few inches above one of the subject's palms. A cardboard screen was used to prevent the subjects from seeing which hand was selected. The practitioners correctly located Emily's hand only 122 (44%) out of 280 trials, which is no better than would be expected by guessing. A score of 50% would be expected through chance alone. George D. Lundberg, M.D., editor of the *Journal of the American Medical Association* (*JAMA*), believes that TT practitioners now have an ethical duty to disclose the results of this study to potential patients and that third-party payers should question whether they should pay for TT procedures. Lundberg also believes that patients should "refuse to pay for this procedure until or unless additional honest experimentation demonstrates an actual effect."

While Emily hovered her hand over the practitioner's hand, the draped towel prevented peeking. The screen was approximately 3 feet high and 1/8th of an inch think.

In 1996, the James Randi Educational Foundation offered $742,000 to anyone who could demonstrate an ability to detect a "human energy field" under conditions similar to those of our study. Although more than 80,000 American practitioners claim to have such ability, only one person attempted to demonstrate it. She failed, and the offer, now at $1 million, has no further takers despite extensive recruiting efforts, including a direct appeal to Dr. Krieger.

Further Notes on Therapeutic Touch

The woman lying in the bed is in pain. She is just back from major abdominal surgery, and her nurse is working to make her more comfortable. Just then, another staff member comes in the room and announces that she will use Therapeutic Touch to relieve the patient's pain. She waits a moment, then begins moving her hands in the air above the patient's body. She makes numerous passes over the patient, and the patient finally reports that she is feeling more comfortable.

Distracted by the dramatic, sweeping gestures going on over her body, the patient did not notice that her nurse had just increased the rate of her IV pain medication; she assumes the arm waving staff member must be responsible for the relief she now feels. And another believer in the power of Therapeutic Touch has just been created.

A similar scenario may be happening now in a hospital near you. More than 100,000 people have been taught Therapeutic Touch (TT) in the past 20 years, including nearly 50,000 nurses and health care professionals. Practitioners have been aggressively demanding respect for their "art." They have formed TT associations, pushed for insurance coverage, established training centers in more than 100 colleges and universities, and have even convinced the North American Nursing Diagnosis Association to include "Energy Field Disturbance" as an official nursing diagnosis, for which TT is the primary intervention.

What Is TT?

Therapeutic Touch was developed in the early 1970s by Dolores Krieger RN, a professor of nursing. Krieger and co-founder Dora Kunz stated that the human body is kept alive and vital by a force called prana (a Sanskrit term meaning "vital force") and that this energy flows around and through the body and is channeled by chakras, a series of non-physical energy centers in the body. Whereas the original protocol was based on actual physical touch, subsequent research claimed that similar results could be obtained without touching the patient. Current practice is based on the assumption that the physical body is surrounded by an energy field that trained practitioners can detect, assess, and manipulate, and that imbalances in this energy field result in illness or pain, which TT can treat. Imbalances are "felt" using the hands, and are described variously as a sensation of tingling, pressure, pulling, temperature variations, energy "spikes," or the like.

A TT session begins with a centering exercise by the practitioner. This initial step is considered to be similar to a brief period of meditation, where the Therapeutic Touch Practitioner (TTP) focuses "internally" and concentrates on their intent to heal. The second phase is assessment, where the TTP sweeps her hands 2-4 inches over the patient's entire body in an attempt to detect energy imbalances in the patient's Human Energy Field (HEF). The third phase is called unruffling.

During this phase the TTP uses circular sweeping motions with the intent to "decongest" accumulated energy and either redistribute it to areas of lower energy, or rid the HEF of the excess energy by sweeping it down the body and off at the feet, shaking the excess off their hands (a motion similar to shaking water off the fingers) at the foot of the bed or table. It is rumored that at least one disgruntled individual is considering suing a Midwestern hospital because he was hit with what he called the "excess negative energy" from a careless TTP working on a patient in the next bed. The thought of hospital lawyers trying to prove it didn't happen is enough to brighten anyone's day.

Testimonials abound for this practice, and TTPs will eagerly discuss anecdotal evidence supporting the efficacy of their treatment. Indeed, published TT literature claims some remarkable results. It is promoted as being virtually a universal cure: from the mundane "comforting the dying" and "increased relaxation," to the highly speculative "remedies thyroid imbalances," "breaks fevers," "relieves acute pain," and even "brings some dead back to life."

The Roots of Therapeutic Touch

Even though Krieger had published her views previously in *Human Dimensions* (1972) and *Psychoenergetic Systems* (1974), it was the article in the *American Journal of Nursing* (*AJN*) that catapulted her to fame. While some Christians saw biblical roots to Krieger's approach, and considered her study's publication in the *AJN* official permission to bring their religious faith more directly into patient care, others recognized and embraced the Eastern mystical roots to the practice.

The concept of prana is taken from Hinduism, and Krieger admitted that prana was "at the base of the human energy transfer in the healing act." Skeptics remarked on what they saw as connections to the teachings of Anton Mesmer, the 18th century hypnotist and theorizer of "animal magnetism." Mesmer believed that a "subtle magnetic fluid" exists in the body and needs to be controlled or expelled in order for healing to occur. He and his followers believed that obstacles to the free flow of this fluid caused illness, and that skilled healers or "sensitives" could remove these obstructions by making passes over the patient's body with their hands. Dora Kunz, TT's co-founder and President of the religious Theosophical Society of America, claimed to be just such a "fifth-generation sensitive."

Some professional nurses did object when Krieger's article came out. In a letter to the editor in a subsequent edition of *AJN*, nursing instructors from the University of Washington pointed to numerous flaws in Krieger's study. They complained that Krieger gave no indication of how patients were assigned to her groups, and wondered why there was such an uneven distribution of patients, with 19 in the therapy group and 9 in the control group. They questioned whether other treatments or conditions (such as medication use, dietary changes, menstrual cycles, transfusions, etc.) might have influenced the results. They also criticized *AJN* for publishing such a study without a critique, charging the article was dangerously misleading, and reminded readers that the energy field Krieger was postulating had never been shown to exist.

Noting that much of the critical response to her studies centered around the vaguely religious concept of prana, Krieger switched to a seemingly more scientific concept being pioneered by nursing theorist Martha Rogers—that of the Human Energy Field. Rogers postulated that humans not only have an energy field, but that they are an energy field, and that this energy field is constantly interacting with the energy of its environment. She extrapolated from this to theories about the non-linearity of time, how clairvoyance and telepathy occur, and how physical contact is unnecessary for the transfer of energies. This led to a doctoral dissertation by Janet Quinn in 1982, which showed that therapeutic touch need not use physical contact in order to produce results similar to the "touch" version. The non-touch version has been the standard ever since.

Individuals in High Places

Some explanations for the phenomenal growth of TT have been less than favorable. Dr. William Jarvis, president of the National Council Against Health Fraud, stated: "I see therapeutic touch as a form of faith healing that has captured the imagination of a few nurses who happen to be in pretty powerful positions of influence within the nursing profession."

Jarvis has a point. The fact that well respected nursing professors and nursing journals were endorsing TT gave it an instant legitimacy it perhaps did not deserve. Krieger was a Professor Emeritus at New York University's Division of Nursing. Martha Rogers was a well-respected nursing theorist and Dean of Nursing at NYU. Janet Quinn, who studied at NYU, would go on to become Associate Professor of Nursing at the University of Colorado. Jean Watson, Distinguished Professor of Nursing at Colorado, also a supporter of TT, would go on to head the National League for Nursing, the board that accredits nursing schools.

Many feel the psychological climate was also conducive to the spread of TT. Nurses, primarily women, have long felt under-appreciated in the medical profession; a profession whose focus of attention and adoration tended to be riveted on the (mostly male) MD's. TT gave nurses a way to feel they were participating more directly in the "healing" of the patient, rather than just passively carrying out doctor's orders. The nurse could now have secret mystical powers which the doctors did not possess—they could now be the shaman, the healers. Carla Selby, a member of the Rocky Mountain Skeptics who would later challenge the University of Colorado's Healing Touch program, observed, "I'm all for nurses getting out from under the thumbs of doctors. But this is exactly the wrong thing to do."

Follow the Money

Unfortunately, TT has meant big money for some, making it difficult to challenge. Over 100,000 people have been trained in TT. Considering that the cost of a basic TT certification training is frequently in the $250-300 range, this amounts to a multi-million dollar industry.

According to the official "Energy Field Disturbance" nursing diagnosis, you should only perform TT if you have had a minimum of 12 hours of instruction and received a certificate. The protocol goes on to note that you should be supervised by a nurse who has a master's degree in nursing and has had 30 hours of instruction in TT theory, and 30 hours of supervised TT practice. Such advanced training can cost thousands. With these criteria officially in place, the TT training mill should stay profitable for a long time.

In Colorado, however, a local skeptics group challenged the State Board of Nursing for its decision to issue continuing education credits for TT. They also challenged the University of Colorado to justify its nursing program's Healing Touch (HT) training. As a result of this pressure, Colorado State University established a blue-ribbon panel in 1994 to investigate TT, and its inclusion in the CU School of Nursing program. The panel consisted of 3 CU faculty members outside the School of Nursing, and two nursing professors from outside CU. It was chaired by Dr. Henry Claman, a distinguished professor and chairman of the department of immunology at CU. This was probably the first scientific jury to sit in judgment on the merits of TT. Despite considerable pressure from the entrenched TT interests in the nursing department, and the obvious financial gain of the TT classes for the school, the panel issued a blistering report critical of TT and the School of Nursing's misleading marketing of the courses. The panel concluded: To date, there is not a sufficient body of data, both in quality and quantity, to establish TT as a unique and efficacious healing modality. If an effect is observable, it can be measured. It is not adequate to state that TT involves mechanisms which exist beyond the five senses and which therefore cannot be proven by ordinary methods. Such comments are a disservice to science and the practice of healing and demonstrate a commitment to metaphysics and the mystical view of life rather than to a scientific or rational view of life. Although TT practitioners state that the existence and nature of the [human] energy field is an hypothesis which has not been confirmed in over 20 years, in practice they behave as if the energy field were a perceptible reality. There is virtually no acceptable scientific evidence concerning the existence or nature of these energy fields.

Despite such a clearly negative finding, the review board voted to allow the school of nursing to continue its Healing Touch focus. The report itself gives us a clue as to the justification for this decision: "TT is potentially a source of considerable income. Training in TT is not complex and arduous and the practice of TT does not require a large investment in equipment or personnel." Indeed, Quinn's Healing Touch training brings in a substantial amount of money for the nursing school. A set of three HT videotapes featuring Quinn sells for $675. Healing Touch classes cost $225 each for the first three levels and $325 each for the next two levels.

But training is not the only cash cow associated with TT. Recently, over half a million dollars of public tax money has been spent on Therapeutic Touch research. The National Institutes of Health has given $150,000 in grants, the Department of Health and Human Services has granted $200,000, and most recently the Department of Defense granted $355,000 to the University of Alabama at Birmingham—all for studies of TT. The study at UAB, to be conducted on burn patients, was billed as being the study that would finally settle the question as to the effectiveness of TT.

The Critics Grow Louder

Nursing theorist Myra Levine has noted: The pretense of the healers that they perform scientific therapies is unconscionable. In our struggle to achieve academic recognition as a profession, we simply cannot afford to indulge in this kind of charlatanism. Therapeutic Touch challenges the validity of modern nursing research, teaching and practice. If its practitioners insist on their healing roles, let them honestly call themselves faith healers and stop claiming they are nurses who heal.

A growing chorus of dissent has, in the past four to five years, finally found its voice. In November 1994, *TIME* magazine featured an article that articulated the concerns of the skeptics. The author of the article scoffed at the research that had been done on TT, noting that, "As proof of TT's efficacy, they cite "scientific" reports in such obscure journals as *Subtle Energies and Psychoenergetic Systems*, as well as stories in popular magazines." Vern Bullough, a retired professor of nursing at the State University of New York was quoted as saying, "None of the research demonstrated that there's any effect, and many of the conclusions are subjective."

In 1994, Linda Rosa RN, Chair of the Questionable Nursing Practices Taskforce of the National Council Against Health Fraud, compiled a thorough review of the TT literature. Presented in her 180-page Survey of Therapeutic Touch "Research," the report presents an abstract of virtually every study done on TT, along with an analysis of the results and the methodological critiques mentioned subsequently by other authors.

Rosa's report states, for example, that when the original "healing" studies were done on plants, there were no controls for heat from the healer's hands which naturally increased enzyme production in the plants, and caused them to grow faster. When appropriate controls were instituted, the healer's effect vanished.

Dolores Krieger's early research studied a healer's powers applied to people. Assuming that plant chlorophyll and human hemoglobin were somehow similar, she decided to measure the subjects' hemoglobin levels before and after TT. She claimed to find increased hemoglobin following TT. Practitioners still excitedly talk about these studies as if they were a scientific breakthrough. But even TT proponent, researcher, and former Krieger student Therese C. Meehan has admitted: Methodological problems preclude scientific support for an increase in hemoglobin values. Subsequent studies have found no significant relationship between TT and increased hemoglobin values or transcutaneous oxygen blood gas pressure.

Yet another study that had a major impact on the nursing practice of TT was the 1984 study on premature newborns in the intensive care unit. The use of TT was evaluated as a stress-reduction intervention for these critically ill newborns. Stress was measured during the routine nursing procedure of taking vital signs by scores on an Infant Behavior Inventory and by measuring the amount of oxygen in their blood. The infants were treated with TT, mock TT (in which a nurse would simply wave their hands over the infant without the intention to "heal" or calm them), and No Touch. Interestingly, TT was declared to be an effective method for reducing the behavioral stress when measured by researchers' scores on the infant behavior rating inventory, but ineffective for reducing physiologic stress as measured by blood oxygen levels. Mock TT actually seemed to increase behavioral stress.

But as Linda Rosa's survey points out, virtually every cardinal sin of research was committed in this severely flawed study. The investigator and her assistant knew which infants were treated with TT and which were treated with mock TT, yet they served as the sole data collectors and the raters of infant behavior. Notably, the unbiased physiologic indicator, the oxygen level in the blood, seemed curiously unimpressed by the TT intervention when compared to the human researchers. Despite its obvious flaws, this study has nurses all over the country waving their hands over critically ill newborns, possibly increasing the infants' stress levels by their bizarre and threatening behavior.

Perhaps the most cited of the TT studies was done by Wirth in 1990. Wirth inflicted volunteers with a full thickness dermal wound (upper arm area) and then applied TT to half the group and no intervention to the other half. The interventions were done behind a screen so the subjects would not be able to tell which group they were in. The results were remarkable for TT. By day 16, half the wounds treated with TT had completely healed, while none of the control group's wounds had.

This study provided TT proponents with the data they needed to claim near miraculous healing power from the use of TT. But true science is not built on one study, and Wirth laboriously continued what would be a series of five trials of this experiment. After the fifth attempt to replicate his original results, Wirth noted: The results of the experiments indicated significance for the treatment group in the initial 2 studies in the series, and non- and reverse-significant results for the control group in the remaining 3 experiments. Although the 5 studies represent a seminal research effort within the field of complementary healing, the overall results of the series are inconclusive in establishing the efficacy of the treatment interventions examined.

In other words, overall, the control group fared as well or better than the group treated with TT. TT proponents often only quote Wirth's first study, which seemed quite promising. Critics have noted that in that first study, subjects in the treatment group were wounded and treated on a different day than the control group, introducing the possibility that non-uniform wound depths between the two groups might have caused the dramatic difference seen in the first study.

When another pro-TT article appeared in the *AJN* in April 1995, claiming supportive evidence from a recent study, the primary researcher for the study wrote to the journal in protest. "The effects of TT on pain are unclear and replication studies are needed before any conclusions can be drawn," she stated. "There is no convincing evidence that TT promotes relaxation and decreases anxiety beyond a placebo effect," she continued. "Other claims about outcomes are, in fact, speculation."

By 1996, staff nurses began calling the bluff of practitioners of TT. Reading one glowing article after another on TT in their professional journals, one group of Emergency and Operating Room nurses in Philadelphia invited a TTP into their ER for a demonstration. The practitioner, who had studied with Dolores Krieger, explained how she could feel a person's energy through clothes, a chair, or even a cast. She stated she could tell the difference between the energy of animate vs. inanimate objects, or between a child and an adult.

The nurses then suggested a demonstration of this claimed ability. They would have the healer assess the energy patterns of several individuals, including an elderly man with heart disease and two healthy girls. From these, she would pick the individual she felt most sure of being able to identify. The nurses would then cover up one of the test subjects with blankets, and the healer would have to identify whether it was the subject she had chosen. She declined. She did recommend that they all take her introductory course ($125) so they could learn to do it themselves. They declined.

The UAB Burn Study Crashes and Burns

The Department of Defense grant of $355,000 to the University of Alabama at Birmingham for the study of TT on burn patients was to be "the first real scientific evidence there is for Therapeutic Touch" according to the primary researcher Joan Turner. Aside from illustrating a potentially problematic researcher bias, this is an accurate assessment of the TT research to date; despite over 20 years of research, remarkably, this would have been the first real evidence. The study was designed to show the effectiveness of TT on both pain relief and the prevention of infections for hospitalized burn patients, with the secondary goal of arriving at a working TT protocol for use in the army. The study tested TT against "mock" TT in which nurses simply mimicked the movements of "real" TT.

The results, as usual, were mixed. When using a verbal pain measurement scale, the TT group seemed to have less pain, however on a visual pain measurement scale there no statistical difference between the groups. Turner reported that when pain was measured on day 3, subjects in the TT group showed a slightly better outcome. Contrary to this assertion, however, and possibly a better indicator of relative pain relief, the TT group actually used slightly more pain medication than the sham control group. And the infection rate, arguably the most serious problem in burn treatment, was found to be three times higher in the TT group than in the mock TT group. Oddly, this fact was left out of the final official report to the Department of Defense.

This was a dismal failure for the TT proponents. On most measures, no significant differences were found between the group receiving "real" TT and the group receiving "mock" TT. In the researcher's own words: The greatest lesson learned from this process is that the inclusion of a true control group in addition to a sham and treatment group is required because a strong placebo effect occurs from the special attention given to patients in the 'sham' treatment.

But the truly astounding aspect of this study is that it was approved at all. One would assume that the Department of Defense has actual scientists working for them who would have reviewed the literature prior to approving this study. If they had, they would have found Janet Quinn's 1989 study, which attempted to show that TT was not merely a placebo or relaxation effect caused by the relationship of focused attention between the client and the practitioner, but an actual physical energy transfer process, independent of the more superficial aspects of the interaction. To prove this, Quinn eliminated eye contact when administering TT. In her own tersely worded conclusion, Quinn states: The theorem that eye and facial contact between TT practitioners and subjects should not be necessary to produce the effect of anxiety reduction was deduced from the Rogerian conceptual system and tested. This theorem was not supported.

If TT alone couldn't even decrease simple anxiety in this study, how could DOD scientists have thought it would be effective on the severe intractable pain of burn patients? Was this really an appropriate use of tax dollars?

More importantly, what Quinn's study (and indirectly, the UAB burn study) had inadvertently shown was simply that patients respond positively to extended, caring, interpersonal contact with their nurse. This is very likely the key element responsible for producing whatever positive results have been observed during TT research. If TTP's would devote half as much energy to lobbying for increased nurse/patient ratios as they do cheerleading for TT, perhaps every staff nurse could spend the time needed to positively influence their patients' outcomes.

The Final Straw

It was 1996 when Linda Rosa's daughter Emily was preparing her fourth-grade science fair entry. She was working on an exhibit with M&Ms that would illustrate the probability of picking out a certain color when one reached blindly into a bowl and plucked one. While she was working out the details, she noticed her mom watching a video on Therapeutic Touch. She said, "I wonder if they can really do that?" Suddenly her science fair project took a different form. After discussing several different possibilities with her mom, Emily decided that instead of having volunteers reach in and grab an M&M, she would invite Therapeutic Touch "healers" to reach through her screen and see whether they could detect which of their hands Emily was holding her hand over. She designed and constructed the screen herself, tested it out on a few school buddies, and then made further modifications to ensure the screen would insulate her from her subjects. She was ready.

James Randi, the famous magician and skeptic, has a standing offer of over $1 million dollars to anyone who can prove they can accurately detect an energy field. Despite publicly offering the challenge to Dolores Krieger and the other 100,000 people who claim to have this ability, Randi has only had one person make the attempt—and she failed. Unlike Randi, however, Emily was able to recruit 21 experienced TT practitioners for her experiment. The TTP's were allowed to "feel" Emily's hands prior to the test, and choose which one they felt the strongest energy radiating from. With the TTP seated behind the screen, Emily then placed her hand over one of the TTP's hands. After 20 trials, these experienced TTP's, some of whom had even published articles on TT, could only sense Emily's hand correctly 44% of the time. By chance alone, they should have guessed correctly 50% of the time. Clearly, except in their own mind, they were not sensing an energy field.

In 1998, the results of Emily's study were published in *JAMA*, the prestigious *Journal of the American Medical Association*. Anticipating criticism about the author's age, *JAMA* editor George Lundberg stated, "Age doesn't matter. All we care about is good science. This was good science." With that, Emily became the youngest author to be published in the journal.

The Response from TT Practitioners

"I do hope it's an April fool's joke," stated Dolores Krieger when informed that the official report of Emily Rosa's research was to be published in *JAMA* on April 1st. She attacked Emily, saying she "completely misunderstood what the nature of basic research is." That's quite an accusation coming from someone who has never been published in a peer-reviewed journal of the stature of *JAMA*. Editor George Lundberg said *JAMA*'s statisticians "were amazed by its simplicity and by the clarity of its results."

Janet Quinn's Healing Touch program in Colorado had an immediate response also. Researcher Cynthia Poznanski Hutchison admitted that for the first several years of her practice of TT touch, she could not sense anyone's energy field. But she kept on practicing anyway. She attempts to justify what might otherwise be called medical fraud by claiming that "Being able to sense another person's energy is an aid in guiding one's treatment, but it is not an essential ingredient."

Fellow TT practitioner and instructor Marilee Tolin agrees, and expands the definition even further. Tolin says that practitioners rely on more than just touch to sense the human energy field. They also use "the sense of intuition and even a sense of sight." What's missing from all of this, of course, is any statement by Krieger and her disciples about how the existence of their energy field can be demonstrated by scientifically accepted methods.

Conclusion

Some 2400 years ago, in *The Sacred Disease*, Hippocrates observed: They who first referred [epilepsy] to the gods appear to me to have been just such persons as the conjurors and charlatans now are, who give themselves out for being excessively religious, and as knowing more than other people. By such sayings and doings, they deceive mankind by [performing] lustrations and purifications upon them, while their discourse turns upon the divinity and the godhead.

Therapeutic Touch practitioners would like to keep us in similar ignorance about the nature of TT by maintaining its "divine" metaphysical nature. They are attempting to shift their practice into a realm where we can no longer test it. They had been content up until now to base their practice on their presumed ability to detect and manipulate the otherwise undetectable "human energy field." This was supposed to be a simple technique that anyone could learn, one that involved the transfer and balancing of actual physical energy. But then James Randi and Emily Rosa came by and showed us that we can test this claim about their practice, and they found that the practitioners tested were unable to feel the energy field they had previously claimed to be detecting, assessing, manipulating, and correcting. Practitioners are now shifting the TT paradigm into an area they hope we cannot test: the healer's "intentionality," or the use of "intuition" as a diagnostic tool.

In their attempt to create a non-disproveable theory of TT, they have instead created a religion; and they expect nurses to believe on faith that this method works despite its lack of scientific credibility. Their fundamentalist stance encourages disdain for science and rationalism, and betrays the basic tenets of modern nursing. They have used their positions of power in the nursing profession to spread their religion, and have craftily used the political dynamics of the late 20th century to stage their holy war as a post-modern feminist cause, rather than a treatment intervention whose effectiveness can be determined scientifically. Early in the Colorado State University investigation, the panel heard testimony from the school of nursing that a negative finding on TT would be viewed as male-dominated medical imperialism against female-dominated nursing. They warned the committee that nurses would not sit still for one more instance of men attempting to keep women in their place, this time denying women the all-important opportunity to be "healers." The goal is to keep the discussion out of the realm of science, where a measure of validity and proof of efficacy could be determined, and plant it firmly in the realm of politics and belief. We should not accept this subterfuge.

Most RNs have taken TT classes because they sincerely desire to help their patients and wish to add another nursing tool to their patient-intervention strategies. They were no doubt led to believe that there was scientific proof of the efficacy of this treatment. But they have been misled. After 25 years of research, there is virtually no evidence for an effect beyond that of a placebo or relaxation response. And as Linda Rosa stated, "We owe our patients more than simply the suggestion that they will improve."

In an editorial titled "Our Naked Emperor" published in *Research in Nursing and Health*, editor Marilyn Oberst criticized the skeptical majority in the nursing research field for not speaking out against TT. Referring to the paucity of valid research supporting TT, Oberst noted, "Like the citizens in the fairy tale, we seem curiously unwilling to go on record about the emperor's obvious nakedness." While supportive of alternative and complementary medicine, Oberst urged nursing researchers "to carefully consider the scientific and practical limits of diversity, and to set some standards for acceptable practice. At the moment we seem to have at least one naked emperor, and I think it's time for the reputable scientists among [us] to say so—loudly, repeatedly, and in public." We can no longer afford to placidly allow those in positions of authority to redirect the field of nursing away from the scientific method and reliable research.

Like the snake-oil salesmen of the last century who, after listening to their customers' stories of miraculous cures, began to believe in the product themselves, modern TT proponents may have become overly influenced by anecdotal evidence. Such case histories are valuable in terms of pointing out a direction for research, but are virtually meaningless for determining the real efficacy of an intervention. Proof of efficacy, according to the principles of the scientific method, requires well designed research that can be independently verified by other researchers. The literature for TT is filled with poorly designed, and non-replicable studies. In responding to Oberst's "Naked Emperor" editorial, Therese C. Meehan, perhaps the most thorough of the TT researchers, noted that, "It appears that many proponents of TT are both clothesless and clueless when it comes to reading research critically." Noting that letter writers had cited studies as evidence for TT that were of notoriously poor quality, Meehan frankly admitted: "The Kramer (1990) study [on TT with children], while no doubt conducted with sincere intent, contains so many flaws in its design and analysis that it would be soundly trounced by a class of undergraduates engaged in their first research critique."

As nurses, we are held responsible by our state Nurse Practice Acts to protect our patients' best interests and report medical malpractice. When "healers" make claims, when questionable treatments are offered as reliable, or when our hospital administrators decide to make major changes in the way we deliver care, we should insist on a scientific evaluation. If the claims do not hold up, or if the plan jeopardizes patient care, we should speak out and make our data available to the public. The public trusts nurses to protect them, but unless we continue to speak out, we may lose that trust.

It is estimated that over a billion dollars a year is spent on cancer quackery alone. When a cancer patient is faced with the difficult decision of choosing chemotherapy or surgery to treat their cancer, they might think back to their last hospital stay when an RN performed TT on them, explaining that this non-invasive technique balances their energy fields, allowing the body to heal itself. Might this encourage them to seek out a "healer" rather than treatment that is known to be effective, possibly with fatal results? The National Council Against Health Fraud recently received a report of a case in which signs of appendicitis were ignored, TT was substituted for proper care, and the patient died. If we continue to allow TT to be practiced in our hospitals, should administrators of those hospitals be held accountable for such fatalities?

In his book *Demon-Haunted World*, Carl Sagan worried that "especially as the Millennium edges nearer, pseudoscience and superstition will seem year by year more tempting, the siren song of unreason more sonorous and attractive." Nurses must continue to be a voice for reason. We must shine the light of science into the darkness of nursing practices based on wishful thinking or fraud. We must expose pseudo-science, and we must do so "loudly, repeatedly, and in public."

Chapter 61

Avoiding "Quackery"

Modern health quacks are supersalesmen. They play on fear. They cater to hope. And once they have you, they'll keep you coming back for more . . . and more . . . and more. Seldom do their victims realize how often or how skillfully they are cheated. Does the mother who feels good as she hands her child a vitamin think to ask herself whether he really needs it? Do subscribers to "health food" publications realize that articles are slanted to stimulate business for their advertisers? Not usually.

Most people think that quackery is easy to spot. Often it is not. Its promoters wear the cloak of science. They use scientific terms and quote (or misquote) scientific references. Talk show hosts may refer to them as experts or as "scientists ahead of their time." The very word "quack" helps their camouflage by making us think of an outlandish character selling snake oil from the back of a covered wagon—and, of course, no intelligent people would buy snake oil nowadays, would they? Well, maybe snake oil isn't selling so well, lately. But "Organic" foods? Hair analysis? The latest diet book? Megavitamins? "Stress formulas?" Cholesterol-lowering teas? Homeopathic remedies? Magnets?

Excerpted from "How Quackery Sells," by William T. Jarvis, Ph.D. and Stephen Barrett, M.D., and "Twenty-Five Ways to Spot Quacks and Vitamin Pushers," by Stephen Barrett, M.D. and Victor Herbert, M.D., J.D., © 2000 Quackwatch, available online at http://www.quackwatch.com; reprinted with permission; and under heading "About Quackwatch," from "Mission Statement," © 2001 Quackwatch, Inc., available online at http://www.quackwatch.com; reprinted with permission.

Nutritional "cures" for AIDS? Or shots to pep you up? Business is booming for health quacks. Their annual take is in the billions. Spot reducers, "immune boosters," water purifiers, "ergogenic aids," systems to "balance body chemistry," special diets for arthritis. Their product list is endless.

What sells is not the quality of their products, but their ability to influence their audience. To those in pain, they promise relief. To the incurable, they offer hope. To the nutrition-conscious, they say, "Make sure you have enough." To a public worried about pollution, they say, "Buy natural." To one and all, they promise better health and a longer life. Modern quacks can reach people emotionally.

Appeals to Vanity

An attractive young airline stewardess once told a physician that she was taking more than 20 vitamin pills a day. "I used to feel rundown all the time," she said, "but now I feel really great!" "Yes," the doctor replied, "but there is no scientific evidence that extra vitamins can do that. Why not take the pills one month on, one month off, to see whether they really help you or whether it's just a coincidence. After all, $300 a year is a lot of money to be wasting." "Look, doctor," she said. "I don't care what you say. I KNOW the pills are helping me."

How was this bright young lady converted into a true believer? First, an appeal to her curiosity persuaded her to try and see. Then an appeal to her vanity convinced her to disregard scientific evidence in favor of personal experience—to think for herself. Supplementation is encouraged by a distorted concept of biochemical individuality—that everyone is unique enough to disregard the Recommended Dietary Allowances (RDAs). Quacks won't tell you that scientists deliberately set the RDAs high enough to allow for individual differences. A more dangerous appeal of this type is the suggestion that although a remedy for a serious disease has not been shown to work for other people, it still might work for you. (You are extraordinary.)

A more subtle appeal to your vanity underlies the message of the TV ad quack: Do it yourself—be your own doctor. "Anyone out there have tired blood?" he used to wonder. (Don't bother to find out what's wrong with you, however. Just try my tonic.) "Troubled with irregularity?" he asks. (Pay no attention to the doctors who say you don't need a daily movement. Just use my laxative.) "Want to kill germs on contact?" (Never mind that mouthwash doesn't prevent colds.) "Trouble sleeping?" (Don't bother to solve the underlying problem. Just try my sedative.)

Turning Customers into Salespeople

Most people who think they have been helped by an unorthodox method enjoy sharing their success stories with their friends. People who give such testimonials are usually motivated by a sincere wish to help their fellow humans. Rarely do they realize how difficult it is to evaluate a "health" product on the basis of personal experience. Like the airline stewardess, the average person who feels better after taking a product will not be able to rule out coincidence—or the placebo effect (feeling better because he thinks he has taken a positive step). Since we tend to believe what others tell us of personal experiences, testimonials can be powerful persuaders. Despite their unreliability, they are the cornerstone of the quack's success.

Multilevel companies that sell nutritional products systematically turn their customers into salespeople. "When you share our products," says the sales manual of one such company, "you're not just selling. You're passing on news about products you believe in to people you care about. Make a list of people you know; you'll be surprised how long it will be. This list is your first source of potential customers." A sales leader from another company suggests, "Answer all objections with testimonials. That's the secret to motivating people."

Don't be surprised if one of your friends or neighbors tries to sell you vitamins. Millions of Americans have signed up as multilevel distributors. Like many drug addicts, they become suppliers to support their habit. A typical sales pitch goes like this: "How would you like to look better, feel better and have more energy? Try my vitamins for a few weeks." People normally have ups and downs, and a friend's interest or suggestion, or the thought of taking a positive step, may actually make a person feel better. Many who try the vitamins will mistakenly think they have been helped—and continue to buy them, usually at inflated prices.

The Use of Fear

The sale of vitamins has become so profitable that some otherwise reputable manufacturers are promoting them with misleading claims. For example, for many years, Lederle Laboratories (makers of Stresstabs) and Hoffmann-La Roche advertised in major magazines that stress "robs" the body of vitamins and creates significant danger of vitamin deficiencies.

Another slick way for quackery to attract customers is the invented disease. Virtually everyone has symptoms of one sort or another—

minor aches or pains, reactions to stress or hormone variations, effects of aging, etc. Labeling these ups and downs of life as symptoms of disease enables the quack to provide "treatment."

Some practitioners claim to detect "deficiencies" (or "imbalances" or "toxins," etc.) before any symptoms appear or before they can be detected by conventional means. Then they can sell you supplements (or balance you, or remove toxins, etc.). And when the terrible consequences they warn about don't develop, they can claim success.

Food safety and environmental protection are important issues in our society. But rather than approach them logically, the food quacks exaggerate and oversimplify. To promote "organic" foods, they lump all additives into one class and attack them as "poisonous." They never mention that natural toxicants are prevented or destroyed by modern food technology. Nor do they let on that many additives are naturally occurring substances.

Sugar has been subject to particularly vicious attack, being (falsely) blamed for most of the world's ailments. But quacks do more than warn about imaginary ailments. They sell "antidotes" for real ones. Care for some vitamin C to reduce the danger of smoking? Or some vitamin E to combat air pollutants? See your local supersalesperson.

Quackery's most serious form of fear-mongering has been its attack on water fluoridation. Although fluoridation's safety is established beyond scientific doubt, well-planned scare campaigns have persuaded thousands of communities not to adjust the fluoride content of their water to prevent cavities. Millions of innocent children have suffered as a result.

Hope for Sale

Since ancient times, people have sought at least four different magic potions: the love potion, the fountain of youth, the cure-all, and the athletic superpill. Quackery has always been willing to cater to these desires. It used to offer unicorn horn, special elixirs, amulets, and magical brews. Today's products are vitamins, bee pollen, ginseng, Gerovital, pyramids, "glandular extracts," biorhythm charts, and many more. Even reputable products are promoted as though they are potions. Toothpastes and colognes will improve our love life. Hair preparations and skin products will make us look "younger than our years." Olympic athletes tell us that breakfast cereals will make us champions. And youthful models reassure us that cigarette smokers are sexy and have fun.

False hope for the seriously ill is the cruelest form of quackery because it can lure victims away from effective treatment. Even when death is inevitable, however, false hope can do great damage. Experts who study the dying process tell us that while the initial reaction is shock and disbelief, most terminally ill patients will adjust very well as long as they do not feel abandoned. People who accept the reality of their fate not only die psychologically prepared, but also can put their affairs in order. On the other hand, those who buy false hope can get stuck in an attitude of denial. They waste not only financial resources but what little remaining time they have left.

How to Avoid Being Tricked

The best way to avoid being tricked is to stay away from tricksters. Unfortunately, in health matters, this is no simple task. Quackery is not sold with a warning label. Moreover, the dividing line between what is quackery and what is not is by no means sharp. A product that is effective in one situation may be part of a quack scheme in another. (Quackery lies in the promise, not the product.) Practitioners who use effective methods may also use ineffective ones. For example, they may mix valuable advice to stop smoking with unsound advice to take vitamins. Even outright quacks may relieve some psychosomatic ailments with their reassuring manner.

How can food quacks and other vitamin pushers be recognized? Here are 25 signs that should arouse suspicion.

When Talking about Nutrients, They Tell Only Part of the Story.

Quacks tell you all the wonderful things that vitamins and minerals do in your body and/or all the horrible things that can happen if you don't get enough. Many claim that their products or programs offer "optimal nutritional support." But they conveniently neglect to tell you that a balanced diet provides the nutrients people need and that the USDA food-group system makes balancing your diet simple.

They Claim That Most Americans Are Poorly Nourished.

This is an appeal to fear that is not only untrue, but ignores the fact that the main forms of bad nourishment in the United States are overweight in the population at large, particularly the poor, and undernourishment among the poverty-stricken. Poor people can ill afford to waste money on unnecessary vitamin pills. Their food money should be spent on nourishing food.

It is falsely alleged that Americans are so addicted to "junk" foods that an adequate diet is exceptional rather than usual. While it is true that some snack foods are mainly "naked calories" (sugars and/or fats without other nutrients), it is not necessary for every morsel of food we eat to be loaded with nutrients. In fact, no normal person following the U.S. Dietary Guidelines is in any danger of vitamin deficiency.

They Recommend "Nutrition Insurance" for Everyone.

Most vitamin pushers suggest that everyone is in danger of deficiency and should therefore take supplements as "insurance." Some suggest that it is difficult to get what you need from food, while others claim that it is impossible. Their pitch resembles that of the door-to-door huckster who states that your perfectly good furnace is in danger of blowing up unless you replace it with his product. Vitamin pushers will never tell you who doesn't need their products. Their "be wary of deficiency" claims may not be limited to essential nutrients. It can also include nonessential chemicals that nobody needs to worry about because the body makes its own supply.

They Say That Most Diseases Are Due to Faulty Diet and Can Be Treated with "Nutritional" Methods.

This simply isn't so. Consult your doctor or any recognized textbook of medicine. They will tell you that although diet is a factor in some diseases (most notably coronary heart disease), most diseases have little or nothing to do with diet. Common symptoms like malaise (feeling poorly), fatigue, lack of pep, aches (including headaches) or pains, insomnia, and similar complaints are usually the body's reaction to emotional stress. The persistence of such symptoms is a signal to see a doctor to be evaluated for possible physical illness. It is not a reason to take vitamin pills.

They Allege That Modern Processing Methods and Storage Remove all Nutritive Value from Our Food.

It is true that food processing can change the nutrient content of foods. But the changes are not so drastic as the quack, who wants you to buy supplements, would like you to believe. While some processing methods destroy some nutrients, others add them. A balanced variety of foods will provide all the nourishment you need.

Quacks distort and oversimplify. When they say that milling removes B-vitamins, they don't bother to tell you that enrichment puts them back. When they tell you that cooking destroys vitamins, they omit the fact that only a few vitamins are sensitive to heat. Nor do they tell you that these vitamins are easily obtained by consuming a portion of fresh uncooked fruit, vegetable, or fresh or frozen fruit juice each day. Any claims that minerals are destroyed by processing or cooking are pure lies. Heat does not destroy minerals.

They Claim That Diet Is a Major Factor in Behavior.

Food quacks relate diet not only to disease but to behavior. Some claim that adverse reactions to additives and/or common foods cause hyperactivity in children and even criminal behavior in adolescents and adults. These claims are based on a combination of delusions, anecdotal evidence, and poorly designed research.

They Claim That Fluoridation Is Dangerous.

Curiously, quacks are not always interested in real deficiencies. Fluoride is necessary to build decay-resistant teeth and strong bones. The best way to obtain adequate amounts of this important nutrient is to augment community water supplies so their fluoride concentration is about one part fluoride for every million parts of water. But quacks usually oppose water fluoridation, and some advocate water filters that remove fluoride. It seems that when they cannot profit from something, they may try to make money by opposing it.

They Claim That Soil Depletion and the Use of Pesticides and "Chemical" Fertilizers Result in Food That Is Less Safe and Less Nourishing.

These claims are used to promote the sale of so-called "organically grown" foods. If an essential nutrient is missing from the soil, a plant simply doesn't grow. Chemical fertilizers counteract the effects of soil depletion. Quacks also lie when they claim that plants grown with natural fertilizers (such as manure) are nutritionally superior to those grown with synthetic fertilizers. Before they can use them, plants convert natural fertilizers into the same chemicals that synthetic fertilizers supply. The vitamin content of a food is determined by its genetic makeup.

Fertilizers can influence the levels of certain minerals in plants, but this is not a significant factor in the American diet. The pesticide residue of our food supply is extremely small and poses no health threat to the consumer. Foods "certified" as "organic" are not safer or more nutritious than other foods. In fact, except for their high price, they are not significantly different.

They Claim You Are in Danger of Being "Poisoned" by Ordinary Food Additives and Preservatives.

This is another scare tactic designed to undermine your confidence in food scientists and government protection agencies as well as our food supply itself. Quacks want you to think they are out to protect you. They hope that if you trust them, you will buy their "natural" food products. The fact is that the tiny amounts of additives used in food pose no threat to human health. Some actually protect our health by preventing spoilage, rancidity, and mold growth.

They Charge That the Recommended Dietary Allowances (RDAs) Have Been Set Too Low.

The RDAs have been published by the National Research Council approximately every five years since 1943. They are defined as "the levels of intake of essential nutrients that, on the basis of scientific knowledge, are judged by the Food and Nutrition Board to be adequate to meet the known nutrient needs of practically all healthy persons." Neither the RDAs nor the Daily Values listed on food labels are "minimums" or "requirements." They are deliberately set higher than most people need. The reason quacks charge that the RDAs are too low is obvious: if you believe you need more than can be obtained from food, you are more likely to buy supplements.

They Claim That under Everyday Stress, and in Certain Diseases, Your Need for Nutrients Is Increased.

Many vitamin manufacturers have advertised that "stress robs the body of vitamins." One company has asserted that, "if you smoke, diet, or happen to be sick, you may be robbing your body of vitamins." Another has warned that "stress can deplete your body of water-soluble vitamins . . . and daily replacement is necessary." Other products are touted to fill the "special needs of athletes."

While it is true that the need for vitamins may rise slightly under physical stress and in certain diseases, this type of advertising is fraudulent. The average American—stressed or not—is not in danger of vitamin deficiency. The increased needs to which the ads refer are not higher than the amounts obtainable by proper eating. Someone who is really in danger of deficiency due to an illness would be very sick and would need medical care, probably in a hospital. But these promotions are aimed at average Americans who certainly don't need vitamin supplements to survive the common cold, a round of golf, or a jog around the neighborhood. Athletes get more than enough vitamins when they eat the food needed to meet their caloric requirements.

Many vitamin pushers suggest that smokers need vitamin C supplements. Although it is true that smokers in North America have somewhat lower blood levels of this vitamin, these levels are still far above deficiency levels. In America, cigarette smoking is the leading cause of death preventable by self-discipline. Rather than seeking false comfort by taking vitamin C, smokers who are concerned about their health should stop smoking. Suggestions that "stress vitamins" are helpful against emotional stress are also fraudulent.

They Recommend "Supplements" and "Health Foods" for Everyone.

Food quacks belittle normal foods and ridicule the food-group systems of good nutrition. They may not tell you they earn their living from such pronouncements—via public appearance fees, product endorsements, sale of publications, or financial interests in vitamin companies, health-food stores, or organic farms.

The very term "health food" is a deceptive slogan. Judgments about individual foods should take into account how they contribute to an individual's overall diet. All food is health food in moderation; any food is junk food in excess. Did you ever stop to think that your corner grocery, fruit market, meat market, and supermarket are also health-food stores? They are—and they generally charge less than stores that use the slogan.

By the way, have you ever wondered why people who eat lots of "health foods" still feel they must load themselves up with vitamin supplements? Or why so many "health food" shoppers complain about ill health?

They Claim That "Natural" Vitamins are Better than "Synthetic" Ones.

This claim is a flat lie. Each vitamin is a chain of atoms strung together as a molecule. With minor exception, molecules made in the "factories" of nature are identical to those made in the factories of chemical companies. Does it make sense to pay extra for vitamins extracted from foods when you can get all you need from the foods themselves?

They Suggest That a Questionnaire Can Be Used to Indicate Whether You Need Dietary Supplements.

No questionnaire can do this. A few entrepreneurs have devised lengthy computer-scored questionnaires with questions about symptoms that could be present if a vitamin deficiency exists. But such symptoms occur much more frequently in conditions unrelated to nutrition. Even when a deficiency actually exists, the tests don't provide enough information to discover the cause so that suitable treatment can be recommended. That requires a physical examination and appropriate laboratory tests. Many responsible nutritionists use a computer to help evaluate their clients' diet. But this is done to make dietary recommendations, such as reducing fat content or increasing fiber content. Supplements are seldom necessary unless the person is unable (or unwilling) to consume an adequate diet.

Be wary, too, of questionnaires purported to determine whether supplements are needed to correct "nutrient deficiencies" or "dietary inadequacies." These questionnaires are scored so that everyone who takes the test is judged deficient. Responsible dietary analyses compare the individual's average daily food consumption with the recommended numbers of servings from each food group. The safest and best way to get nutrients is generally from food, not pills. So even if a diet is deficient, the most prudent action is usually diet modification rather than supplementation with pills.

They Say It Is Easy to Lose Weight.

Diet quacks would like you to believe that special pills or food combinations can cause "effortless" weight loss. But the only way to lose weight is to burn off more calories than you eat. This requires self-discipline: eating less, exercising more, or preferably doing both. There are about 3,500 calories in a pound of body weight. To lose one pound a week (a safe amount that is not just water), you must eat about five hundred fewer calories per day than you burn up. The most sensible diet for losing weight is one that is nutritionally balanced in carbohydrates, fats, and proteins. Most fad diets "work" by producing temporary weight loss—as a result of calorie restriction. But they are invariably too monotonous and are often too dangerous for long-term use. Unless a dieter develops and maintains better eating and exercise habits, weight lost on a diet will soon return.

The term "cellulite" is sometimes used to describe the dimpled fat found on the hips and thighs of many women. Although no medical evidence supports the claim, cellulite is represented as a special type of fat that is resistant to diet and exercise. Sure-fire cellulite remedies include creams (to "dissolve" it), brushes, rollers, "loofah" sponges, body wraps, and vitamin-mineral supplements with or without herbs. The cost of various treatment plans runs from a few dollars for a bottle of vitamins to many hundreds of dollars at a salon that offers heat treatments, massage, enzyme injections, and/or treatment with various gadgets. The simple truth about "cellulite" is that it is ordinary fat that can be lost only as part of an overall reducing program.

They Promise Quick, Dramatic, Miraculous Results.

Often the promises are subtle or couched in "weasel words" that create an illusion of a promise, so promoters can deny making them when the "feds" close in. False promises of cure are the quacks' most immoral practice. They don't seem to care how many people they break financially or in spirit—by elation over their expected good fortune followed by deep depression when the "treatment" fails. Nor do quacks keep count—while they fill their bank accounts—of how many people they lure away from effective medical care into disability or death.

Quacks will tell you that "megavitamins" (huge doses of vitamins) can prevent or cure many different ailments, particularly emotional ones. But they won't tell you that the "evidence" supporting such claims is unreliable because it is based on inadequate investigations, anecdotes, or testimonials. Nor do quacks inform you that megadoses may be harmful. Megavitamin therapy (also called orthomolecular therapy) is nutritional roulette, and only the house makes the profit.

They Routinely Sell Vitamins and Other "Dietary Supplements" as Part of Their Practice.

Although vitamins are useful as therapeutic agents for certain health problems, the number of such conditions is small. Practitioners who sell supplements in their offices invariably recommend them inappropriately. In addition, such products tend to be substantially more expensive than similar ones in drugstores—or even health-food stores. You should also disregard any publication whose editor or publisher sells dietary supplements.

They Use Disclaimers Couched in Pseudomedical Jargon.

Instead of promising to cure your disease, some quacks will promise to "purify," or "revitalize" your body; "balance" its chemistry or "electromagnetic energy"; bring it in harmony with nature; "stimulate" or "strengthen" your immune system; "support" or "rejuvenate" various organs in your body; or stimulate your body's power to heal itself. Of course, they never identify or make valid before-and-after measurements of any of these processes. These disclaimers serve two purposes. First, since it is impossible to measure the processes quacks allege, it may be difficult to prove them wrong. Moreover, if a quack is not a physician, the use of nonmedical terminology may help to avoid prosecution for practicing medicine without a license—although it shouldn't.

They Use Anecdotes and Testimonials to Support Their Claims.

We all tend to believe what others tell us about personal experiences. But separating cause and effect from coincidence can be difficult. If people tell you that product X has cured their cancer, arthritis, or whatever, be skeptical. They may not actually have had the condition. If they did, their recovery most likely would have occurred without the help of product X. Most single episodes of disease end with just the passage of time, and most chronic ailments have symptom-free periods.

Establishing medical truths requires careful and repeated investigation—with well-designed experiments, not reports of coincidences misperceived as cause-and-effect. That's why testimonial evidence is forbidden in scientific articles, is usually inadmissible in court, and is not used to evaluate whether or not drugs should be legally marketable. (Imagine what would happen if the FDA decided that clinical trials were too expensive and therefore drug approval would be based on testimonial letters or interviews with a few patients.)

Never underestimate the extent to which people can be fooled by a worthless remedy. During the early 1940s, many thousands of people became convinced that "glyoxylide" could cure cancer. Yet analysis showed that it was simply distilled water.[1] Many years before that, when arsenic was used as a "tonic," countless numbers of people swore by it even as it slowly poisoned them.

Symptoms that are psychosomatic (bodily reactions to tension) are often relieved by anything taken with a suggestion that it will work. Tiredness and other minor aches and pains may respond to any enthusiastically recommended nostrum. For these problems, even physicians may prescribe a placebo. A placebo is a substance that has no pharmacological effect on the condition for which it is used, but is given to satisfy a patient who supposes it to be a medicine. Vitamins (such as B12 shots) are commonly used in this way.

Placebos act by suggestion. Unfortunately, some doctors swallow the advertising hype or become confused by their own observations and "believe in vitamins" beyond those supplied by a good diet. Those who share such false beliefs do so because they confuse coincidence or placebo action with cause and effect.

They Claim That Sugar Is a Deadly Poison.

Many vitamin pushers would have us believe that refined [white] sugar is "the killer on the breakfast table" and is the underlying cause of everything from heart disease to hypoglycemia. The fact is, however, that when sugar is used in moderation as part of a normal, balanced diet, it is a perfectly safe source of calories and eating pleasure. Sugar is a factor in the tooth decay process, but what counts is not merely the amount of sugar in the diet but how long any digestible carbohydrate remains in contact with the teeth. This, in turn, depends on such factors as the stickiness of the food, the type of bacteria on the teeth, and the extent of oral hygiene practiced by the individual.

They Display Credentials Not Recognized by Responsible Scientists or Educators.

The backbone of educational integrity in America is a system of accreditation by agencies recognized by the U.S. Secretary of Education or the Council on Higher Education Accreditation (CHEA), which is a nongovernmental coordinating agency. "Degrees" from nonaccredited schools are rarely worth the paper they are printed on. In the health field, there is no such thing as a reliable school that is not accredited.

Unfortunately, possession of an accredited degree does not guarantee reliability. Some schools that teach unscientific methods have achieved accreditation. Worse yet, a small percentage of individuals trained in reputable institutions (such as medical or dental schools or accredited universities) have strayed from scientific thought.

531

Since quacks operate outside of the scientific community, they also tend to form their own "professional" organizations. In some cases, the only membership requirement is payment of a fee. We and others we know have secured fancy "professional member" certificates for household pets by merely submitting the pet's name, address, and a check for $50. Don't assume that all groups with scientific-sounding names are respectable. Find out whether their views are scientifically based.

Some quacks are promoted with superlatives like "the world's foremost nutritionist" or "America's leading nutrition expert." There is no law against this tactic, just as there is none against calling oneself the "World's Foremost Lover." However, the scientific community recognizes no such titles. The designation "Nobel Prize Nominee" is also bogus and can be assumed to mean that someone has either nominated himself or had a close associate do so.

Some entrepreneurs claim to have degrees and/or affiliations to schools, hospitals, and/or professional that actually don't exist. The modern champion of this approach appears to be Gregory E. Caplinger, who claims to have acquired a medical degree, specialty training, board certification, and scores of professional affiliations— all from bogus or nonexistent sources.

Even legitimate credentials can be used to mislead. The American Medical Association's "Physician's Recognition Award" requires participation in 150 hours of continuing education over a three-year period and payment of a small fee. Most practicing physicians meet this educational standard because it is necessary to study to keep up-to-date. Accredited hospitals require this amount of continuing education to maintain staff privileges, and some states require it for license renewal. However, most physicians who do this don't bother to get the AMA certificate. Since the award reflects no special accomplishment or expertise, using it for promotional purposes is not appropriate behavior.

They Offer to Determine Your Body's Nutritional State with a Laboratory Test or a Questionnaire.

Various health-food industry members and unscientific practitioners utilize tests that they claim can determine your body's nutritional state and—of course—what products you should buy from them. One favorite method is hair analysis. For $35 to $75 plus a lock of your hair, you can get an elaborate computer printout of vitamins and minerals you supposedly need. Hair analysis has limited value (mainly in forensic medicine) in the diagnosis of heavy metal poisoning, but it is worthless as a screening device to detect nutritional problems.[2] If a hair analysis laboratory recommends supplements, you can be sure that its computers are programmed to recommend them to everyone. Other tests used to hawk supplements include amino acid analysis of urine, muscle-testing (applied kinesiology), iridology, blood typing, "nutrient-deficiency" and/or lifestyle questionnaires, and "electrodiagnostic" gadgets.

They Claim They Are Being Persecuted by Orthodox Medicine and That Their Work Is Being Suppressed Because It's Controversial.

The "conspiracy charge" is an attempt to gain sympathy by portraying the quack as an "underdog." Quacks typically claim that the American Medical Association is against them because their cures would cut into the incomes that doctors make by keeping people sick. Don't fall for such nonsense. Reputable physicians are plenty busy. Moreover, many doctors engaged in prepaid health plans, group practice, full-time teaching, and government service receive the same salary whether or not their patients are sick—so keeping their patients healthy reduces their workload, not their income.

Quacks also claim there is a "controversy" about facts between themselves and "the bureaucrats," organized medicine, or "the establishment." They clamor for medical examination of their claims, but ignore any evidence that refutes them. The gambit "Do you believe in vitamins?" is another tactic used to increase confusion. Everyone knows that vitamins are needed by the human body. The real question is "Do you need additional vitamins beyond those in a well-balanced diet?" For most people, the answer is no. Nutrition is a science, not a religion. It is based upon matters of fact, not questions of belief.

Any physician who found a vitamin or other preparation that could cure sterility, heart disease, arthritis, cancer, or the like, could make an enormous fortune. Patients would flock to such a doctor (as they now do to those who falsely claim to cure such problems), and colleagues would shower the doctor with awards—including the extremely lucrative Nobel Prize. And don't forget, doctors get sick, too. Do you believe they would conspire to suppress cures for diseases that also afflict them and their loved ones? When polio was conquered, iron lungs became virtually obsolete, but nobody resisted this advancement because it would force hospitals to change. And neither will scientists mourn the eventual defeat of cancer.

They Warn You Not to Trust Your Doctor.

Quacks, who want you to trust them, suggest that most doctors are "butchers" and "poisoners." They exaggerate the shortcomings of our healthcare delivery system, but completely disregard their own—and those of other quacks. For the same reason, quacks also claim that doctors are nutrition illiterates. This, too, is untrue. The principles of nutrition are those of human biochemistry and physiology, courses required in every medical school. Some medical schools don't teach a separate required course labeled "Nutrition" because the subject is included in other courses at the points where it is most relevant. For example, nutrition in growth and development is taught in pediatrics, nutrition in wound healing is taught in surgery, and nutrition in pregnancy is covered in obstetrics. In addition, many medical schools do offer separate instruction in nutrition.

A physician's training, of course, does not end on the day of graduation from medical school or completion of specialty training. The medical profession advocates lifelong education, and some states require it for license renewal. Physicians can further their knowledge of nutrition by reading medical journals and textbooks, discussing cases with colleagues, and attending continuing education courses. Most doctors know what nutrients can and cannot do and can tell the difference between a real nutritional discovery and a piece of quack nonsense. Those who are unable to answer questions about dietetics (meal planning) can refer patients to someone who can—usually a registered dietitian.

Like all human beings, doctors sometimes make mistakes. However, quacks deliver mistreatment most of the time.

They Encourage Patients to Lend Political Support to Their Treatment Methods.

A century ago, before scientific methodology was generally accepted, valid new ideas were hard to evaluate and were sometimes rejected by a majority of the medical community, only to be upheld later. But today, treatments demonstrated as effective are welcomed by scientific practitioners and do not need a group to crusade for them. Quacks seek political endorsement because they can't prove that their methods work. Instead, they may seek to legalize their treatment and force insurance companies to pay for it. One of the surest signs that a treatment doesn't work is a political campaign to legalize its use.

About Quackwatch

Quackwatch, Inc., a member of Consumer Federation of America, is a nonprofit corporation whose purpose is to combat health-related frauds, myths, fads, and fallacies. Its primary focus is on quackery-related information that is difficult or impossible to get elsewhere. Founded by Dr. Stephen Barrett in 1969 as the Lehigh Valley Committee Against Health Fraud, it was incorporated in 1970. In 1997, it assumed its current name and began developing a worldwide network of volunteers and expert advisors and assumed its current name. Our activities include:

- Investigating questionable claims
- Answering inquiries
- Distributing reliable publications
- Reporting illegal marketing
- Generating consumer-protection lawsuits
- Improving the quality of health information on the Internet
- Attacking misleading advertising on the Internet

Web Sites

The Quackwatch Web site was launched December 1996. In October 1998, it initiated Chirobase, a guide to the history, theories, and current practices of chiropractors. Chirobase is cosponsored by the National Council Against Health Fraud, Inc., and Victims of Chiropractic.

Research Projects

Quackwatch has five research projects underway:

- Alternative Cancer Treatment Registry
- Dubious Advertising
- Multilevel Marketing through the Internet
- Quackery for Pets
- Questionable Methods Project

The following task forces are being organized:

- Anti-Biotechnology Quackery
- Antifluoridation Quackery
- Anti-Immunization Quackery

- Book Evaluation
- Cancer Quackery
- Dental Quackery
- Dietary Supplements
- Multilevel Marketing
- Mental Health Quackery
- Mental Retardation Quackery
- Physical Therapy Quackery
- Special Education Quackery

Affiliations

Quackwatch is a participant member of the Fraud Defense Network, an Internet-based alliance of insurance companies, government agencies, and other interested parties working to prevent, detect, and investigate fraudulent activity.

It's database provides a consensus of scientific information on herbal products and dietary supplements. Each month, Quackwatch posts one monograph. The entire database is available by subscription, both online (updated daily) and in print format.

Quackwatch is part of the Skeptic Ring, an alliance of sites that examine claims about paranormal phenomena and fringe science from a skeptical point of view.

Quackwatch.com

To find more information about Quackwatch search their website at: http://www.quackwatch.com

References

1. Young JH, McFayden RE. The Koch Cancer Treatment. *Journal of the History of Medicine* 53:254-284, 1998.

2. Hambidge KM. Hair analyses: Worthless for vitamins, limited for minerals. *American Journal of Clinical Nutrition* 36:943-949, 1983.

Part Nine

Additional Help and Information

Chapter 62

CAM-Related Terms

The terms in this glossary explain some concepts related to complementary and alternative medicine. To aid people who may be seeking to understand varying options, some traditional terms for common medications and treatments that are often used by physicians and other health care practitioners are also included.

abdominal: Having to do with the abdomen, which is the part of the body between the chest and the hips that contains the pancreas, stomach, intestines, liver, gallbladder, and other organs.

acetaminophen: Relieves fever and pain by blocking pain centers in the central nervous system. Examples of brand names include Tylenol, Panadol, and Datril.

active treatment: In a clinical trial, the treatment being tested by the experiment.

Terms included in this glossary were excerpted from "Acupuncture Information and Resources," National Center for Complementary and Alternative Medicine, 1999; "Cartilage (Shark and Bovine)," National Cancer Institute (NCI), 2000; "Harmful Effects of Medicines on the Adult Digestive System," National Institute of Diabetes and Digestive and Kidney Diseases, NIH Publication No. 95-3421; "Headache—Hope through Research," National Institute of Neurological Disorders and Stroke, originally printed in 1996 and updated in July 2001; and "Hepatitis C: Treatment Alternatives," 2000 National Center for Complementary and Alternative Medicine (NCCAM), Publication Z-04, May 2000.

acupuncture: An ancient Chinese health practice that involves puncturing the skin with hair-thin needles at particular locations, called acupuncture points, on the patient's body. Acupuncture is believed to help reduce pain or change a body function. Sometimes the needles are twirled, given a slight electric charge, or warmed.

alternative medicine: Medical systems, therapies, and techniques that mainstream Western (conventional) medicine does not commonly use, accept, study, understand, or make available. Alternative medicine includes practices usually used instead of conventional medical practices. Alternative health care practices include a vast array of treatments and beliefs, which may be well known, exotic, mysterious, or even dangerous. They are based on no common or consistent philosophy or school of thought. A few of the many alternative medicine practices include the use of acupuncture, homeopathy, herbs, therapeutic massage, and traditional oriental medicine to promote well being or treat health conditions.

amino acid sequence: The arrangement of amino acids in a protein. Proteins can be made from 20 different kinds of amino acids, and the structure and function of each type of protein are determined by the kinds of amino acids used to make it and how they are arranged.

antacids: relieve heartburn, acid indigestion, sour stomach, and symptoms of peptic ulcer. They work by neutralizing stomach acid. Aluminum hydroxide antacids include Alu-Tab and Amphojel; calcium carbonate antacids include Tums, Alka Mints, and Rolaids Calcium Rich; magnesium antacids include Mylanta and Maalox.

antibiotics: Destroy or block the growth of bacteria that cause infection. Hundreds of antibiotics are available, including penicillins (Amoxil, Amcil, and Augmentin), clindamycin, cephalosporins (Keflex and Ceclor), tetracyclines (Minocin, Sumycin, and Vibramycin), quinolones (Cipro), and sulfa drugs (Bactrim).

antibody: A type of protein produced by certain white blood cells in response to a foreign substance (antigen). Each antibody can bind to only a specific antigen. The purpose of this binding is to help destroy the antigen. Antibodies can work in several ways, depending on the nature of the antigen. Some antibodies disable antigens directly. Others make the antigen more vulnerable to destruction by white blood cells.

anticholinergics: Medicines that affect the nerve cells or nerve fibers and includes drugs for depression, anxiety, and nervousness. Examples of anticholinergics include propantheline (Pro-banthine) and dicyclomine (Bentyl). Examples of antidepressants include amitriptyline (Elavil and Endep), and nortriptyline (Aventyl and Pamelor).

anticonvulsants: Medicines that control epilepsy and other types of seizure disorders. They act by lessening overactive nerve impulses in the brain. Examples of this class of medicines include phenytoin (Dilantin) and valproic acid (Dalpro).

antihypertensives: Medicines that lower high blood pressure. They act by relaxing blood vessels, which makes blood flow more easily. Examples of antihypertensives include methyldopa (Aldomet) and clonidine hydrochloride (Catapres).

anti-inflammatory: Refers to reducing inflammation.

aqueous: Having to do with water.

arthritis: A disease marked by inflammation and pain in the joints.

B cells: White blood cells that develop from bone marrow and produce antibodies. Also called B lymphocytes.

binding agent: A substance that makes a loose mixture stick together. For example, binding agents can be used to make solid pills from loose powders.

bioavailable: The ability of a drug or other substance to be absorbed and used by the body. Orally bioavailable means that a drug or other substance that is taken by mouth can be absorbed and used by the body.

biofeedback: A technique in which patients are trained to gain some voluntary control over certain physiological conditions, such as blood pressure and muscle tension, to promote relaxation.

carcinoma: Cancer that begins in skin or in tissues that line or cover internal organs.

541

cartilage: A type of connective tissue that contains cells (chondrocytes) surrounded by a tough but flexible matrix. The cartilage matrix is made of several types of the protein collagen and several types of proteoglycans, which are combinations of protein and long sugar molecules called glycosaminoglycans. Chondroitin sulfate is the major glycosaminoglycan in cartilage.

case series: A group or series of case reports involving patients who were given similar treatment. Reports of case series usually contain detailed information about the individual patients. This includes demographic information (for example, age, gender, ethnic origin) and information on diagnosis, treatment, response to treatment, and follow-up after treatment.

chondrocytes: Cartilage cells. They make the structural components of cartilage.

chondroitin sulfate: The major glycosaminoglycan (a type of sugar molecule) in cartilage.

chorioallantoic membrane: The membrane in hen's eggs that helps chicken embryos get enough oxygen and calcium for development. The calcium comes from the egg shell.

circulatory system: The system that contains the heart and the blood vessels and moves blood throughout the body. This system helps tissues get enough oxygen and nutrients, and it helps them get rid of waste products. The lymph system, which connects with the blood system, is often considered part of the circulatory system.

clinical study: A research study in which patients receive treatment in a clinic or other medical facility. Clinical study reports can contain results for single patients (case reports) or many patients (case series or clinical trials).

clinical trial: A research study that evaluates the effectiveness of new interventions in people. Each study is designed to evaluate new methods of screening, prevention, diagnosis, or treatment of a disease.

collagen: A fibrous protein found in cartilage and other connective tissue.

complementary and alternative medicine (CAM): Forms of treatment in addition to (complementary) or instead of (alternative) standard treatments. These practices include dietary supplements, megadose vitamins, herbal preparations, special teas, massage therapy, magnet therapy, spiritual healing, and meditation.

control group: In a clinical trial, the group that does not receive the new treatment being studied. This group is compared to the group that receives the new treatment, to see if the new treatment works.

controlled study: An experiment or clinical trial that includes a comparison (control) group.

conventional therapy: A currently accepted and widely used treatment for a certain type of disease, based on the results of past research. Also called conventional treatment.

cytotoxic: Cell-killing.

double-blind: A type of study in which neither the participants nor the doctors giving the treatments know who is getting the active treatment and who is getting the placebo.

dysgeusia: A bad taste in the mouth. Also called parageusia.

dyspepsia: Upset stomach.

electroacupuncture: A variation of traditional acupuncture treatment in which acupuncture or needle points are stimulated electronically.

electroencephalogram (EEG): A technique for recording electrical activity in the brain.

electromagnetic signals: The minute electrical impulses that transmit information through and between nerve cells. For example, electromagnetic signals convey information about pain and other sensations within the body's nervous system.

electromyography (EMG): A special recording technique that detects electric activity in muscle. Patients are sometimes offered a type of biofeedback called EMG training, in which they learn to control muscle tension in the face, neck, and shoulders.

endorphins: Naturally occurring painkilling chemicals. Some scientists theorize that people who suffer from severe headache have lower levels of endorphins than people who are generally pain free.

enema: The injection of a liquid through the anus into the large bowel.

enzyme: A protein that speeds up the rate at which chemical reactions take place in the body.

hepatitis: Inflammation of the liver.

holistic: Describes therapies based on facts about the "whole person," including spiritual and mental aspects, not only the specific part of the body being treated. Holistic practitioners may advise changes in diet, physical activity, and other lifestyle factors to help treat a patient's condition.

hormone therapy: Treatment of cancer by removing, blocking, or adding hormones. Also called hormone therapy or endocrine therapy.

inflammation: A response of redness, swelling, pain, and a feeling of heat in certain areas, which is meant to protect tissues affected by injury or disease.

iron: A mineral the body needs to produce red blood cells. Iron supplements are used to treat iron deficiency or iron-deficiency anemia.

keratan sulfate: A glycosaminoglycan (a type of polysaccharide) found in cartilage and in the cornea of the eye.

laxatives: For relieving constipation. Common brand names of laxatives include Phillips' Milk of Magnesia, Citroma, Epsom salts, Correctol, and ExLax.

liver: A large gland in the upper abdomen that is essential to life. Important liver functions include: helping the body produce or make use of the fats, sugars, proteins, vitamins, and most other compounds it needs; and reducing the ill effects of poisons, such as alcohol and nicotine, in the body.

magnetic resonance imaging (MRI): An imaging technique that uses radio waves, magnetic fields, and computer analysis to provide a picture of body tissues and structures.

malignant: Cancerous; a growth with a tendency to invade and destroy nearby tissue and spread to other parts of the body.

meridians: A traditional Chinese medicine term for the 14 pathways throughout the body for the flow of qi, or vital energy, accessed through acupuncture points.

metastasis: The spread of cancer from one part of the body to another. Tumors formed from cells that have spread are called "secondary tumors," and contain cells that are like those in the original (primary) tumor. The plural is metastases.

moxibustion: The use of dried herbs in acupuncture. The herbs are placed on top of acupuncture needles and burned. This method is believed to be more effective at treating some health conditions than using acupuncture needles alone.

neurohormones: Chemical substances made by tissue in the body's nervous system that can change the structure or function or direct the activity of an organ or organs.

neurological: A term referring to the body's nervous system, which starts, oversees, and controls all body functions.

neurotransmitters: Biochemical substances that stimulate or inhibit nerve impulses in the brain that relay information about external stimuli and sensations, such as pain.

nociceptors: The endings of pain-sensitive nerves that, when stimulated by stress, muscular tension, dilated blood vessels, or other triggers, send messages up the nerve fibers to nerve cells in the brain, signaling that a part of the body hurts.

nonsteroidal anti-inflammatory drugs (NSAIDs): These drugs block the body's production of prostaglandins, substances that mediate pain and inflammation. NSAIDs relieve the pain from chronic and acute inflammatory conditions, including arthritis and other rheumatic conditions, and pain associated with injuries, bursitis, tendinitis, and

545

dental problems. NSAIDs also relieve pain associated with noninflammatory conditions. Generic and brand names of NSAIDs include aspirin (Bayer and Bufferin), ibuprofen (Advil, Nuprin, and Motrin), tometin (Tolectin), naproxen (Naprosyn), and piroxicam (Feldene).

opioids: Synthetic or naturally occurring chemicals in the brain that may reduce pain and induce sleep.

oral: By or having to do with the mouth.

osteoporosis: A condition that is characterized by a decrease in bone mass and density, causing bones to become fragile.

pancreas: A glandular organ located in the abdomen. It makes pancreatic juices, which contain enzymes that aid in digestion, and it produces several hormones, including insulin. The pancreas is surrounded by the stomach, intestines, and other organs.

placebo: An inactive substance that looks the same as, and is administered in the same way as, a drug in a clinical trial.

placebo-controlled: A type of study of usually one group of subjects to distinguish the specific and nonspecific effects of the active treatment. Randomized Study participants are assigned without bias to particular arms of a study.

polysaccharide: A type of carbohydrate. It contains sugar molecules that are linked together chemically.

preclinical studies: Tests performed after a treatment has been shown in laboratory studies to have a desirable effect. Preclinical studies provide information about a treatment's harmful side effects and safety at different doses in animals.

qi: Pronounced "chee." The Chinese term for vital energy or life force.

randomized controlled clinical trials: A type of clinical study that is designed to provide information about whether a treatment is safe and effective in humans. These trials generally use two groups of people; one group receives the treatment and the other does not. The participants being studied do not know which group receives the actual treatment.

response: In medicine, an improvement related to treatment.

retrospective: Looking back at events that have already taken place.

side effects: Unintended, and usually undesirable, reactions that result from a treatment.

therapeutic: Used to treat disease and help healing take place.

thermography: A technique sometimes used for diagnosing headache in which an infrared camera converts skin temperature into a color picture, called a thermogram, with different degrees of heat appearing as different colors.

topical: On the surface of the body.

traditional Chinese medicine: An ancient system of medicine and health care that is based on the concept of balanced qi, or vital energy, that flows throughout the body. Components of traditional Chinese medicine include herbal and nutritional therapy, restorative physical exercises, meditation, acupuncture, acupressure, and remedial massage.

virus: A tiny organism that can only grow in the cells of an animal or a person. Several hundred viruses have been found to cause diseases in people.

vitamins: Compounds that serve as nutritional supplements in people with poor diets, in people recovering from surgery, or in people with special health problems.

- Niacin helps the body break down food for energy and is used to treat niacin deficiency and to lower levels of fats and cholesterol.
- Vitamin A is necessary for normal growth and for healthy eyes and skin.
- Vitamin C is necessary for healthy function of cells.

yang: The Chinese concept of positive energy and forces in the universe and human body. Acupuncture is believed to remove yang imbalances and bring the body into balance.

yin: The Chinese concept of negative energy and forces in the universe and human body. Acupuncture is believed to remove yin imbalances and bring the body into balance.

Chapter 63

Acupuncture Resources

The National Institutes of Health (NIH) does not endorse any of the following resources. You, as a health care consumer, are encouraged to explore these resources fully to determine their relevancy, position on treatment, relative cost, and background of authors or staff. You may wish to discuss this information with your doctor, who can assist you in critically evaluating all resources for their relevance to your diagnoses and circumstances.

National Institutes of Health

Combined Health Information Database (CHID)
7830 Old Georgetown Road
Suite 204
Bethesda, MD 20814
Internet: http://chid.nih.gov
E-Mail: chid@aerie.com

CHID Online is a searchable and user-friendly database produced by more than a dozen health-related agencies of the Federal Government. This database provides titles, abstracts, and availability information for health information and health education resources, including acupuncture and Chinese medicine.

"Acupuncture Information and Resources," Publication Number Z-01, National Center for Complementary and Alternative Medicine (NCCAM), NCCAM Clearinghouse, April 1999, updated March 2001.

National Center for Complementary and Alternative Medicine (NCCAM) Clearinghouse
P.O. Box 7923
Gaithersburg, MD 20898
Toll Free: 888-644-6226
TTY: 866-464-3615
Fax: 866-464-3616
Internet: http://nccam.nih.gov
E-Mail: nccam-info@nccam.nih.gov

The NCCAM Clearinghouse, the information arm of NIH's NCCAM, provides information about complementary and alternative medicine (CAM), including acupuncture, and the activities of the NCCAM. The NCCAM Web site has acupuncture information and provides links to the Web sites of nine CAM research centers (sponsored by the NCCAM), some of which are conducting acupuncture research.

NIH Consensus Program Information Center
P.O. Box 2577
Kensington, MD 20891
Toll Free: 888-644-2667
Fax: 301-593-9485
E-Mail: consensus_statement@nih.gov

The NIH organized a conference that produced a consensus statement about acupuncture (November 3-5, 1997).

U.S. National Library of Medicine (NLM)
MEDLINE
8600 Rockville Pike
Bethesda, MD 20894
Tel: 888-346-3656
Fax: 301-402-1384
Internet: http://www.nlm.nih.gov/
E-Mail: custserv@nlm.nih.gov

An online consumer health information tool.

Publications

A Manual of Acupuncture
by Peter Deadman and Mazin Al-Khafaji, East Sussex, England, *Journal of Chinese Medicine Publications*, 1998.

A detailed guidebook to descriptions of the theories and actual specific methods of acupuncture. It provides information on the channels, collaterals, point categories, point selection methods, point location, and needling.

Basics of Acupuncture
by Gabriel Stux (Editor) and Bruce Pomerantz, Berlin, Germany: Springer Verlag, 1995.

The most recent of several widely used texts by acupuncture researchers.

Between Heaven and Earth: A Guide to Chinese Medicine
by Harriet Beinfield and Efrem Korngold, New York, NY: Ballantine Books, 1991.

An overview of Chinese medicine, with case histories of treatments and illustrated explanations of philosophy, components, and treatments.

Principles and Practice of Contemporary Acupuncture
by Sung J. Liao, Matthew Lee, and Lorenz K.Y. Ng, New York, NY: Marcel Dekker, 1994.

Contains translations of ancient Chinese medical classics previously unavailable in English. Compares and contrasts traditional Chinese and Western scientific medicine.

The Chinese Way to Healing: Many Paths to Wholeness
by Misha Ruth Cohen, New York, NY: The Berkeley Publishing Group, 1996.

A guidebook to Chinese medicine in the United States, with information about diet, herbs, acupuncture, and finding qualified practitioners.

The Web That Has No Weaver
by Ted Kaptchuk, New York, NY: Congdon and Weed, 1992.

An introduction to traditional Chinese medicine, with comparisons of Eastern and Western medical treatments.

The Yellow Emperor's Classic of Internal Medicine
by Maoshing Ni, Boston, MA: Shambala Press, 1995.

A contemporary translation of the classic traditional Chinese medicine text that dates from 2000 B.C.

Periodicals

These periodicals contain information about acupuncture research studies, techniques, effects, and use. Look for "peer reviewed" journals, which publish studies reviewed by researchers in the field to ensure suitability for publication.

Acupuncture and Electro-Therapeutics Research
Cognizant Communications Corporation
3 Hartsdale Road
Elmsford, NY 10523-3701
Tel: 914-592-7720
Fax: 914-592-8981
Internet: http://www.cognizantcommunication.com
E-Mail: cogcomm@aol.com

A peer-reviewed quarterly in its 23rd year and indexed/abstracted in MEDLINE.

Alternative Medicine Review:
A Journal of Clinical Therapeutics
Thorne Research, Inc.
P.O. Box 3200
Sandpoint, ID 83864
Tel: 208-263-1337
Fax: 208-265-2488

A peer-reviewed quarterly indexed/abstracted in MEDLINE.

American Journal of Acupuncture
1840 41st Avenue, Suite 102
Capitola, CA 95010
Tel: 831-475-1700
Fax: 831-475-1439
Internet: http://www.acupuncturejournal.com

A quarterly peer-reviewed journal.

European Journal of Oriental Medicine
63 Jeddo Rd
London W12 9HQ
England
Tel: 011-44 20-8749-1300
Fax: 011-44 20-8749-1301

A quarterly research journal.

Guideposts: *Acupuncture in Recovery*
J&M Reports
7402 NE 58th Street
Vancouver, WA 98662-5207
Tel: 360-254-0186
Fax: 360-260-8620

A newsletter concerning acupuncture used to treat addiction, alcoholism, and mental health problems.

Journal of *Alternative and Complementary Medicine*
Research on Paradigm, Practice and Policy
Mary Ann Liebert, Publisher
2 Madison Avenue
Larchmont, NY 10538
Toll Free: 800-654-3278
Tel: 914-834-3100
Fax: 914-834-3688
E-Mail: mailto:info@liebertpub.com
Internet: http://www.liebertpub.com

A quarterly journal abstracted/indexed in MEDLINE.

Journal of *Chinese Medicine*
22 Cromwell Road
Hove BN3 3EB
England
Tel: 011-44 1273 748588
Fax: 011-44 1273 748588
Email: info@jcm.co.uk

A professional journal published three times a year.

Journal of *Traditional Chinese Medicine*
Co-sponsored by the China Association of Traditional Chinese Medicine and Pharmacy and the China Academy of Traditional Chinese Medicine. Distributed by the American Center of Chinese Medicine
3121 Park Avenue, Suite J
Soquel, CA 95073

A quarterly journal on clinical and theoretical research that is indexed/abstracted in MEDLINE.

Organizations

American Academy of Medical Acupuncture
Medical Acupuncture Research Organization
5820 Wilshire Boulevard, Suite 500
Los Angeles, CA 90036
Toll Free: 800-521-2262
Tel: 323-937-5514
Fax: 323-937-0959
Internet: http://www.medicalacupuncture.org

A professional association of medical doctors who practice acupuncture. The academy provides a referral list of doctors who practice acupuncture. It also provides general information about acupuncture, legislative representation, publications, meetings, and proficiency examinations.

American Association of Oriental Medicine
433 Front Street
Catasauqua, PA 18032
Toll Free: 888-500-7999
Tel: 610-266-1433
Fax: 610-264-2768
E-Mail: aaom1@aol.com
Internet: http://www.aaom.org

A nonprofit professional organization of acupuncturists and practitioners of Oriental medicine. The association determines standards of practice and education through the National Certification Commission for Acupuncture and Oriental Medicine. It also funds research and provides a list of acupuncturists and Oriental medicine practitioners by geographic area. The association provides articles and fact sheets, membership and licensing information, a list of acupuncture schools, and a list of state acupuncture associations.

British Medical Acupuncture Society
12 Marbury House, Higher Whitley
Warrington, Cheshire WA4 4WQ
England
Tel: 011-44 1925 730727
Fax: 011-44 1925 730492
E-Mail: bmasadmin@aol.com
Internet: http://www.medical-acupuncture.co.uk

A group of doctors who practice acupuncture with more conventional treatments. The Society produces the journal *Acupuncture in Medicine*, published twice per year, covering original research and reviews.

Foundation for Traditional Chinese Medicine
122A Acomb Road
York YO2 4EY
England
Tel: 011-44 1904 785120
Fax: 011-44 1904 784828
Internet: http://www.demon.co.uk/acupuncture/index.html

The Foundation funds the Acupuncture Research Resource Center and provides information about acupuncture research listed by condition, including migraine and lower back pain.

International Council of Medical Acupuncture and Related Techniques
Rue de l'Amazone 62
1060 Brussels
Belgium
Tel: 011-32 2 539 39 00
Fax: 011-32 2 539 36 92
Internet: http://users.med.auth.gr/~karanik/english/icmart/intro.html

A nonprofit organization created in 1983 of more than 40 national acupuncture-related associations of medical doctors practicing acupuncture and/or related techniques.

National Acupuncture and Oriental Medicine Alliance
14637 Starr Road SE
Olalla, WA 98359
Tel: 253-851-6896
Fax: 253-851-6883
Internet: http://www.acuall.org

A professional society of state-licensed, registered, or certified acupuncturists, with membership open to consumers, schools, organizations, corporate sponsors, and health care providers. The Alliance lists thousands of acupuncturists across the country on its Web site and provides information about them to callers to their information and referral line. The Alliance requires documentation of state license or national board certification from all acupuncturists it lists.

National Acupuncture Detoxification Association

P.O. Box 1927
Vancouver, WA 98668-1927
Tel: 888-765-6232
Fax: 805-969-6051
Email: email@acupuncture.com

A nonprofit organization that provides training and consultation for more than 500 drug and alcohol acupuncture treatment programs run by local agencies. The organization's clearinghouse provides a library of audiotapes, videotapes, and literature on using acupuncture to treat addiction and mental disorders.

National Acupuncture Foundation

P.O. Box 2271
Gig Harbor, WA 98335-4271
Tel: 253-851-6538
Fax: 253-851-6538

The Foundation publishes books, including the Acupuncture and Oriental Medicine Law Book and the Clean Needle Technique Manual. The Foundation filed the U.S. Food and Drug Administration needle reclassification petition of 1996.

Society for Acupuncture Research

6900 Wisconsin Avenue, Suite 700
Bethesda, MD 20815
Tel: 301-571-0624
Fax: 301-961-5340

A nonprofit organization that facilitates the scientific evaluation of acupuncture.

Training and Credentialing Organizations

Accreditation Commission for Acupuncture and Oriental Medicine

1010 Wayne Avenue, Suite 1270
Silver Spring, MD 20910
Tel: 301-608-9680
Fax: 301-608-9576

The Commission, established in 1982, evaluates professional master's degree and first professional master's-level certificate and diploma programs in acupuncture and Oriental medicine, with concentrations in both acupuncture and herbal therapy.

Council of Colleges of Acupuncture and Oriental Medicine
7501 Greenway Center Dr.
Suite 820
Greenbelt, MD 20770
Tel: 301-313-0868
Fax: 301-313-0869
Internet: http://www.ccaom.org

This Council was formed in 1982 and has developed academic and clinical guidelines and core curriculum requirements for master's and doctoral programs in acupuncture as well as acupuncture and Oriental medicine.

NAFTA Acupuncture Commission
Standards Management, Inc.
14637 Starr Road SE
Olalla, WA 98359
Tel: 253-851-6896
Fax: 253-851-6883

This group of educators, acupuncturists, medical doctors, and naturopathic doctors meet to exchange information and discuss training standards of competence for the practice of acupuncture and Oriental medicine in North America, including Mexico and Canada.

National Certification Commission for Acupuncture and Oriental Medicine
11 Canal Center Plaza
Suite 300
Alexandria, VA 22314
Tel: 703-548-9004
Fax: 703-548-9079
E-Mail: info@nccaom.org
Internet: http://www.nccaom.org

This Commission was established in 1982 to implement nationally recognized standards of competence for the practice of acupuncture and Oriental medicine. It provides information and programs on certification standards for acupuncturists.

Online Resources

The Internet is one of the fastest ways to access health information, but much of this information is not controlled or reviewed by qualified health professionals. Approach information from the Internet with caution, as it may be misleading, incorrect, or even dangerous.

Acuall.org
Internet: http://www.acuall.org

A site sponsored by the National Acupuncture and Oriental Medicine Alliance with general information on acupuncture and Oriental medicine, referrals to practitioners, legislative status, national issues, conferences and workshops, publications, and information for potential students.

Acupuncture.com
Internet: http://www.acupuncture.com

Describes and summarizes acupuncture procedures, areas of research, and other pertinent information from multiple sources.

Medical Matrix
Internet: http://www.medmatrix.org

A gateway to clinical medical resources, including numerous medical journals.

National Library of Medicine. Current Bibliographies in Medicine: Acupuncture
Internet: http://www.nlm.nih.gov/pubs/cbm/acupuncture.html

Bibliographies to 2,302 scientific papers collected between January 1970 and October 1997.

Chapter 64

Clinical Homeopathy Programs

There are a number of searchable online databases and lists now available to help you to locate a homeopathic practitioner in your area.

The NCH Directory of Practitioners (Searchable)
Internet: http://homeopathic.org/NCHSearch.htm

The NCH State by State Resources Page
Internet: http://www.homeopathic.org/resources.htm

The NASH Directory of Registered Homeopaths
Internet: http://www.homeopathy.org/directory.htm

The HANP Searchable Database of Members and Practitioners
Internet: http://www.healthy.net/HANP/HANPSearch.htm

The CHC Searchable Database of Certified Practitioners
Internet: http://www.homeopathicdirectory.com

The Database of Classical Homeopaths Maintained by Steven Waldstein
Internet: http://www.nccn.net/~wwithin/STEVELIST.htm

"Clinical Homeopathy Programmes: USA Organisations," © 2001 Homeopathy Home (www.homeopathyhome.net); reprinted with permission.

List of Homeopathic Physicians (MD's and DO's) Maintained by William F. McCoy, M.D, and List of Veterinary Homeopaths by the AVH.
Internet: http://www.homeopathic-md-do.com

The following organizations can also help you locate a homeopathic physician in your area.

The National Center for Homeopathy
801 North Fairfax Street
Suite 306
Alexandria VA 22314
Toll Free: 877-624-0613
Tel: 703-548-7790
Fax: 703-548-7792
Internet: http://www.homeopathic.org
E-Mail: nchinfo@igc.apc.org

A non-profit membership organization dedicated to promoting homeopathy in the United States through education, publication, research, and membership services. Membership is $40/year and includes the Directory of Practitioners and Study Groups, and the monthly magazine *Homeopathy Today*. An information packet, including the Directory, is available for $6.

North American Society of Homeopaths (NASH)
1122 East Pike Street, # 1122
Seattle, WA 98122
Tel: 206-720-7000
Fax: 208-248-1942
Internet: http://www.homeopathy.org
E-Mail: nashinfo@aol.com

American Institute of Homeopathy
801 North Fairfax Street
Suite 306
Alexandria, VA 22314
Toll Free: 888-445-9988
Tel: 703-246-9501
Internet: http://www.homeopathyusa.org
E-Mail: aih@homeopathyusa.org
Conferences, journal, referrals.

Homeopathic Academy of Naturopathic Physicians
12132 SE Foster Place
Portland, OR 97266
Tel: 503-761-3298
Fax: 503-762-1929
Internet: http://www.healthy.net/pan/pa/homeopathic/hanp/index.html
E-Mail: hanp@igc.apc.org

Council for Homeopathic Certification
PO Box 12180
La Crescenta, CA 91224
Toll Free: 866-242-3399
Tel: 818-541-9172
Fax: 818-541-9173
Internet: http://www.homeopathicdirectory.com/old/index.htm
E-Mail: hswope@igc.org

Hahnemann Medical Clinic
1918 Bonita Ave.
Berkeley, CA 94704
Tel: 510-524-3117

Consultations, training.

The National Board of Homeopathic Examiners
6536 Stadium Drive
Zephyrhills, Florida 33540
Tel: 813-782-2690
Fax: 813-782-3275
Internet: http://www.nbhe.com

Homeopathic Nurses Association
HC 81 Box 6023
Questa , NM 87556
Tel: 505-586-1166
Internet: http://www.homeopathicnurses.org

An international support organization for nurses who are studying homeopathy and using it in their client's healthcare and education.

The American Association of Naturopathic Physicians
8201 Greensboro Drive
Suite 300
McLean, VA 98102
Toll Free: 877-969-2267
Tel: 703-610-9037
Fax: 703-610-9005
Internet: http://www.naturopathic.org

The Arizona Homeopathic Medical Association
2525 West Greenway Road
Suite 300
Phoenix, Arizona 85023
Tel: 602-978-1722
Fax: 602-942-3787

Atlanta Homeopathy Study Group
Sage Hill Chiropractic
Sage Hill Shopping Center
1799 Briarcliff Rd. NE
Suite X
Atlanta, GA 30306
Tel: 404-607-7625
Fax: 404-607-1399
Internet: http://www.accessatlanta.com/community/groups/homeopathy/index.html

Connecticut Homeopathic Association
P.O. Box 1055
Greens Farms, CT 06436
Tel: 203-327-6525
E-Mail: cha@simile.org

The Academy of Veterinary Homeopathy
751 N.E. 168th St.
N. Miami, FL 33162-2427
Tel: 305-652-1590
Fax: 305-653-7244
Internet: http://www.acadvethom.org
E-Mail: avh@naturalholistic.com

Chapter 65

National Center for Complementary and Alternative Medicine (NCCAM)

Introduction

This chapter provides general information about complementary and alternative medicine (CAM) and the National Center for Complementary and Alternative Medicine (NCCAM). It is designed to give you a quick overview of NCCAM efforts to advance CAM research. When possible, this chapter includes the names and telephone numbers of resources that can give you more information.

What Is the NCCAM?

In 1998, the Congress established the NCCAM at the National Institutes of Health (NIH) to stimulate, develop, and support research on CAM for the benefit of the public. The NCCAM is an advocate for quality science, rigorous and relevant research, and open and objective inquiry into which CAM practices work, which do not, and why. Its overriding mission is to give the American public reliable information about the safety and effectiveness of CAM practices.

The NCCAM is one of more than 20 Institutes and Centers (ICs) composing the NIH. The NIH is one of eight health agencies within the Public Health Service of the U.S. Department of Health and Human Services (DHHS). The NIH is among the world's foremost biomedical

"General Information about CAM and the NCCAM," Publication Number M-42, National Center for Complementary and Alternative Medicine (NCCAM), NCCAM Clearinghouse, June 2000, updated February 2001.

research institutions and is the Federal Government's focal point for biomedical research in the United States.

NCCAM's Purpose and Mission

The NCCAM conducts and supports basic and applied (clinical) research and research training on CAM. Basic research generally refers to investigations, such as test-tube studies, that take place under controlled conditions in scientific laboratories. Clinical research refers to medical studies of new treatments in people that take place in health care settings, such as hospitals or medical clinics. Scientific inquiry into CAM is a relatively new area of research.

The NCCAM provides information about CAM to health care providers and the public. The Center also develops other programs to further the investigation and application of CAM treatments that show promise.

The NCCAM focuses on the following efforts:

- Evaluating the safety and efficacy of widely used natural products, such as herbal remedies and nutritional and food supplements (e.g., mega-doses of vitamins);

- Supporting pharmacological studies to determine the potential interactive effects of CAM products with standard treatment medications; and

- Evaluating CAM practices, such as acupuncture and chiropractic.

The director of the NCCAM is appointed by the Secretary of the DHHS and reports to the director of the NIH. In 1999, Stephen E. Straus, M.D., an internationally recognized expert in clinical research, was named the director of the NCCAM.

Since Fiscal Year (FY) 1993, NCCAM's budget has steadily risen from $2 million to $68.7 million in FY 2000. This funding increase reflects the public's growing need for CAM information that is based on rigorous scientific research.

The Center is located on the NIH campus in Bethesda, Maryland.

NCCAM's Objectives

The NCCAM works toward the following goals, grouped under three main headings:

Research

- Collaborate with other NIH Institutes and Centers (ICs) and other Federal agencies to advance CAM scientific study.

- Identify and investigate promising, understudied areas.

- Establish a global network for CAM research.

Research Training

- Implement a comprehensive research training plan.

- Provide research training and clinical fellowships.

- Educate CAM scientists about biomedical research methods.

- Educate conventional researchers about the nature and principles of CAM.

Communications

- Establish effective partnerships with CAM researchers, health professionals, and the public.

- Collaborate on CAM information dissemination with other NIH ICs and other Federal agencies.

- Distribute scientifically based information about CAM research, practices, and findings to health care providers and consumers.

NCCAM's History and Related Legislation

The NCCAM was initiated through a congressional mandate under the FY 1999 Omnibus appropriations bill signed by President Bill Clinton on October 21, 1998. Before that time, the NCCAM was the Office of Alternative Medicine (OAM). The OAM, established in 1992 within the NIH Office of the Director, facilitated and coordinated the evaluation of alternative medical treatment modalities through research projects and other initiatives with NIH's ICs.

At that time, OAM's primary role was to emphasize the rigorous scientific evaluation of CAM treatments, develop a solid infrastructure to coordinate and conduct research at the NIH, and establish a clearinghouse to provide information to the public.

OAM's expansion into a Center gives the NCCAM greater ability to initiate and fund additional research projects and to provide more information to the public at a time when a growing number of people are interested in CAM therapies and systems of practice.

The 1999 Omnibus legislation also established a White House Commission on Complementary and Alternative Medicine Policy. This Commission will study issues regarding research; training and certification of CAM practitioners; insurance coverage; and other alternative medicine issues. The DHHS will make appointments to and oversee the Commission.

NCCAM's Program Advisory Council

The National Institutes of Health Revitalization Act of 1993 provided for the establishment of a Program Advisory Council to advise the OAM director. The Council officially was formed in the summer of 1994, and its first meeting was held in September of that year.

The Council, now called the National Advisory Council on Complementary and Alternative Medicine (NACCAM), meets 3 times a year and currently has 17 members. According to the 1999 Omnibus legislation, at least half of the members are practitioners licensed in one or more of the main subsystems of CAM with which the NCCAM is concerned, and at least three members are consumer representatives. Council members are appointed by the Secretary of the DHHS for overlapping terms up to 4 years.

NCCAM Programs

Underlying NCCAM's programs is the congressional mandate to study and disseminate information about the safety and effectiveness of CAM therapies and facilitate the integration of safe and effective treatments into an interdisciplinary health care delivery system.

To accomplish such a broad mandate, NCCAM programs support rigorous scientific review, tapping the expertise of scientists from other NIH ICs and other Federal agencies. NCCAM's programs incorporate input from the NACCAM.

Following, we have organized the description of NCCAM's programs into the following five functional areas: extramural research, intramural research training, scientific databases, public information clearinghouse, and liaison with CAM stakeholders.

Extramural Research (Grants)

The Extramural Research Program helps design, develop, review, fund, and implement specific CAM research projects and training that occur outside the NIH, in addition to coordinating grants with other NIH ICs.

The goals of this program are to increase the number of NCCAM-supported grants, increase co-funding of the CAM-related activities of other NIH ICs, streamline the management of extramural grants and IC cooperative activities, and maintain information on the status and results of NCCAM-supported research.

The program awards National Research Service Award Institutional Training Grants (T32) to eligible institutions to develop or enhance research training opportunities for individuals, selected by the institution, who are training for careers in specified areas of biomedical and behavioral research. The program supports CAM research-related training of pre-doctoral and post-doctoral students.

A great challenge of the program is to educate potential researchers in CAM to follow methodological procedures that have been long established in the biomedical research communities.

At the same time, conventional researchers interested in CAM need information about the nature, principles, and practices of CAM systems and modalities and their linkage to NCCAM research priorities. In this way, scientific research standards can be applied to CAM research to provide valid and reliable results.

For information about specific extramural research projects, call the NCCAM Clearinghouse at 301-589-5367, or toll-free at 888-644-6226.

The NCCAM funds several CAM Research Centers outside the NIH. For up-to-date contact information, specialty areas, and brief descriptions of the Centers, visit NCCAM's Web site http://nccam.nih.gov/nccam/fi/research/centers.html, or call the NCCAM Clearinghouse at 301-589-5367, or toll-free at 888-644-6226.

Intramural Research Training

The Intramural Research Program supports the work of CAM researchers at scientific laboratories within the NIH. This program provides a foundation for NIH scientists to conduct basic and clinical research in CAM.

The program funds individual post-doctoral fellowships. These fellowships are designed to train a group of investigators who have the skills needed to conduct systematic studies of the safety, efficacy, cost-effectiveness, or mechanisms of action of unconventional methods for treating major diseases and promoting well-being.

Scientific Databases

The Scientific Databases Program provides an infrastructure for identifying, organizing, and appraising the scientific literature on CAM practices. The goal is to establish comprehensive, electronic, bibliographic databases of this literature. The literature in these databases is designed to serve as an ongoing source of CAM information for scientists, researchers, practitioners, and the public.

The program also evaluates the scientific literature on CAM practices in conjunction with DHHS's Agency for Healthcare Research and Quality (AHRQ), provides research-based information about CAM practices for dissemination to health professionals and the public, and continues development of a classification system specific for CAM practices. Additionally, the program enhances existing indexing and retrieval capabilities of bibliographic databases for information about CAM practices.

Through the use of rigorous techniques to appraise CAM scientific literature, this program is implementing a process with the AHRQ for developing systematic reviews and meta-analyses of the scientific literature. A systematic review is a report on the science in a particular area of health care. In a meta-analysis, a number of research papers on a specific topic are collected and evaluated scientifically.

To date, this program includes the following two bibliographic databases of CAM information for dissemination to the public via the Internet:

- **CAM on PubMed.** CAM on PubMed, developed jointly by the National Library of Medicine and the National Center for Complementary and Alternative Medicine, contains bibliographic citations (1966-present) related to complementary and alternative medicine. These citations are a subset of the National Library of Medicine's PubMed system that contains over 11 million journal citations from the MEDLINE database and additional life science journals important to health researchers, practitioners and consumers. CAM on PubMed also displays links to publisher web sites offering full text of articles.

- **AM Database of CHID.** Through its Public Information Clearinghouse, the NCCAM maintains the Complementary and Alternative Medicine (AM) Database of the Combined Health Information Database (CHID). The AM Database contains bibliographic summaries of books, journal articles, research reports, audiovisuals, and other materials about CAM. As a single source of information from the Federal Government about a wide range of health topics, CHID is a convenient reference tool for health professionals, patients, and the public.

Public Information Clearinghouse

The NCCAM Clearinghouse, established in 1996, is the public's point of contact and access to information about CAM and NCCAM's programs, conferences, and research activities. Services include a toll-free information line (888-644-6226), publications, referrals to other information resources, and the AM Database of CHID. The Clearinghouse is located in Maryland near the NIH campus.

The Clearinghouse collects and disseminates information to the public, media, and health care professionals to promote awareness and education about CAM research and the NCCAM. The Clearinghouse disseminates CAM information that focuses on the scientific research funded, conducted, or collected by the NCCAM, other NIH ICs, and their grantees. The Clearinghouse does not provide medical referrals, medical advice, or recommendations for specific CAM therapies.

NCCAM Clearinghouse information specialists respond in English and Spanish to inquiries for information by calling 301-589-5367, or toll-free telephone (888-644-6226), TTY/TDY for the hearing impaired (888-644-6226), fax (301-495-4957), e-mail (nccam-info@nccam.nih.gov), and postal mail (NCCAM Clearinghouse, P.O. Box 8218, Silver Spring, MD 20907-8218). They answer calls Monday through Friday, from 8:30 a.m. to 5:00 p.m., Eastern time.

After regular business hours, callers either may leave their names and telephone numbers or request fact sheets and other information through the Clearinghouse's Fax-On-Demand system, available through the toll-free number (888-644-6226).

The NCCAM is not a referral agency for alternative medical treatments or individual practitioners. Therefore, the NCCAM Clearinghouse does not provide medical advice to patients, and it does not provide referrals to alternative health care practitioners.

NCCAM Clearinghouse information specialists are not health care professionals. The information they provide cannot substitute for the medical expertise and advice of a doctor. The NCCAM encourages all patients to talk with their primary health care practitioner about the advantages and risks of CAM treatments.

The NCCAM Clearinghouse processes requests for general information within 2 business days upon receipt of the requests.

NCCAM Clearinghouse staff members strive to give you quality service. Constructive feedback is welcomed. Please mail comments in writing to the NCCAM Clearinghouse Project Director at the NCCAM Clearinghouse, P.O. Box 8218, Silver Spring, MD 20907-8218. For more information about the NCCAM Clearinghouse, call the NCCAM Clearinghouse at 301-589-5367, or toll-free at 1-888-644-6226 and ask for a copy of the Clearinghouse's brochure, "Want Information About Alternative Medicine?"

In addition to maintaining the AM Database of CHID, the NCCAM Clearinghouse produces fact sheets, a newsletter, and other publications that provide information about CAM research supported by the NCCAM and other ICs of the NIH. The information is free of charge. For a list of our publications, call the NCCAM Clearinghouse at 301-589-5367, or toll-free at 888-644-6226, and ask for a copy of our publications order form.

The Clearinghouse produces NCCAM's newsletter that features CAM updates, NIH research news, and information from the NCCAM. The newsletter is available to the public through the NCCAM Clearinghouse or on NCCAM's Web site http://nccam.nih.gov/nccam/ne/newsletter/index.html.

NCCAM's Media Relations—NCCAM's Media Relations area facilitates accurate coverage of relevant stories with the news media, and provides information about the NCCAM and its current activities to mass media audiences.

Liaison with CAM Stakeholders

The International and Professional Liaison Program supports and facilitates cooperative efforts in research and education in CAM approaches worldwide and with professional organizations across the United States. In November 1996, the NCCAM, then the OAM, was designated a World Health Organization Collaborating Center in Traditional Medicine. The 4-year designation includes the NCCAM as part of an international network of 19 established institutions, located in national governments or universities worldwide, that focus on traditional medicine and CAM.

Other NCCAM Activities

A major function of the NCCAM is to facilitate the evaluation of various alternative treatment modalities through ICs within the NIH. This cooperation is based on well-established expertise and encourages collaboration on projects of mutual interest. The NCCAM has identified a network of coordinators at the NIH to assist with issues related to researching alternative medical practices and treatments. In addition, the NCCAM facilitates CAM data review and research with other agencies of the Federal Government.

NCCAM's Web Site

The NCCAM maintains a Web site http://nccam.nih.gov/ to give you CAM information. Topics on NCCAM's Web site include: the NCCAM; frequently asked questions; Clearinghouse publications; CAM databases; NCCAM research; clinical trial opportunities; research policies, applications, and guidelines; NCCAM's newsletter; press releases; and minutes of NCCAM-sponsored meetings.

Town Meetings

The NCCAM plans to convene a series of regional town meetings for CAM consumers, researchers, practitioners, and the public. The first town meeting, on March 15, 2000, at Harvard University in Boston, Massachusetts, was sponsored in collaboration with the Center for Alternative Medicine Research, Beth Israel Deaconess Medical Center.

The town meetings offer an opportunity for input from professionals, patients, advocacy groups, and local residents who have an interest in CAM, the NCCAM, or other ICs of the NIH.

CAM Conferences and Education. The NCCAM collaborates with other ICs of the NIH to sponsor CAM-related conferences and educational programs. Separate topics covered to date include acupuncture, behavioral treatments, chronic pain, health insurance issues, liver disease, and nursing education.

Cancer Advisory Panel for CAM Research

The Cancer Advisory Panel for Complementary and Alternative Medicine (CAPCAM) is a 15-member panel created in 1998 that includes patient advocates, researchers, and administrators from conventional biomedical and CAM communities. The CAPCAM facilitates the joint review of data from cancer research projects through the NCCAM and National Cancer Institute, another NIH IC. CAPCAM's mission is to review and assess clinical data submitted by CAM cancer researchers and to advise the NCCAM on the next research steps.

571

The CAPCAM held its first meeting on July 8-9, 1999, in Bethesda, Maryland. The agenda enabled panel members to explore the scope of their advisory role and to hear presentations of two Best Case Series. The term "Best Case Series" refers to precise clinical information—collected while patients undergo treatment—that indicates some benefit to the patients being studied.

The second CAPCAM meeting was held on December 13, 1999, in Bethesda, Maryland. Speakers from within the NCCAM and NIH discussed the Best Case program for analyzing data from CAM cancer medicine practitioners. Guest speakers discussed the benefits of psychosocial treatment (e.g., group therapy) to patients with certain types of cancer and the current efforts to study the use of CAM as a complement to standard radiation oncology procedures.

Trans-Agency CAM Coordinating Committee

NCCAM's Trans-Agency CAM Coordinating Committee is a group of representatives of several other Federal agencies and departments. The Committee is designed to help the NCCAM coordinate scientific input for CAM research and explore research partnerships.

For More Information

Please send requests for information about complementary or alternative medicine to:

NCCAM Clearinghouse
P.O. Box 7923
Gaithersburg, MD 20898
Toll Free: 888-644-6226
TTY:866-464-3615
Fax: 866-464-3616
Internet: http://nccam.nih.gov
E-Mail: nccam-info@nccam.nih.gov

Chapter 66

Health Insurance for Alternative Medicine

For information regarding insurance benefits for alternative medicine, contact:

Alternative Health Benefit Services
P.O. Box 5167
West Hills, CA 91308
Tel: 818-226-9829
Fax: 818-226-9820
Internet: http://www.alternativeinsurance.com
E-Mail: HealthyIns@AOL.com

The Mission of Alternative Health Benefit Services is to create greater credibility and access for less invasive, more natural healthcare, and to enable all Americans to select the type of medical care and physician/medical provider of their choice.

This Mission is being accomplished through the efforts of compatible businesses working with the business community, the insurance industry, the medical community (medical doctors and complementary/alternative healthcare practitioners), the American labor movement, and other entities that may support these goals.

Holistic Health Insurance & Financial Services was created by the employees of Alternative Health Insurance Services, which was

From "Alternative Health Benefit Services," and undated document cited January 2002 © The Alternative Health Group (Thousand Oaks, CA); reprinted with permission.

established in 1985 and incorporated in 1988. The company is a managing general agency, general agent, and personal producer for various traditional health insurance products.

Alternative Health Insurance Administrators was established in 1999 to provide expertise in the administration of complementary and alternative health benefits provided through insurance companies and other third party payers.

Several associations have been formed to provide benefits to health conscious consumers and to promote programs that support the mission of Alternative Health Benefit Services. Natural Marketing Association was established in 1983, Alliance for Alternatives in Healthcare was established in 1990 (incorporated in 1991), Alliance for Natural Health was established in 1997, and Natural Health Alliance was established in 1999 These organizations negotiate with providers of health care (insurers, labor unions, and other third party payers) to obtain benefits that include alternative and complementary medicine.

Actuarially Sound Benefit Consultants was established in 1991 to work with associations, labor unions, or other entities seeking assistance to develop health plans that include alternative and complementary medicine.

The Holistic Health Network contracts with complementary and alternative medical providers (CAM providers) to provide greater access for CAM services to the consumer, and to participants of subscribing employers, associations, or other groups.

Index

Index

Page numbers followed by 'n' indicate a footnote. Page numbers in *italics* indicate a table or illustration.

A

abdominial, defined 539
abetalipoproteinemia 273
ABNOBAviscum 490
"About Chiropractic" (ACA) 97n
absinthe *104*
ACA *see* American Chiropractic Association
The Academy of Veterinary Homeopathy, contact information 562
Accreditation Commission for Acupuncture and Oriental Medicine, contact information 556
Accutane (isotretinoin) 246
acetaminophen, defined 539
active treatment, defined 539
Acuall.org, Web site address 558
acupressure
  defined 376
  naturopathic medicine 125
  nausea 42, 43–44
acupuncture
  alternative therapy 32
  bioenergetic medicine 349

acupuncture, continued
  Chinese traditional medicine 74
  complications 47
  defined 540
  described 35–55
  diabetes mellitus 401
  headache treatment 412
  naturopathic medicine 32, 125
  needles, described 51
  physician attitudes survey 18, *20, 22*
  resource information 549–58
  theories 36
  see also electroacupuncture
Acupuncture and Electro-Therapeutics Research 552
Acupuncture.com, Web site address 558
"Acupuncture Information and Resources" (NCCAM) 35n, 539n
addiction
  acupuncture 49
  detoxification 285–306
  see also alcohol abuse; drug abuse; substance abuse
AE-941/Neovastat 457, 459, 462–63
aerobic metabolism 465
aerobic respiration 465
afferent, described 58

577

anticholinergics, defined 541
anticonvulsants, defined 541
antidepressant medications 232–33
  see also St. John's wort
antiemetics, acupuncture 42
antihypertensives, defined 541
anti-inflammatory, defined 541
antineoplastons 433, 449–50
antioxidants
  described 198, 225, 465
  vitamin E 271
apa dhatu, described 66
apana, described 71
aparigraha, described 148–49
appendix, described 78
aqueous, defined 541
The Arizona Homeopathic Medical
  Association, contact information
  562
aromatherapy
  headache treatment 415
  overview 341–44
"Aromatherapy - Frequently Asked
  Questions" (Atlantic Institute of
  Aromatherapy) 341n
arthritis
  defined 541
  selenium 230
art therapy
  mind-body intervention 33
  overview 345–47
asanas, described 142, 154–56
The Association for Applied Psycho-
  physiology and Biofeedback, contact
  information 165–66
Association of Reflexologists 381n
asteya, described 146–47
asthma, acupuncture 41–42
astragalus 200–201
atap-seva, described 68, 70
Atlanta Homeopathy Study Group,
  contact information 562
Atlantic Institute of Aromatherapy
  341n
attention deficit hyperactivity disorder, acupuncture 49
aureomycin 352
auscultation, Chinese traditional
  medicine 81–82

ayurveda
  described 32, 57–72
  naturopathic medicine 125
The Ayurvedic Institute
  contact information 57n
  publication 57n

B

back pain
  acupuncture 41
  chiropractic 98
BAL *see* British antiLewisite
balance, Native American medicine
  113–14
Barrett, Stephen 431n, 497n, 503n,
  519n
"Basic Explanation of the Electrodermal Screening Test and the Concepts of Bio-Energetic Medicine"
  (American Association of Acupuncture and Bio-Energetic Medicine)
  349n
"The Basic Principles of Chinese Traditional Medicine" (Lewith) 73n
basil 343
basti, described 67
B cells, defined 541
BeneFin 462
Benson, Herbert 180–81, 183, 184
benzoic acid 301
benzoquinone compound 465, 467
Bersworth, Frederick 358
Best Case Series Program 398
beta-blockers 471
beta-carotene
  environmental damage 198
  overview 239–48
biapigenin 233
binding agent, defined 541
bioavailable, defined 541
bioelectromagnetic based therapies,
  described 34
bioenergetic medicine, overview 349–
  56
biofeedback
  defined 541
  diabetes mellitus 401–2

National Institute of Neurological Disorders and Stroke (NINDS), headache research publication 539n

National Institutes of Health (NIH), contact information 4, 549–50

National Toxicology Program 101–4

Native American medicine, overview 113–20

natulan 474

naturopathic medicine
alternative therapy 32
described 32
manipulative therapy, described 127
overview 121–38

nausea
acupuncture 42–44
hypnosis 178

NCATA *see* National Coalition of Arts Therapies Association

NCCAM *see* National Center for Complementary and Alternative Medicine

NCCAM Clearinghouse, contact information 572

The NCH Directory of Practitioners, Web site address 559

The NCH State by State Resources Page, Web site address 559

NCI *see* National Cancer Institute

neck pain, acupuncture 39–40

Nelson, Mildred 437

nervous system, vitamin B6 251–52

neurohormones, defined 545

neurological, defined 545

neurotransmitters
acupuncture 37
defined 545

niacin
detoxification 301
Greek cancer cure 437
vitamin B6 249

NIDDK *see* National Institute of Diabetes and Digestive Diseases

NIH *see* National Institutes of Health

NIH Consensus Program Information Center, contact information 550

niyamas, described 142, 149–54

NLM *see* U.S. National Library of Medicine

nociceptors, defined 545

nonsteroidal anti-inflammatory drugs (NSAID), defined 545–46

North American Society of Homeopaths (NASH), contact information 560

nosodes, described 353

nourishing qi, described 75

NSAID *see* nonsteroidal anti-inflammatory drugs

nutrition *see* diet and nutrition

"Nutrition: The Science behind the Fiction" (Friedman) 197n

O

Oberst, Marilyn 517

obesity, fasting 312

ODS *see* Office of Dietary Supplements

Office of Dietary Supplements, National Institutes of Health (ODS-NIH), publications
dietary supplements 203n
folate 207n
magnesium 217n
selenium 225n
vitamin B6 249n
vitamin B12 257n
vitamin D 263n
vitamin E 271n
zinc 279n

oil drop test, described 66–67

olfaction, described 342–43

omega-3 fatty acids 198

126-F *see* cancell

opioids
acupuncture 37, 44–45
defined 546

Optifast 312

oral, defined 546

oriental massage, alternative therapy 32

Ornish, Dean 127–28

orthomolecular therapies, descibed 33

osteoarthritis
acupuncture 40, 48–49
chelation 359

osteopathy, body-based therapy 33

Voll, Reinhold 349–52
vomiting
  acupuncture 42–44
  hypnosis 178
VRT *see* vegetative reflex test
vyayama, described 68, 69–70
Vysorel 490

W

Waldstein, Steven 559
warfarin 235, 471
water
  described 59
  detoxification 301
Watson, Jean 508
"What are Dietary Supplements?"
  (ODS) 203n
"What Is Biofeedback?" (Runck) 161n
"What Is Complementary and Alter-
  native Medicine?" (NCCAM) 3n
"What Is Imagery, and How Does It
  Work?" (Rossman) 167n
"What Is Yoga?" (Farhi) 139n
Wills, Lucy 207
workplace, massage therapy 375
wormwood *104*
wrist bands, nausea 43

X

xerophthalmia, described 241
xin-heart
  blood 76
  described 74–75
  syndromes 83–85
xu nature, described 74
xu pulse, described 79

Y

yagyakunda, described 69
yamas, described 142, 144–49
yang
  defined 547
  described 36, 73–74
  see also Chinese traditional medi-
    cine; yin
yantra, described 71
Yarbrough, Lynne 17n
yin
  defined 548
  described 36, 73–74
  see also Chinese traditional medi-
    cine; yang
ylang-ylang 343
yoga
  ayurveda 69–70
  detoxification 300
  overview 139–58
*Yoga Mind, Body and Spirit: A Re-
  turn to Wholeness* (Farhi) 139n
Yogananda, Paramahansa 309
yoga sutras, described 141
Yogi, Mahesh 184
yo-yo syndrome 312

Z

zang channels, described 74
zang organs, described 74–75
Zeff, Jared 125, 128, 130–31, 133, 135
zhong qi, described 75
zinc
  food sources 279, *282*
  overview 279–84
zone therapy 381

Health Reference Series
COMPLETE CATALOG

Adolescent Health Sourcebook

Basic Consumer Health Information about Common Medical, Mental, and Emotional Concerns in Adolescents, Including Facts about Acne, Body Piercing, Mononucleosis, Nutrition, Eating Disorders, Stress, Depression, Behavior Problems, Peer Pressure, Violence, Gangs, Drug Use, Puberty, Sexuality, Pregnancy, Learning Disabilities, and More

Along with a Glossary of Terms and Other Resources for Further Help and Information

Edited by Chad T. Kimball. 658 pages. 2002. 0-7808-0248-9. $78.

AIDS Sourcebook, 1st Edition

Basic Information about AIDS and HIV Infection, Featuring Historical and Statistical Data, Current Research, Prevention, and Other Special Topics of Interest for Persons Living with AIDS

Along with Source Listings for Further Assistance

Edited by Karen Bellenir and Peter D. Dresser. 831 pages. 1995. 0-7808-0031-1. $78.

"One strength of this book is its practical emphasis. The intended audience is the lay reader . . . useful as an educational tool for health care providers who work with AIDS patients. Recommended for public libraries as well as hospital or academic libraries that collect consumer materials."
— *Bulletin of the Medical Library Association, Jan '96*

"This is the most comprehensive volume of its kind on an important medical topic. Highly recommended for all libraries." — *Reference Book Review, '96*

"Very useful reference for all libraries."
— *Choice, Association of College and Research Libraries, Oct '95*

"There is a wealth of information here that can provide much educational assistance. It is a must book for all libraries and should be on the desk of each and every congressional leader. Highly recommended."
— *AIDS Book Review Journal, Aug '95*

"Recommended for most collections."
— *Library Journal, Jul '95*

AIDS Sourcebook, 2nd Edition

Basic Consumer Health Information about Acquired Immune Deficiency Syndrome (AIDS) and Human Immunodeficiency Virus (HIV) Infection, Featuring Updated Statistical Data, Reports on Recent Research and Prevention Initiatives, and Other Special Topics of Interest for Persons Living with AIDS, Including New Antiretroviral Treatment Options, Strategies for Com-

bating Opportunistic Infections, Information about Clinical Trials, and More

Along with a Glossary of Important Terms and Resource Listings for Further Help and Information

Edited by Karen Bellenir. 751 pages. 1999. 0-7808-0225-X. $78.

"Highly recommended."
— *American Reference Books Annual, 2000*

"Excellent sourcebook. This continues to be a highly recommended book. There is no other book that provides as much information as this book provides."
— *AIDS Book Review Journal, Dec-Jan 2000*

"Recommended reference source."
— *Booklist, American Library Association, Dec '99*

"A solid text for college-level health libraries."
— *The Bookwatch, Aug '99*

Cited in *Reference Sources for Small and Medium-Sized Libraries, American Library Association, 1999*

Alcoholism Sourcebook

Basic Consumer Health Information about the Physical and Mental Consequences of Alcohol Abuse, Including Liver Disease, Pancreatitis, Wernicke-Korsakoff Syndrome (Alcoholic Dementia), Fetal Alcohol Syndrome, Heart Disease, Kidney Disorders, Gastrointestinal Problems, and Immune System Compromise and Featuring Facts about Addiction, Detoxification, Alcohol Withdrawal, Recovery, and the Maintenance of Sobriety

Along with a Glossary and Directories of Resources for Further Help and Information

Edited by Karen Bellenir. 613 pages. 2000. 0-7808-0325-6. $78.

"This title is one of the few reference works on alcoholism for general readers. For some readers this will be a welcome complement to the many self-help books on the market. Recommended for collections serving general readers and consumer health collections."
— *E-Streams, Mar '01*

"This book is an excellent choice for public and academic libraries."
— *American Reference Books Annual, 2001*

"Recommended reference source."
— *Booklist, American Library Association, Dec '00*

"Presents a wealth of information on alcohol use and abuse and its effects on the body and mind, treatment, and prevention." — *SciTech Book News, Dec '00*

"Important new health guide which packs in the latest consumer information about the problems of alcoholism." — *Reviewer's Bookwatch, Nov '00*

SEE ALSO *Drug Abuse Sourcebook, Substance Abuse Sourcebook*

Allergies Sourcebook, 1st Edition

Basic Information about Major Forms and Mechanisms of Common Allergic Reactions, Sensitivities, and Intolerances, Including Anaphylaxis, Asthma, Hives and Other Dermatologic Symptoms, Rhinitis, and Sinusitis

Along with Their Usual Triggers Like Animal Fur, Chemicals, Drugs, Dust, Foods, Insects, Latex, Pollen, and Poison Ivy, Oak, and Sumac; Plus Information on Prevention, Identification, and Treatment

Edited by Allan R. Cook. 611 pages. 1997. 0-7808-0036-2. $78.

Allergies Sourcebook, 2nd Edition

Basic Consumer Health Information about Allergic Disorders, Triggers, Reactions, and Related Symptoms, Including Anaphylaxis, Rhinitis, Sinusitis, Asthma, Dermatitis, Conjunctivitis, and Multiple Chemical Sensitivity

Along with Tips on Diagnosis, Prevention, and Treatment, Statistical Data, a Glossary, and a Directory of Sources for Further Help and Information

Edited by Annemarie S. Muth. 598 pages. 2002. 0-7808-0376-0. $78.

Alternative Medicine Sourcebook, First Edition

Basic Consumer Health Information about Alternatives to Conventional Medicine, Including Acupressure, Acupuncture, Aromatherapy, Ayurveda, Bioelectromagnetics, Environmental Medicine, Essence Therapy, Food and Nutrition Therapy, Herbal Therapy, Homeopathy, Imaging, Massage, Naturopathy, Reflexology, Relaxation and Meditation, Sound Therapy, Vitamin and Mineral Therapy, and Yoga, and More

Edited by Allan R. Cook. 737 pages. 1999. 0-7808-0200-4. $78.

"Recommended reference source."
—Booklist, American Library Association, Feb '00

"A great addition to the reference collection of every type of library." —American Reference Books Annual, 2000

Alternative Medicine Sourcebook, Second Edition

Basic Consumer Health Information about Alternative and Complementary Medical Practices, Including Acupuncture, Chiropractic, Herbal Medicine, Homeopathy, Naturopathic Medicine, Mind-Body Interventions, Ayurveda, and Other Non-Western Medical Traditions

Along with Facts about such Specific Therapies as Massage Therapy, Aromatherapy, Qigong, Hypnosis, Prayer, Dance, and Art Therapies, a Glossary, and Resources for Further Information

Edited by Dawn D. Matthews. 618 pages. 2002. 0-7808-0605-0. $78.

Alzheimer's, Stroke & 29 Other Neurological Disorders Sourcebook, 1st Edition

Basic Information for the Layperson on 31 Diseases or Disorders Affecting the Brain and Nervous System, First Describing the Illness, Then Listing Symptoms, Diagnostic Methods, and Treatment Options, and Including Statistics on Incidences and Causes

Edited by Frank E. Bair. 579 pages. 1993. 1-55888-748-2. $78.

"Nontechnical reference book that provides reader-friendly information."
—Family Caregiver Alliance Update, Winter '96

"Should be included in any library's patient education section." —American Reference Books Annual, 1994

"Written in an approachable and accessible style. Recommended for patient education and consumer health collections in health science center and public libraries." —Academic Library Book Review, Dec '93

"It is very handy to have information on more than thirty neurological disorders under one cover, and there is no recent source like it." —Reference Quarterly, American Library Association, Fall '93

SEE ALSO Brain Disorders Sourcebook

Alzheimer's Disease Sourcebook, 2nd Edition

Basic Consumer Health Information about Alzheimer's Disease, Related Disorders, and Other Dementias, Including Multi-Infarct Dementia, AIDS-Related Dementia, Alcoholic Dementia, Huntington's Disease, Delirium, and Confusional States

Along with Reports Detailing Current Research Efforts in Prevention and Treatment, Long-Term Care Issues, and Listings of Sources for Additional Help and Information

Edited by Karen Bellenir. 524 pages. 1999. 0-7808-0223-3. $78.

"Provides a wealth of useful information not otherwise available in one place. This resource is recommended for all types of libraries."
—American Reference Books Annual, 2000

"Recommended reference source."
—Booklist, American Library Association, Oct '99

Arthritis Sourcebook

Basic Consumer Health Information about Specific Forms of Arthritis and Related Disorders, Including Rheumatoid Arthritis, Osteoarthritis, Gout, Polymyalgia Rheumatica, Psoriatic Arthritis, Spondyloarthropathies, Juvenile Rheumatoid Arthritis, and Juvenile Ankylosing Spondylitis

Along with Information about Medical, Surgical, and Alternative Treatment Options, and Including Strategies for Coping with Pain, Fatigue, and Stress

598

Edited by Allan R. Cook. 550 pages. 1998. 0-7808-0201-2. $78.

"... accessible to the layperson."
> —*Reference and Research Book News, Feb '99*

Asthma Sourcebook

Basic Consumer Health Information about Asthma, Including Symptoms, Traditional and Nontraditional Remedies, Treatment Advances, Quality-of-Life Aids, Medical Research Updates, and the Role of Allergies, Exercise, Age, the Environment, and Genetics in the Development of Asthma

Along with Statistical Data, a Glossary, and Directories of Support Groups, and Other Resources for Further Information

Edited by Annemarie S. Muth. 628 pages. 2000. 0-7808-0381-7. $78.

"A worthwhile reference acquisition for public libraries and academic medical libraries whose readers desire a quick introduction to the wide range of asthma information." — *Choice, Association of College & Research Libraries, Jun '01*

"Recommended reference source."
> —*Booklist, American Library Association, Feb '01*

"Highly recommended." — *The Bookwatch, Jan '01*

"There is much good information for patients and their families who deal with asthma daily."
> —*American Medical Writers Association Journal, Winter '01*

"This informative text is recommended for consumer health collections in public, secondary school, and community college libraries and the libraries of universities with a large undergraduate population."
> —*American Reference Books Annual, 2001*

Attention Deficit Disorder Sourcebook, First Edition

Basic Consumer Health Information about Attention Deficit/Hyperactivity Disorder in Children and Adults, Including Facts about Causes, Symptoms, Diagnostic Criteria, and Treatment Options Such as Medications, Behavior Therapy, Coaching, and Homeopathy

Along with Reports on Current Research Initiatives, Legal Issues, and Government Regulations, and Featuring a Glossary of Related Terms, Internet Resources, and a List of Additional Reading Material

Edited by Dawn D. Matthews. 450 pages. 2002. 0-7808-0624-7. $78.

Back & Neck Disorders Sourcebook

Basic Information about Disorders and Injuries of the Spinal Cord and Vertebrae, Including Facts on Chiropractic Treatment, Surgical Interventions, Paralysis, and Rehabilitation

Along with Advice for Preventing Back Trouble

Edited by Karen Bellenir. 548 pages. 1997. 0-7808-0202-0. $78.

"The strength of this work is its basic, easy-to-read format. Recommended."
> —*Reference and User Services Quarterly, American Library Association, Winter '97*

Blood & Circulatory Disorders Sourcebook

Basic Information about Blood and Its Components, Anemias, Leukemias, Bleeding Disorders, and Circulatory Disorders, Including Aplastic Anemia, Thalassemia, Sickle-Cell Disease, Hemochromatosis, Hemophilia, Von Willebrand Disease, and Vascular Diseases

Along with a Special Section on Blood Transfusions and Blood Supply Safety, a Glossary, and Source Listings for Further Help and Information

Edited by Karen Bellenir and Linda M. Shin. 554 pages. 1998. 0-7808-0203-9. $78.

"Recommended reference source."
> —*Booklist, American Library Association, Feb '99*

"An important reference sourcebook written in simple language for everyday, non-technical users. "
> —*Reviewer's Bookwatch, Jan '99*

Brain Disorders Sourcebook

Basic Consumer Health Information about Strokes, Epilepsy, Amyotrophic Lateral Sclerosis (ALS/Lou Gehrig's Disease), Parkinson's Disease, Brain Tumors, Cerebral Palsy, Headache, Tourette Syndrome, and More

Along with Statistical Data, Treatment and Rehabilitation Options, Coping Strategies, Reports on Current Research Initiatives, a Glossary, and Resource Listings for Additional Help and Information

Edited by Karen Bellenir. 481 pages. 1999. 0-7808-0229-2. $78.

"Belongs on the shelves of any library with a consumer health collection." — *E-Streams, Mar '00*

"Recommended reference source."
> —*Booklist, American Library Association, Oct '99*

SEE ALSO *Alzheimer's, Stroke & 29 Other Neurological Disorders Sourcebook, 1st Edition*

Breast Cancer Sourcebook

Basic Consumer Health Information about Breast Cancer, Including Diagnostic Methods, Treatment Options, Alternative Therapies, Self-Help Information, Related Health Concerns, Statistical and Demographic Data, and Facts for Men with Breast Cancer

Along with Reports on Current Research Initiatives, a Glossary of Related Medical Terms, and a Directory of Sources for Further Help and Information

Edited by Edward J. Prucha and Karen Bellenir. 580 pages. 2001. 0-7808-0244-6. $78.

"Recommended reference source."
— *Booklist, American Library Association, Jan '02*

"This reference source is highly recommended. It is quite informative, comprehensive and detailed in nature, and yet it offers practical advice in easy-to-read language. It could be thought of as the 'bible' of breast cancer for the consumer." — *E-Streams, Jan '02*

"The broad range of topics covered in lay language make the *Breast Cancer Sourcebook* an excellent addition to public and consumer health library collections."
— *American Reference Books Annual 2002*

"From the pros and cons of different screening methods and results to treatment options, *Breast Cancer Sourcebook* provides the latest information on the subject."
— *Library Bookwatch, Dec '01*

"This thoroughgoing, very readable reference covers all aspects of breast health and cancer. . . . Readers will find much to consider here. Recommended for all public and patient health collections."
— *Library Journal, Sep '01*

SEE ALSO Cancer Sourcebook for Women, 1st and 2nd Editions, Women's Health Concerns Sourcebook

∎

Breastfeeding Sourcebook

Basic Consumer Health Information about the Benefits of Breastmilk, Preparing to Breastfeed, Breastfeeding as a Baby Grows, Nutrition, and More, Including Information on Special Situations and Concerns Such as Mastitis, Illness, Medications, Allergies, Multiple Births, Prematurity, Special Needs, and Adoption

Along with a Glossary and Resources for Additional Help and Information

Edited by Jenni Lynn Colson. 388 pages. 2002. 0-7808-0332-9. $78.

SEE ALSO Pregnancy & Birth Sourcebook

∎

Burns Sourcebook

Basic Consumer Health Information about Various Types of Burns and Scalds, Including Flame, Heat, Cold, Electrical, Chemical, and Sun Burns

Along with Information on Short-Term and Long-Term Treatments, Tissue Reconstruction, Plastic Surgery, Prevention Suggestions, and First Aid

Edited by Allan R. Cook. 604 pages. 1999. 0-7808-0204-7. $78.

"This is an exceptional addition to the series and is highly recommended for all consumer health collections, hospital libraries, and academic medical centers."
— *E-Streams, Mar '00*

"This key reference guide is an invaluable addition to all health care and public libraries in confronting this ongoing health issue."
— *American Reference Books Annual, 2000*

"Recommended reference source."
— *Booklist, American Library Association, Dec '99*

SEE ALSO Skin Disorders Sourcebook

∎

Cancer Sourcebook, 1st Edition

Basic Information on Cancer Types, Symptoms, Diagnostic Methods, and Treatments, Including Statistics on Cancer Occurrences Worldwide and the Risks Associated with Known Carcinogens and Activities

Edited by Frank E. Bair. 932 pages. 1990. 1-55888-888-8. $78.

Cited in *Reference Sources for Small and Medium-Sized Libraries, American Library Association, 1999*

"Written in nontechnical language. Useful for patients, their families, medical professionals, and librarians."
— *Guide to Reference Books, 1996*

"Designed with the non-medical professional in mind. Libraries and medical facilities interested in patient education should certainly consider adding the *Cancer Sourcebook* to their holdings. This compact collection of reliable information . . . is an invaluable tool for helping patients and patients' families and friends to take the first steps in coping with the many difficulties of cancer."
— *Medical Reference Services Quarterly, Winter '91*

"Specifically created for the nontechnical reader . . . an important resource for the general reader trying to understand the complexities of cancer."
— *American Reference Books Annual, 1991*

"This publication's nontechnical nature and very comprehensive format make it useful for both the general public and undergraduate students."
— *Choice, Association of College and Research Libraries, Oct '90*

∎

New Cancer Sourcebook, 2nd Edition

Basic Information about Major Forms and Stages of Cancer, Featuring Facts about Primary and Secondary Tumors of the Respiratory, Nervous, Lymphatic, Circulatory, Skeletal, and Gastrointestinal Systems, and Specific Organs; Statistical and Demographic Data; Treatment Options; and Strategies for Coping

Edited by Allan R. Cook. 1,313 pages. 1996. 0-7808-0041-9. $78.

"An excellent resource for patients with newly diagnosed cancer and their families. The dialogue is simple, direct, and comprehensive. Highly recommended for

patients and families to aid in their understanding of cancer and its treatment."
— *Booklist Health Sciences Supplement, American Library Association, Oct '97*

"The amount of factual and useful information is extensive. The writing is very clear, geared to general readers. Recommended for all levels." — *Choice, Association of College & Research Libraries, Jan '97*

Cancer Sourcebook, 3rd Edition

Basic Consumer Health Information about Major Forms and Stages of Cancer, Featuring Facts about Primary and Secondary Tumors of the Respiratory, Nervous, Lymphatic, Circulatory, Skeletal, and Gastrointestinal Systems, and Specific Organs

Along with Statistical and Demographic Data, Treatment Options, Strategies for Coping, a Glossary, and a Directory of Sources for Additional Help and Information

Edited by Edward J. Prucha. 1,069 pages. 2000. 0-7808-0227-6. $78.

"This title is recommended for health sciences and public libraries with consumer health collections."
— *E-Streams, Feb '01*

". . . can be effectively used by cancer patients and their families who are looking for answers in a language they can understand. Public and hospital libraries should have it on their shelves."
— *American Reference Books Annual, 2001*

"Recommended reference source."
— *Booklist, American Library Association, Dec '00*

Cancer Sourcebook for Women, 1st Edition

Basic Information about Specific Forms of Cancer That Affect Women, Featuring Facts about Breast Cancer, Cervical Cancer, Ovarian Cancer, Cancer of the Uterus and Uterine Sarcoma, Cancer of the Vagina, and Cancer of the Vulva; Statistical and Demographic Data; Treatments, Self-Help Management Suggestions, and Current Research Initiatives

Edited by Allan R. Cook and Peter D. Dresser. 524 pages. 1996. 0-7808-0076-1. $78.

". . . written in easily understandable, non-technical language. Recommended for public libraries or hospital and academic libraries that collect patient education or consumer health materials."
— *Medical Reference Services Quarterly, Spring '97*

"Would be of value in a consumer health library. . . . written with the health care consumer in mind. Medical jargon is at a minimum, and medical terms are explained in clear, understandable sentences."
— *Bulletin of the Medical Library Association, Oct '96*

"The availability under one cover of all these pertinent publications, grouped under cohesive headings, makes this certainly a most useful sourcebook." — *Choice, Association of College & Research Libraries, Jun '96*

"Presents a comprehensive knowledge base for general readers. Men and women both benefit from the gold mine of information nestled between the two covers of this book. Recommended."
— *Academic Library Book Review, Summer '96*

"This timely book is highly recommended for consumer health and patient education collections in all libraries." — *Library Journal, Apr '96*

SEE ALSO *Breast Cancer Sourcebook, Women's Health Concerns Sourcebook*

Cancer Sourcebook for Women, 2nd Edition

Basic Consumer Health Information about Gynecologic Cancers and Related Concerns, Including Cervical Cancer, Endometrial Cancer, Gestational Trophoblastic Tumor, Ovarian Cancer, Uterine Cancer, Vaginal Cancer, Vulvar Cancer, Breast Cancer, and Common Non-Cancerous Uterine Conditions, with Facts about Cancer Risk Factors, Screening and Prevention, Treatment Options, and Reports on Current Research Initiatives

Along with a Glossary of Cancer Terms and a Directory of Resources for Additional Help and Information

Edited by Karen Bellenir. 604 pages. 2002. 0-7808-0226-8. $78.

SEE ALSO *Breast Cancer Sourcebook, Women's Health Concerns Sourcebook*

Cardiovascular Diseases & Disorders Sourcebook, 1st Edition

Basic Information about Cardiovascular Diseases and Disorders, Featuring Facts about the Cardiovascular System, Demographic and Statistical Data, Descriptions of Pharmacological and Surgical Interventions, Lifestyle Modifications, and a Special Section Focusing on Heart Disorders in Children

Edited by Karen Bellenir and Peter D. Dresser. 683 pages. 1995. 0-7808-0032-X. $78.

". . . comprehensive format provides an extensive overview on this subject." — *Choice, Association of College & Research Libraries, Jun '96*

". . . an easily understood, complete, up-to-date resource. This well executed public health tool will make valuable information available to those that need it most, patients and their families. The typeface, sturdy non-reflective paper, and library binding add a feel of quality found wanting in other publications. Highly recommended for academic and general libraries. "
— *Academic Library Book Review, Summer '96*

SEE ALSO *Healthy Heart Sourcebook for Women, Heart Diseases & Disorders Sourcebook, 2nd Edition*

Caregiving Sourcebook

Basic Consumer Health Information for Caregivers, Including a Profile of Caregivers, Caregiving Responsibilities and Concerns, Tips for Specific Conditions, Care Environments, and the Effects of Caregiving

Along with Facts about Legal Issues, Financial Information, and Future Planning, a Glossary, and a Listing of Additional Resources

Edited by Joyce Brennfleck Shannon. 600 pages. 2001. 0-7808-0331-0. $78.

"Essential for most collections."
— *Library Journal*, Apr 1, 2002

"An ideal addition to the reference collection of any public library. Health sciences information professionals may also want to acquire the *Caregiving Sourcebook* for their hospital or academic library for use as a ready reference tool by health care workers interested in aging and caregiving." —*E-Streams*, Jan '02

"Recommended reference source."
—*Booklist, American Library Association*, Oct '01

■

Colds, Flu & Other Common Ailments Sourcebook

Basic Consumer Health Information about Common Ailments and Injuries, Including Colds, Coughs, the Flu, Sinus Problems, Headaches, Fever, Nausea and Vomiting, Menstrual Cramps, Diarrhea, Constipation, Hemorrhoids, Back Pain, Dandruff, Dry and Itchy Skin, Cuts, Scrapes, Sprains, Bruises, and More

Along with Information about Prevention, Self-Care, Choosing a Doctor, Over-the-Counter Medications, Folk Remedies, and Alternative Therapies, and Including a Glossary of Important Terms and a Directory of Resources for Further Help and Information

Edited by Chad T. Kimball. 638 pages. 2001. 0-7808-0435-X. $78.

"A good starting point for research on common illnesses. It will be a useful addition to public and consumer health library collections."
— *American Reference Books Annual 2002*

"Will prove valuable to any library seeking to maintain a current, comprehensive reference collection of health resources. . . . Excellent reference."
— *The Bookwatch*, Aug '01

"Recommended reference source."
—*Booklist, American Library Association*, July '01

■

Communication Disorders Sourcebook

Basic Information about Deafness and Hearing Loss, Speech and Language Disorders, Voice Disorders, Balance and Vestibular Disorders, and Disorders of Smell, Taste, and Touch

Edited by Linda M. Ross. 533 pages. 1996. 0-7808-0077-X. $78.

"This is skillfully edited and is a welcome resource for the layperson. It should be found in every public and medical library." — *Booklist Health Sciences Supplement, American Library Association*, Oct '97

■

Congenital Disorders Sourcebook

Basic Information about Disorders Acquired during Gestation, Including Spina Bifida, Hydrocephalus, Cerebral Palsy, Heart Defects, Craniofacial Abnormalities, Fetal Alcohol Syndrome, and More

Along with Current Treatment Options and Statistical Data

Edited by Karen Bellenir. 607 pages. 1997. 0-7808-0205-5. $78.

"Recommended reference source."
— *Booklist, American Library Association*, Oct '97

SEE ALSO Pregnancy & Birth Sourcebook

■

Consumer Issues in Health Care Sourcebook

Basic Information about Health Care Fundamentals and Related Consumer Issues, Including Exams and Screening Tests, Physician Specialties, Choosing a Doctor, Using Prescription and Over-the-Counter Medications Safely, Avoiding Health Scams, Managing Common Health Risks in the Home, Care Options for Chronically or Terminally Ill Patients, and a List of Resources for Obtaining Help and Further Information

Edited by Karen Bellenir. 618 pages. 1998. 0-7808-0221-7. $78.

"Both public and academic libraries will want to have a copy in their collection for readers who are interested in self-education on health issues."
—*American Reference Books Annual*, 2000

"The editor has researched the literature from government agencies and others, saving readers the time and effort of having to do the research themselves. Recommended for public libraries."
— *Reference and User Services Quarterly, American Library Association*, Spring '99

"Recommended reference source."
— *Booklist, American Library Association*, Dec '98

■

Contagious & Non-Contagious Infectious Diseases Sourcebook

Basic Information about Contagious Diseases like Measles, Polio, Hepatitis B, and Infectious Mononucleosis, and Non-Contagious Infectious Diseases like Tetanus and Toxic Shock Syndrome, and Diseases Occurring as Secondary Infections Such as Shingles and Reye Syndrome

Along with Vaccination, Prevention, and Treatment Information, and a Section Describing Emerging Infectious Disease Threats

Edited by Karen Bellenir and Peter D. Dresser. 566 pages. 1996. 0-7808-0075-3. $78.

Death & Dying Sourcebook

Basic Consumer Health Information for the Layperson about End-of-Life Care and Related Ethical and Legal Issues, Including Chief Causes of Death, Autopsies, Pain Management for the Terminally Ill, Life Support Systems, Insurance, Euthanasia, Assisted Suicide, Hospice Programs, Living Wills, Funeral Planning, Counseling, Mourning, Organ Donation, and Physician Training

Along with Statistical Data, a Glossary, and Listings of Sources for Further Help and Information

Edited by Annemarie S. Muth. 641 pages. 1999. 0-7808-0230-6. $78.

"Public libraries, medical libraries, and academic libraries will all find this sourcebook a useful addition to their collections."
— American Reference Books Annual, 2001

"An extremely useful resource for those concerned with death and dying in the United States."
— Respiratory Care, Nov '00

"Recommended reference source."
—Booklist, American Library Association, Aug '00

"This book is a definite must for all those involved in end-of-life care." *— Doody's Review Service, 2000*

■

Diabetes Sourcebook, 1st Edition

Basic Information about Insulin-Dependent and Non-insulin-Dependent Diabetes Mellitus, Gestational Diabetes, and Diabetic Complications, Symptoms, Treatment, and Research Results, Including Statistics on Prevalence, Morbidity, and Mortality

Along with Source Listings for Further Help and Information

Edited by Karen Bellenir and Peter D. Dresser. 827 pages. 1994. 1-55888-751-2. $78.

". . . very informative and understandable for the layperson without being simplistic. It provides a comprehensive overview for laypersons who want a general understanding of the disease or who want to focus on various aspects of the disease."
— Bulletin of the Medical Library Association, Jan '96

■

Diabetes Sourcebook, 2nd Edition

Basic Consumer Health Information about Type 1 Diabetes (Insulin-Dependent or Juvenile-Onset Diabetes), Type 2 (Noninsulin-Dependent or Adult-Onset Diabetes), Gestational Diabetes, and Related Disorders, Including Diabetes Prevalence Data, Management Issues, the Role of Diet and Exercise in Controlling Diabetes, Insulin and Other Diabetes Medicines, and Complications of Diabetes Such as Eye Diseases, Periodontal Disease, Amputation, and End-Stage Renal Disease

Along with Reports on Current Research Initiatives, a Glossary, and Resource Listings for Further Help and Information

Edited by Karen Bellenir. 688 pages. 1998. 0-7808-0224-1. $78.

"An invaluable reference." *—Library Journal, May '00*

Selected as one of the 250 "Best Health Sciences Books of 1999." *—Doody's Rating Service, Mar-Apr 2000*

"This comprehensive book is an excellent addition for high school, academic, medical, and public libraries. This volume is highly recommended."
—American Reference Books Annual, 2000

"Provides useful information for the general public."
— Healthlines, University of Michigan Health Management Research Center, Sep/Oct '99

". . . provides reliable mainstream medical information . . . belongs on the shelves of any library with a consumer health collection." *— E-Streams, Sep '99*

"Recommended reference source."
— Booklist, American Library Association, Feb '99

■

Diet & Nutrition Sourcebook, 1st Edition

Basic Information about Nutrition, Including the Dietary Guidelines for Americans, the Food Guide Pyramid, and Their Applications in Daily Diet, Nutritional Advice for Specific Age Groups, Current Nutritional Issues and Controversies, the New Food Label and How to Use It to Promote Healthy Eating, and Recent Developments in Nutritional Research

Edited by Dan R. Harris. 662 pages. 1996. 0-7808-0084-2. $78.

"Useful reference as a food and nutrition sourcebook for the general consumer." *— Booklist Health Sciences Supplement, American Library Association, Oct '97*

"Recommended for public libraries and medical libraries that receive general information requests on nutrition. It is readable and will appeal to those interested in learning more about healthy dietary practices."
— Medical Reference Services Quarterly, Fall '97

"An abundance of medical and social statistics is translated into readable information geared toward the general reader." *— Bookwatch, Mar '97*

"With dozens of questionable diet books on the market, it is so refreshing to find a reliable and factual reference book. Recommended to aspiring professionals, librarians, and others seeking and giving reliable dietary advice. An excellent compilation." *— Choice, Association of College and Research Libraries, Feb '97*

SEE ALSO *Digestive Diseases & Disorders Sourcebook, Gastrointestinal Diseases & Disorders Sourcebook*

■

Diet & Nutrition Sourcebook, 2nd Edition

Basic Consumer Health Information about Dietary Guidelines, Recommended Daily Intake Values, Vitamins, Minerals, Fiber, Fat, Weight Control, Dietary Supplements, and Food Additives

Along with Special Sections on Nutrition Needs throughout Life and Nutrition for People with Such Spe-

cific *Medical Concerns as Allergies, High Blood Cho-lesterol, Hypertension, Diabetes, Celiac Disease, Seizure Disorders, Phenylketonuria (PKU), Cancer, and Eating Disorders, and Including Reports on Current Nutrition Research and Source Listings for Additional Help and Information*

Edited by Karen Bellenir. 650 pages. 1999. 0-7808-0228-4. $78.

"This book is an excellent source of basic diet and nutrition information." — *Booklist Health Sciences Supplement, American Library Association, Dec '00*

"This reference document should be in any public library, but it would be a very good guide for beginning students in the health sciences. If the other books in this publisher's series are as good as this, they should all be in the health sciences collections."
— *American Reference Books Annual, 2000*

"This book is an excellent general nutrition reference for consumers who desire to take an active role in their health care for prevention. Consumers of all ages who select this book can feel confident they are receiving current and accurate information." — *Journal of Nutrition for the Elderly, Vol. 19, No. 4, '00*

"Recommended reference source."
— *Booklist, American Library Association, Dec '99*

SEE ALSO *Digestive Diseases & Disorders Sourcebook, Gastrointestinal Diseases & Disorders Sourcebook*

∎

Digestive Diseases & Disorders Sourcebook

Basic Consumer Health Information about Diseases and Disorders that Impact the Upper and Lower Digestive System, Including Celiac Disease, Constipation, Crohn's Disease, Cyclic Vomiting Syndrome, Diarrhea, Diverticulosis and Diverticulitis, Gallstones, Heartburn, Hemorrhoids, Hernias, Indigestion (Dyspepsia), Irritable Bowel Syndrome, Lactose Intolerance, Ulcers, and More

Along with Information about Medications and Other Treatments, Tips for Maintaining a Healthy Digestive Tract, a Glossary, and Directory of Digestive Diseases Organizations

Edited by Karen Bellenir. 335 pages. 2000. 0-7808-0327-2. $78.

"This title would be an excellent addition to all public or patient-research libraries."
— *American Reference Books Annual, 2001*

"This title is recommended for public, hospital, and health sciences libraries with consumer health collections." — *E-Streams, Jul-Aug '00*

"Recommended reference source."
— *Booklist, American Library Association, May '00*

SEE ALSO *Diet & Nutrition Sourcebook, 1st and 2nd Editions, Gastrointestinal Diseases & Disorders Sourcebook*

Disabilities Sourcebook

Basic Consumer Health Information about Physical and Psychiatric Disabilities, Including Descriptions of Major Causes of Disability, Assistive and Adaptive Aids, Workplace Issues, and Accessibility Concerns

Along with Information about the Americans with Disabilities Act, a Glossary, and Resources for Additional Help and Information

Edited by Dawn D. Matthews. 616 pages. 2000. 0-7808-0389-2. $78.

"It is a must for libraries with a consumer health section." — *American Reference Books Annual 2002*

"A much needed addition to the Omnigraphics *Health Reference Series*. A current reference work to provide people with disabilities, their families, caregivers or those who work with them, a broad range of information in one volume, has not been available until now. . . . It is recommended for all public and academic library reference collections." — *E-Streams, May '01*

"An excellent source book in easy-to-read format covering many current topics; highly recommended for all libraries." — *Choice, Association of College and Research Libraries, Jan '01*

"Recommended reference source."
— *Booklist, American Library Association, Jul '00*

"An involving, invaluable handbook."
— *The Bookwatch, May '00*

∎

Domestic Violence & Child Abuse Sourcebook

Basic Consumer Health Information about Spousal/ Partner, Child, Sibling, Parent, and Elder Abuse, Covering Physical, Emotional, and Sexual Abuse, Teen Dating Violence, and Stalking; Includes Information about Hotlines, Safe Houses, Safety Plans, and Other Resources for Support and Assistance, Community Initiatives, and Reports on Current Directions in Research and Treatment

Along with a Glossary, Sources for Further Reading, and Governmental and Non-Governmental Organizations Contact Information

Edited by Helene Henderson. 1,064 pages. 2001. 0-7808-0235-7. $78.

"This is important information. The Web has many resources but this sourcebook fills an important societal need. I am not aware of any other resources of this type." — *Doody's Review Service, Sep '01*

"Recommended for all libraries, scholars, and practitioners." — *Choice, Association of College & Research Libraries, Jul '01*

"Recommended reference source."
— *Booklist, American Library Association, Apr '01*

"Important pick for college-level health reference libraries." — *The Bookwatch, Mar '01*

"Because this problem is so widespread and because this book includes a lot of issues within one volume, this work is recommended for all public libraries."
— *American Reference Books Annual, 2001*

Drug Abuse Sourcebook

Basic Consumer Health Information about Illicit Substances of Abuse and the Diversion of Prescription Medications, Including Depressants, Hallucinogens, Inhalants, Marijuana, Narcotics, Stimulants, and Anabolic Steroids

Along with Facts about Related Health Risks, Treatment Issues, and Substance Abuse Prevention Programs, a Glossary of Terms, Statistical Data, and Directories of Hotline Services, Self-Help Groups, and Organizations Able to Provide Further Information

Edited by Karen Bellenir. 629 pages. 2000. 0-7808-0242-X. $78.

"Containing a wealth of information, this book will be useful to the college student just beginning to explore the topic of substance abuse. This resource belongs in libraries that serve a lower-division undergraduate or community college clientele as well as the general public." — *Choice, Association of College and Research Libraries, Jun '01*

"Recommended reference source." — *Booklist, American Library Association, Feb '01*

"Highly recommended." — *The Bookwatch, Jan '01*

"Even though there is a plethora of books on drug abuse, this volume is recommended for school, public, and college libraries." — *American Reference Books Annual, 2001*

SEE ALSO *Alcoholism Sourcebook, Substance Abuse Sourcebook*

Ear, Nose & Throat Disorders Sourcebook

Basic Information about Disorders of the Ears, Nose, Sinus Cavities, Pharynx, and Larynx, Including Ear Infections, Tinnitus, Vestibular Disorders, Allergic and Non-Allergic Rhinitis, Sore Throats, Tonsillitis, and Cancers That Affect the Ears, Nose, Sinuses, and Throat

Along with Reports on Current Research Initiatives, a Glossary of Related Medical Terms, and a Directory of Sources for Further Help and Information

Edited by Karen Bellenir and Linda M. Shin. 576 pages. 1998. 0-7808-0206-3. $78.

"Overall, this sourcebook is helpful for the consumer seeking information on ENT issues. It is recommended for public libraries." — *American Reference Books Annual, 1999*

"Recommended reference source." — *Booklist, American Library Association, Dec '98*

Eating Disorders Sourcebook

Basic Consumer Health Information about Eating Disorders, Including Information about Anorexia Nervosa, Bulimia Nervosa, Binge Eating, Body Dysmorphic Disorder, Pica, Laxative Abuse, and Night Eating Syndrome

Along with Information about Causes, Adverse Effects, and Treatment and Prevention Issues, and Featuring a

Section on Concerns Specific to Children and Adolescents, a Glossary, and Resources for Further Help and Information

Edited by Dawn D. Matthews. 322 pages. 2001. 0-7808-0335-3. $78.

"Recommended for health science libraries that are open to the public, as well as hospital libraries. This book is a good resource for the consumer who is concerned about eating disorders." — *E-Streams, Mar '02*

"This volume is another convenient collection of excerpted articles. Recommended for school and public library patrons; lower-division undergraduates; and two-year technical program students." — *Choice, Association of College & Research Libraries, Jan '02*

"Recommended reference source." — *Booklist, American Library Association, Oct '01*

Endocrine & Metabolic Disorders Sourcebook

Basic Information for the Layperson about Pancreatic and Insulin-Related Disorders Such as Pancreatitis, Diabetes, and Hypoglycemia; Adrenal Gland Disorders Such as Cushing's Syndrome, Addison's Disease, and Congenital Adrenal Hyperplasia; Pituitary Gland Disorders Such as Growth Hormone Deficiency, Acromegaly, and Pituitary Tumors; Thyroid Disorders Such as Hypothyroidism, Graves' Disease, Hashimoto's Disease, and Goiter; Hyperparathyroidism; and Other Diseases and Syndromes of Hormone Imbalance or Metabolic Dysfunction

Along with Reports on Current Research Initiatives

Edited by Linda M. Shin. 574 pages. 1998. 0-7808-0207-1. $78.

"Omnigraphics has produced another needed resource for health information consumers." — *American Reference Books Annual, 2000*

"Recommended reference source." — *Booklist, American Library Association, Dec '98*

Environmentally Induced Disorders Sourcebook

Basic Information about Diseases and Syndromes Linked to Exposure to Pollutants and Other Substances in Outdoor and Indoor Environments Such as Lead, Asbestos, Formaldehyde, Mercury, Emissions, Noise, and More

Edited by Allan R. Cook. 620 pages. 1997. 0-7808-0083-4. $78.

"Recommended reference source." — *Booklist, American Library Association, Sep '98*

"This book will be a useful addition to anyone's library." — *Choice Health Sciences Supplement, Association of College and Research Libraries, May '98*

"... a good survey of numerous environmentally induced physical disorders ... a useful addition to anyone's library."
— *Doody's Health Sciences Book Reviews, Jan '98*

"... provide[s] introductory information from the best authorities around. Since this volume covers topics that potentially affect everyone, it will surely be one of the most frequently consulted volumes in the *Health Reference Series*." — *Rettig on Reference, Nov '97*

∎

Ethnic Diseases Sourcebook

Basic Consumer Health Information for Ethnic and Racial Minority Groups in the United States, Including General Health Indicators and Behaviors, Ethnic Diseases, Genetic Testing, the Impact of Chronic Diseases, Women's Health, Mental Health Issues, and Preventive Health Care Services

Along with a Glossary and a Listing of Additional Resources

Edited by Joyce Brennfleck Shannon. 664 pages. 2001. 0-7808-0336-1. $78.

"Recommended for health sciences libraries where public health programs are a priority."
— *E-Streams, Jan '02*

"Not many books have been written on this topic to date, and the *Ethnic Diseases Sourcebook* is a strong addition to the list. It will be an important introductory resource for health consumers, students, health care personnel, and social scientists. It is recommended for public, academic, and large hospital libraries."
— *American Reference Books Annual 2002*

"Recommended reference source."
— *Booklist, American Library Association, Oct '01*

"Will prove valuable to any library seeking to maintain a current, comprehensive reference collection of health resources.... An excellent source of health information about genetic disorders which affect particular ethnic and racial minorities in the U.S."
— *The Bookwatch, Aug '01*

∎

Family Planning Sourcebook

Basic Consumer Health Information about Planning for Pregnancy and Contraception, Including Traditional Methods, Barrier Methods, Hormonal Methods, Permanent Methods, Future Methods, Emergency Contraception, and Birth Control Choices for Women at Each Stage of Life

Along with Statistics, a Glossary, and Sources of Additional Information

Edited by Amy Marcaccio Keyzer. 520 pages. 2001. 0-7808-0379-5. $78.

"Recommended for public, health, and undergraduate libraries as part of the circulating collection."
— *E-Streams, Mar '02*

"Information is presented in an unbiased, readable manner, and the sourcebook will certainly be a neces-

sary addition to those public and high school libraries where Internet access is restricted or otherwise problematic." — *American Reference Books Annual 2002*

"Recommended reference source."
— *Booklist, American Library Association, Oct '01*

"Will prove valuable to any library seeking to maintain a current, comprehensive reference collection of health resources.... Excellent reference."
— *The Bookwatch, Aug '01*

SEE ALSO Pregnancy & Birth Sourcebook

∎

Fitness & Exercise Sourcebook, 1st Edition

Basic Information on Fitness and Exercise, Including Fitness Activities for Specific Age Groups, Exercise for People with Specific Medical Conditions, How to Begin a Fitness Program in Running, Walking, Swimming, Cycling, and Other Athletic Activities, and Recent Research in Fitness and Exercise

Edited by Dan R. Harris. 663 pages. 1996. 0-7808-0186-5. $78.

"A good resource for general readers." — *Choice, Association of College and Research Libraries, Nov '97*

"The perennial popularity of the topic ... make this an appealing selection for public libraries."
— *Rettig on Reference, Jun/Jul '97*

∎

Fitness & Exercise Sourcebook, 2nd Edition

Basic Consumer Health Information about the Fundamentals of Fitness and Exercise, Including How to Begin and Maintain a Fitness Program, Fitness as a Lifestyle, the Link between Fitness and Diet, Advice for Specific Groups of People, Exercise as It Relates to Specific Medical Conditions, and Recent Research in Fitness and Exercise

Along with a Glossary of Important Terms and Resources for Additional Help and Information

Edited by Kristen M. Gledhill. 646 pages. 2001. 0-7808-0334-5. $78.

"This work is recommended for all general reference collections."
— *American Reference Books Annual 2002*

"Highly recommended for public, consumer, and school grades fourth through college."
— *E-Streams, Nov '01*

"Recommended reference source." — *Booklist, American Library Association, Oct '01*

"The information appears quite comprehensive and is considered reliable.... This second edition is a welcomed addition to the series."
— *Doody's Review Service, Sep '01*

"This reference is a valuable choice for those who desire a broad source of information on exercise, fitness, and chronic-disease prevention through a healthy lifestyle." *—American Medical Writers Association Journal, Fall '01*

"Will prove valuable to any library seeking to maintain a current, comprehensive reference collection of health resources. . . . Excellent reference." *— The Bookwatch, Aug '01*

■

Food & Animal Borne Diseases Sourcebook

Basic Information about Diseases That Can Be Spread to Humans through the Ingestion of Contaminated Food or Water or by Contact with Infected Animals and Insects, Such as Botulism, E. Coli, Hepatitis A, Trichinosis, Lyme Disease, and Rabies

Along with Information Regarding Prevention and Treatment Methods, and Including a Special Section for International Travelers Describing Diseases Such as Cholera, Malaria, Travelers' Diarrhea, and Yellow Fever, and Offering Recommendations for Avoiding Illness

Edited by Karen Bellenir and Peter D. Dresser. 535 pages. 1995. 0-7808-0033-8. $78.

"Targeting general readers and providing them with a single, comprehensive source of information on selected topics, this book continues, with the excellent caliber of its predecessors, to catalog topical information on health matters of general interest. Readable and thorough, this valuable resource is highly recommended for all libraries." *—Academic Library Book Review, Summer '96*

"A comprehensive collection of authoritative information." *— Emergency Medical Services, Oct '95*

■

Food Safety Sourcebook

Basic Consumer Health Information about the Safe Handling of Meat, Poultry, Seafood, Eggs, Fruit Juices, and Other Food Items, and Facts about Pesticides, Drinking Water, Food Safety Overseas, and the Onset, Duration, and Symptoms of Foodborne Illnesses, Including Types of Pathogenic Bacteria, Parasitic Protozoa, Worms, Viruses, and Natural Toxins

Along with the Role of the Consumer, the Food Handler, and the Government in Food Safety; a Glossary, and Resources for Additional Help and Information

Edited by Dawn D. Matthews. 339 pages. 1999. 0-7808-0326-4. $78.

"This book is recommended for public libraries and universities with home economic and food science programs." *— E-Streams, Nov '00*

"Recommended reference source." *—Booklist, American Library Association, May '00*

"This book takes the complex issues of food safety and foodborne pathogens and presents them in a easily understood manner. [It does] an excellent job of covering a large and often confusing topic." *—American Reference Books Annual, 2000*

Forensic Medicine Sourcebook

Basic Consumer Information for the Layperson about Forensic Medicine, Including Crime Scene Investigation, Evidence Collection and Analysis, Expert Testimony, Computer-Aided Criminal Identification, Digital Imaging in the Courtroom, DNA Profiling, Accident Reconstruction, Autopsies, Ballistics, Drugs and Explosives Detection, Latent Fingerprints, Product Tampering, and Questioned Document Examination

Along with Statistical Data, a Glossary of Forensics Terminology, and Listings of Sources for Further Help and Information

Edited by Annemarie S. Muth. 574 pages. 1999. 0-7808-0232-2. $78.

"Given the expected widespread interest in its content and its easy to read style, this book is recommended for most public and all college and university libraries." *— E-Streams, Feb '01*

"Recommended for public libraries." *—Reference & User Services Quarterly, American Library Association, Spring 2000*

"Recommended reference source." *—Booklist, American Library Association, Feb '00*

"A wealth of information, useful statistics, references are up-to-date and extremely complete. This wonderful collection of data will help students who are interested in a career in any type of forensic field. It is a great resource for attorneys who need information about types of expert witnesses needed in a particular case. It also offers useful information for fiction and nonfiction writers whose work involves a crime. A fascinating compilation. All levels." *— Choice, Association of College and Research Libraries, Jan 2000*

"There are several items that make this book attractive to consumers who are seeking certain forensic data. . . . This is a useful current source for those seeking general forensic medical answers." *—American Reference Books Annual, 2000*

■

Gastrointestinal Diseases & Disorders Sourcebook

Basic Information about Gastroesophageal Reflux Disease (Heartburn), Ulcers, Diverticulosis, Irritable Bowel Syndrome, Crohn's Disease, Ulcerative Colitis, Diarrhea, Constipation, Lactose Intolerance, Hemorrhoids, Hepatitis, Cirrhosis, and Other Digestive Problems, Featuring Statistics, Descriptions of Symptoms, and Current Treatment Methods of Interest for Persons Living with Upper and Lower Gastrointestinal Maladies

Edited by Linda M. Ross. 413 pages. 1996. 0-7808-0078-8. $78.

". . . very readable form. The successful editorial work that brought this material together into a useful and understandable reference makes accessible to all readers information that can help them more effectively understand and obtain help for digestive tract problems." *— Choice, Association of College & Research Libraries, Feb '97*

SEE ALSO *Diet & Nutrition Sourcebook, 1st and 2nd Editions, Digestive Diseases & Disorders*

Genetic Disorders Sourcebook, 1st Edition

Basic Information about Heritable Diseases and Disorders Such as Down Syndrome, PKU, Hemophilia, Von Willebrand Disease, Gaucher Disease, Tay-Sachs Disease, and Sickle-Cell Disease, Along with Information about Genetic Screening, Gene Therapy, Home Care, and Including Source Listings for Further Help and Information on More Than 300 Disorders

Edited by Karen Bellenir. 642 pages. 1996. 0-7808-0034-6. $78.

"Recommended for undergraduate libraries or libraries that serve the public."
—Science & Technology Libraries, Vol. 18, No. 1, '99

"Provides essential medical information to both the general public and those diagnosed with a serious or fatal genetic disease or disorder." —Choice, Association of College and Research Libraries, Jan '97

"Geared toward the lay public. It would be well placed in all public libraries and in those hospital and medical libraries in which access to genetic references is limited." —Doody's Health Sciences Book Review, Oct '96

∎

Genetic Disorders Sourcebook, 2nd Edition

Basic Consumer Health Information about Hereditary Diseases and Disorders, Including Cystic Fibrosis, Down Syndrome, Hemophilia, Huntington's Disease, Sickle Cell Anemia, and More; Facts about Genes, Gene Research and Therapy, Genetic Screening, Ethics of Gene Testing, Genetic Counseling, and Advice on Coping and Caring

Along with a Glossary of Genetic Terminology and a Resource List for Help, Support, and Further Information

Edited by Kathy Massimini. 768 pages. 2001. 0-7808-0241-1. $78.

"Recommended for public libraries and medical and hospital libraries with consumer health collections."
—E-Streams, May '01

"Recommended reference source."
—Booklist, American Library Association, Apr '01

"Important pick for college-level health reference libraries." —The Bookwatch, Mar '01

∎

Head Trauma Sourcebook

Basic Information for the Layperson about Open-Head and Closed-Head Injuries, Treatment Advances, Recovery, and Rehabilitation

Along with Reports on Current Research Initiatives

Edited by Karen Bellenir. 414 pages. 1997. 0-7808-0208-X. $78.

Headache Sourcebook

Basic Consumer Health Information about Migraine, Tension, Cluster, Rebound and Other Types of Headaches, with Facts about the Cause and Prevention of Headaches, the Effects of Stress and the Environment, Headaches during Pregnancy and Menopause, and Childhood Headaches

Along with a Glossary and Other Resources for Additional Help and Information

Edited by Dawn D. Matthews. 362 pages. 2002. 0-7808-0337-X. $78.

∎

Health Insurance Sourcebook

Basic Information about Managed Care Organizations, Traditional Fee-for-Service Insurance, Insurance Portability and Pre-Existing Conditions Clauses, Medicare, Medicaid, Social Security, and Military Health Care

Along with Information about Insurance Fraud

Edited by Wendy Wilcox. 530 pages. 1997. 0-7808-0222-5. $78.

"Particularly useful because it brings much of this information together in one volume. This book will be a handy reference source in the health sciences library, hospital library, college and university library, and medium to large public library."
—Medical Reference Services Quarterly, Fall '98

Awarded "Books of the Year Award"
—American Journal of Nursing, 1997

"The layout of the book is particularly helpful as it provides easy access to reference material. A most useful addition to the vast amount of information about health insurance. The use of data from U.S. government agencies is most commendable. Useful in a library or learning center for healthcare professional students."
—Doody's Health Sciences Book Reviews, Nov '97

∎

Health Reference Series Cumulative Index 1999

A Comprehensive Index to the Individual Volumes of the Health Reference Series, Including a Subject Index, Name Index, Organization Index, and Publication Index

Along with a Master List of Acronyms and Abbreviations

Edited by Edward J. Prucha, Anne Holmes, and Robert Rudnick. 990 pages. 2000. 0-7808-0382-5. $78.

"This volume will be most helpful in libraries that have a relatively complete collection of the Health Reference Series." —American Reference Books Annual, 2001

"Essential for collections that hold any of the numerous Health Reference Series titles."
—Choice, Association of College and Research Libraries, Nov '00

Healthy Aging Sourcebook

Basic Consumer Health Information about Maintaining Health through the Aging Process, Including Advice on Nutrition, Exercise, and Sleep, Help in Making Decisions about Midlife Issues and Retirement, Guidance Concerning Practical and Informed Choices in Health Consumerism

Along with Data Concerning the Theories of Aging, Different Experiences in Aging by Minority Groups, and Facts about Aging Now and Aging in the Future; and Featuring a Glossary, a Guide to Consumer Help, Additional Suggested Reading, and Practical Resource Directory

Edited by Jenifer Swanson. 536 pages. 1999. 0-7808-0390-6. $78.

"Recommended reference source."
—Booklist, American Library Association, Feb '00

SEE ALSO Physical & Mental Issues in Aging Sourcebook

■

Healthy Heart Sourcebook for Women

Basic Consumer Health Information about Cardiac Issues Specific to Women, Including Facts about Major Risk Factors and Prevention, Treatment and Control Strategies, and Important Dietary Issues

Along with a Special Section Regarding the Pros and Cons of Hormone Replacement Therapy and Its Impact on Heart Health, and Additional Help, Including Recipes, a Glossary, and a Directory of Resources

Edited by Dawn D. Matthews. 336 pages. 2000. 0-7808-0329-9. $78.

"A good reference source and recommended for all public, academic, medical, and hospital libraries."
—Medical Reference Services Quarterly, Summer '01

"Because of the lack of information specific to women on this topic, this book is recommended for public libraries and consumer libraries."
—American Reference Books Annual, 2001

"Contains very important information about coronary artery disease that all women should know. The information is current and presented in an easy-to-read format. The book will make a good addition to any library."
—American Medical Writers Association Journal, Summer '00

"Important, basic reference."
—Reviewer's Bookwatch, Jul '00

SEE ALSO Cardiovascular Diseases & Disorders Sourcebook, 1st Edition, Heart Diseases & Disorders Sourcebook, 2nd Edition, Women's Health Concerns Sourcebook

■

Heart Diseases & Disorders Sourcebook, 2nd Edition

Basic Consumer Health Information about Heart Attacks, Angina, Rhythm Disorders, Heart Failure,

Valve Disease, Congenital Heart Disorders, and More, Including Descriptions of Surgical Procedures and Other Interventions, Medications, Cardiac Rehabilitation, Risk Identification, and Prevention Tips

Along with Statistical Data, Reports on Current Research Initiatives, a Glossary of Cardiovascular Terms, and Resource Directory

Edited by Karen Bellenir. 612 pages. 2000. 0-7808-0238-1. $78.

"This work stands out as an imminently accessible resource for the general public. It is recommended for the reference and circulating shelves of school, public, and academic libraries."
—American Reference Books Annual, 2001

"Recommended reference source."
—Booklist, American Library Association, Dec '00

"Provides comprehensive coverage of matters related to the heart. This title is recommended for health sciences and public libraries with consumer health collections."
—E-Streams, Oct '00

SEE ALSO Cardiovascular Diseases & Disorders Sourcebook, 1st Edition; Healthy Heart Sourcebook for Women

■

Household Safety Sourcebook

Basic Consumer Health Information about Household Safety, Including Information about Poisons, Chemicals, Fire, and Water Hazards in the Home

Along with Advice about the Safe Use of Home Maintenance Equipment, Choosing Toys and Nursery Furniture, Holiday and Recreation Safety, a Glossary, and Resources for Further Help and Information

Edited by Dawn D. Matthews. 606 pages. 2002. 0-7808-0338-8. $78.

■

Immune System Disorders Sourcebook

Basic Information about Lupus, Multiple Sclerosis, Guillain-Barré Syndrome, Chronic Granulomatous Disease, and More

Along with Statistical and Demographic Data and Reports on Current Research Initiatives

Edited by Allan R. Cook. 608 pages. 1997. 0-7808-0209-8. $78.

■

Infant & Toddler Health Sourcebook

Basic Consumer Health Information about the Physical and Mental Development of Newborns, Infants, and Toddlers, Including Neonatal Concerns, Nutrition Recommendations, Immunization Schedules, Common Pediatric Disorders, Assessments and Milestones, Safety Tips, and Advice for Parents and Other Caregivers

Along with a Glossary of Terms and Resource Listings for Additional Help

Edited by Jenifer Swanson. 585 pages. 2000. 0-7808-0246-2. $78.

"As a reference for the general public, this would be useful in any library." — *E-Streams, May '01*

"Recommended reference source."
— *Booklist, American Library Association, Feb '01*

"This is a good source for general use."
— *American Reference Books Annual, 2001*

■

Injury & Trauma Sourcebook

Basic Consumer Health Information about the Impact of Injury, the Diagnosis and Treatment of Common and Traumatic Injuries, Emergency Care, and Specific Injuries Related to Home, Community, Workplace, Transportation, and Recreation

Along with Guidelines for Injury Prevention, a Glossary, and a Directory of Additional Resources

Edited by Joyce Brennfleck Shannon. 696 pages. 2002. 0-7808-0421-X. $78.

■

Kidney & Urinary Tract Diseases & Disorders Sourcebook

Basic Information about Kidney Stones, Urinary Incontinence, Bladder Disease, End Stage Renal Disease, Dialysis, and More

Along with Statistical and Demographic Data and Reports on Current Research Initiatives

Edited by Linda M. Ross. 602 pages. 1997. 0-7808-0079-6. $78.

■

Learning Disabilities Sourcebook

Basic Information about Disorders Such as Dyslexia, Visual and Auditory Processing Deficits, Attention Deficit/Hyperactivity Disorder, and Autism

Along with Statistical and Demographic Data, Reports on Current Research Initiatives, an Explanation of the Assessment Process, and a Special Section for Adults with Learning Disabilities

Edited by Linda M. Shin. 579 pages. 1998. 0-7808-0210-1. $78.

Named "Outstanding Reference Book of 1999."
— *New York Public Library, Feb 2000*

"An excellent candidate for inclusion in a public library reference section. It's a great source of information. Teachers will also find the book useful. Definitely worth reading."
— *Journal of Adolescent & Adult Literacy, Feb 2000*

"Readable . . . provides a solid base of information regarding successful techniques used with individuals who have learning disabilities, as well as practical suggestions for educators and family members. Clear language, concise descriptions, and pertinent information

for contacting multiple resources add to the strength of this book as a useful tool." — *Choice, Association of College and Research Libraries, Feb '99*

"Recommended reference source."
— *Booklist, American Library Association, Sep '98*

"A useful resource for libraries and for those who don't have the time to identify and locate the individual publications." — *Disability Resources Monthly, Sep '98*

■

Liver Disorders Sourcebook

Basic Consumer Health Information about the Liver and How It Works; Liver Diseases, Including Cancer, Cirrhosis, Hepatitis, and Toxic and Drug Related Diseases; Tips for Maintaining a Healthy Liver; Laboratory Tests, Radiology Tests, and Facts about Liver Transplantation

Along with a Section on Support Groups, a Glossary, and Resource Listings

Edited by Joyce Brennfleck Shannon. 591 pages. 2000. 0-7808-0383-3. $78.

"A valuable resource."
— *American Reference Books Annual, 2001*

"This title is recommended for health sciences and public libraries with consumer health collections."
— *E-Streams, Oct '00*

"Recommended reference source."
— *Booklist, American Library Association, Jun '00*

■

Lung Disorders Sourcebook

Basic Consumer Health Information about Emphysema, Pneumonia, Tuberculosis, Asthma, Cystic Fibrosis, and Other Lung Disorders, Including Facts about Diagnostic Procedures, Treatment Strategies, Disease Prevention Efforts, and Such Risk Factors as Smoking, Air Pollution, and Exposure to Asbestos, Radon, and Other Agents

Along with a Glossary and Resources for Additional Help and Information

Edited by Dawn D. Matthews. 678 pages. 2002. 0-7808-0339-6. $78.

■

Medical Tests Sourcebook

Basic Consumer Health Information about Medical Tests, Including Periodic Health Exams, General Screening Tests, Tests You Can Do at Home, Findings of the U.S. Preventive Services Task Force, X-ray and Radiology Tests, Electrical Tests, Tests of Blood and Other Body Fluids and Tissues, Scope Tests, Lung Tests, Genetic Tests, Pregnancy Tests, Newborn Screening Tests, Sexually Transmitted Disease Tests, and Computer Aided Diagnoses

Along with a Section on Paying for Medical Tests, a Glossary, and Resource Listings

Edited by Joyce Brennfleck Shannon. 691 pages. 1999. 0-7808-0243-8. $78.

"Recommended for hospital and health sciences libraries with consumer health collections."
— *E-Streams, Mar '00*

"This is an overall excellent reference with a wealth of general knowledge that may aid those who are reluctant to get vital tests performed."
— *Today's Librarian, Jan 2000*

"A valuable reference guide."
— *American Reference Books Annual, 2000*

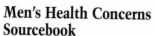

Men's Health Concerns Sourcebook

Basic Information about Health Issues That Affect Men, Featuring Facts about the Top Causes of Death in Men, Including Heart Disease, Stroke, Cancers, Prostate Disorders, Chronic Obstructive Pulmonary Disease, Pneumonia and Influenza, Human Immunodeficiency Virus and Acquired Immune Deficiency Syndrome, Diabetes Mellitus, Stress, Suicide, Accidents and Homicides; and Facts about Common Concerns for Men, Including Impotence, Contraception, Circumcision, Sleep Disorders, Snoring, Hair Loss, Diet, Nutrition, Exercise, Kidney and Urological Disorders, and Backaches

Edited by Allan R. Cook. 738 pages. 1998. 0-7808-0212-8. $78.

"This comprehensive resource and the series are highly recommended."
— *American Reference Books Annual, 2000*

"Recommended reference source."
— *Booklist, American Library Association, Dec '98*

◼

Mental Health Disorders Sourcebook, 1st Edition

Basic Information about Schizophrenia, Depression, Bipolar Disorder, Panic Disorder, Obsessive-Compulsive Disorder, Phobias and Other Anxiety Disorders, Paranoia and Other Personality Disorders, Eating Disorders, and Sleep Disorders

Along with Information about Treatment and Therapies

Edited by Karen Bellenir. 548 pages. 1995. 0-7808-0040-0. $78.

"This is an excellent new book . . . written in easy-to-understand language."
— *Booklist Health Sciences Supplement, American Library Association, Oct '97*

". . . useful for public and academic libraries and consumer health collections."
— *Medical Reference Services Quarterly, Spring '97*

"The great strengths of the book are its readability and its inclusion of places to find more information. Especially recommended."
— *Reference Quarterly, American Library Association, Winter '96*

". . . a good resource for a consumer health library."
— *Bulletin of the Medical Library Association, Oct '96*

"The information is data-based and couched in brief, concise language that avoids jargon. . . . a useful reference source."
— *Readings, Sep '96*

"The text is well organized and adequately written for its target audience."
— *Choice, Association of College and Research Libraries, Jun '96*

". . . provides information on a wide range of mental disorders, presented in nontechnical language."
— *Exceptional Child Education Resources, Spring '96*

"Recommended for public and academic libraries."
— *Reference Book Review, 1996*

◼

Mental Health Disorders Sourcebook, 2nd Edition

Basic Consumer Health Information about Anxiety Disorders, Depression and Other Mood Disorders, Eating Disorders, Personality Disorders, Schizophrenia, and More, Including Disease Descriptions, Treatment Options, and Reports on Current Research Initiatives

Along with Statistical Data, Tips for Maintaining Mental Health, a Glossary, and Directory of Sources for Additional Help and Information

Edited by Karen Bellenir. 605 pages. 2000. 0-7808-0240-3. $78.

"Well organized and well written."
— *American Reference Books Annual, 2001*

"Recommended reference source."
— *Booklist, American Library Association, Jun '00*

◼

Mental Retardation Sourcebook

Basic Consumer Health Information about Mental Retardation and Its Causes, Including Down Syndrome, Fetal Alcohol Syndrome, Fragile X Syndrome, Genetic Conditions, Injury, and Environmental Sources

Along with Preventive Strategies, Parenting Issues, Educational Implications, Health Care Needs, Employment and Economic Matters, Legal Issues, a Glossary, and a Resource Listing for Additional Help and Information

Edited by Joyce Brennfleck Shannon. 642 pages. 2000. 0-7808-0377-9. $78.

"Public libraries will find the book useful for reference and as a beginning research point for students, parents, and caregivers."
— *American Reference Books Annual, 2001*

"The strength of this work is that it compiles many basic fact sheets and addresses for further information in one volume. It is intended and suitable for the general public. This sourcebook is relevant to any collection providing health information to the general public."
— *E-Streams, Nov '00*

"From preventing retardation to parenting and family challenges, this covers health, social and legal issues and will prove an invaluable overview."
— *Reviewer's Bookwatch, Jul '00*

Obesity Sourcebook

Basic Consumer Health Information about Diseases and Other Problems Associated with Obesity, and Including Facts about Risk Factors, Prevention Issues, and Management Approaches

Along with Statistical and Demographic Data, Information about Special Populations, Research Updates, a Glossary, and Source Listings for Further Help and Information

Edited by Wilma Caldwell and Chad T. Kimball. 376 pages. 2001. 0-7808-0333-7. $78.

"The book synthesizes the reliable medical literature on obesity into one easy-to-read and useful resource for the general public."
— *American Reference Books Annual 2002*

"This is a very useful resource book for the lay public."
— *Doody's Review Service, Nov '01*

"Well suited for the health reference collection of a public library or an academic health science library that serves the general population." — *E-Streams, Sep '01*

"Recommended reference source."
— *Booklist, American Library Association, Apr '01*

" Recommended pick both for specialty health library collections and any general consumer health reference collection." — *The Bookwatch, Apr '01*

Ophthalmic Disorders Sourcebook

Basic Information about Glaucoma, Cataracts, Macular Degeneration, Strabismus, Refractive Disorders, and More

Along with Statistical and Demographic Data and Reports on Current Research Initiatives

Edited by Linda M. Ross. 631 pages. 1996. 0-7808-0081-8. $78.

Oral Health Sourcebook

Basic Information about Diseases and Conditions Affecting Oral Health, Including Cavities, Gum Disease, Dry Mouth, Oral Cancers, Fever Blisters, Canker Sores, Oral Thrush, Bad Breath, Temporomandibular Disorders, and other Craniofacial Syndromes

Along with Statistical Data on the Oral Health of Americans, Oral Hygiene, Emergency First Aid, Information on Treatment Procedures and Methods of Replacing Lost Teeth

Edited by Allan R. Cook. 558 pages. 1997. 0-7808-0082-6. $78.

"Unique source which will fill a gap in dental sources for patients and the lay public. A valuable reference tool even in a library with thousands of books on dentistry. Comprehensive, clear, inexpensive, and easy to read and use. It fills an enormous gap in the health care literature." — *Reference and User Services Quarterly, American Library Association, Summer '98*

"Recommended reference source."
— *Booklist, American Library Association, Dec '97*

Osteoporosis Sourcebook

Basic Consumer Health Information about Primary and Secondary Osteoporosis and Juvenile Osteoporosis and Related Conditions, Including Fibrous Dysplasia, Gaucher Disease, Hyperthyroidism, Hypophosphatasia, Myeloma, Osteopetrosis, Osteogenesis Imperfecta, and Paget's Disease

Along with Information about Risk Factors, Treatments, Traditional and Non-Traditional Pain Management, a Glossary of Related Terms, and a Directory of Resources

Edited by Allan R. Cook. 584 pages. 2001. 0-7808-0239-X. $78.

"This would be a book to be kept in a staff or patient library. The targeted audience is the layperson, but the therapist who needs a quick bit of information on a particular topic will also find the book useful."
— *Physical Therapy, Jan '02*

"This resource is recommended as a great reference source for public, health, and academic libraries, and is another triumph for the editors of Omnigraphics."
— *American Reference Books Annual 2002*

"Recommended for all public libraries and general health collections, especially those supporting patient education or consumer health programs."
— *E-Streams, Nov '01*

"Will prove valuable to any library seeking to maintain a current, comprehensive reference collection of health resources. . . . From prevention to treatment and associated conditions, this provides an excellent survey."
— *The Bookwatch, Aug '01*

"Recommended reference source."
— *Booklist, American Library Association, July '01*

SEE ALSO *Women's Health Concerns Sourcebook*

Pain Sourcebook, 1st Edition

Basic Information about Specific Forms of Acute and Chronic Pain, Including Headaches, Back Pain, Muscular Pain, Neuralgia, Surgical Pain, and Cancer Pain

Along with Pain Relief Options Such as Analgesics, Narcotics, Nerve Blocks, Transcutaneous Nerve Stimulation, and Alternative Forms of Pain Control, Including Biofeedback, Imaging, Behavior Modification, and Relaxation Techniques

Edited by Allan R. Cook. 667 pages. 1997. 0-7808-0213-6. $78.

"The text is readable, easily understood, and well indexed. This excellent volume belongs in all patient education libraries, consumer health sections of public libraries, and many personal collections."
— *American Reference Books Annual, 1999*

"A beneficial reference." — *Booklist Health Sciences Supplement, American Library Association, Oct '98*

"The information is basic in terms of scholarship and is appropriate for general readers. Written in journalistic style . . . intended for non-professionals. Quite thorough

612

in its coverage of different pain conditions and summarizes the latest clinical information regarding pain treatment." — *Choice, Association of College and Research Libraries, Jun '98*

"Recommended reference source."
— *Booklist, American Library Association, Mar '98*

■

Pain Sourcebook, 2nd Edition

Basic Consumer Health Information about Specific Forms of Acute and Chronic Pain, Including Muscle and Skeletal Pain, Nerve Pain, Cancer Pain, and Disorders Characterized by Pain, Such as Fibromyalgia, Shingles, Angina, Arthritis, and Headaches

Along with Information about Pain Medications and Management Techniques, Complementary and Alternative Pain Relief Options, Tips for People Living with Chronic Pain, a Glossary, and a Directory of Sources for Further Information

Edited by Karen Bellenir. 670 pages. 2002. 0-7808-0612-3. $78.

■

Pediatric Cancer Sourcebook

Basic Consumer Health Information about Leukemias, Brain Tumors, Sarcomas, Lymphomas, and Other Cancers in Infants, Children, and Adolescents, Including Descriptions of Cancers, Treatments, and Coping Strategies

Along with Suggestions for Parents, Caregivers, and Concerned Relatives, a Glossary of Cancer Terms, and Resource Listings

Edited by Edward J. Prucha. 587 pages. 1999. 0-7808-0245-4. $78.

"An excellent source of information. Recommended for public, hospital, and health science libraries with consumer health collections." — *E-Streams, Jun '00*

"Recommended reference source."
— *Booklist, American Library Association, Feb '00*

"A valuable addition to all libraries specializing in health services and many public libraries."
—*American Reference Books Annual, 2000*

■

Physical & Mental Issues in Aging Sourcebook

Basic Consumer Health Information on Physical and Mental Disorders Associated with the Aging Process, Including Concerns about Cardiovascular Disease, Pulmonary Disease, Oral Health, Digestive Disorders, Musculoskeletal and Skin Disorders, Metabolic Changes, Sexual and Reproductive Issues, and Changes in Vision, Hearing, and Other Senses

Along with Data about Longevity and Causes of Death, Information on Acute and Chronic Pain, Descriptions of Mental Concerns, a Glossary of Terms, and Resource Listings for Additional Help

Edited by Jenifer Swanson. 660 pages. 1999. 0-7808-0233-0. $78.

"This is a treasure of health information for the layperson." — *Choice Health Sciences Supplement, Association of College & Research Libraries, May 2000*

"Recommended for public libraries."
—*American Reference Books Annual, 2000*

"Recommended reference source."
— *Booklist, American Library Association, Oct '99*

SEE ALSO *Healthy Aging Sourcebook*

■

Podiatry Sourcebook

Basic Consumer Health Information about Foot Conditions, Diseases, and Injuries, Including Bunions, Corns, Calluses, Athlete's Foot, Plantar Warts, Hammertoes and Clawtoes, Clubfoot, Heel Pain, Gout, and More

Along with Facts about Foot Care, Disease Prevention, Foot Safety, Choosing a Foot Care Specialist, a Glossary of Terms, and Resource Listings for Additional Information

Edited by M. Lisa Weatherford. 380 pages. 2001. 0-7808-0215-2. $78.

"Recommended reference source."
— *Booklist, American Library Association, Feb '02*

"There is a lot of information presented here on a topic that is usually only covered sparingly in most larger comprehensive medical encyclopedias."
— *American Reference Books Annual 2002*

■

Pregnancy & Birth Sourcebook

Basic Information about Planning for Pregnancy, Maternal Health, Fetal Growth and Development, Labor and Delivery, Postpartum and Perinatal Care, Pregnancy in Mothers with Special Concerns, and Disorders of Pregnancy, Including Genetic Counseling, Nutrition and Exercise, Obstetrical Tests, Pregnancy Discomfort, Multiple Births, Cesarean Sections, Medical Testing of Newborns, Breastfeeding, Gestational Diabetes, and Ectopic Pregnancy

Edited by Heather E. Aldred. 737 pages. 1997. 0-7808-0216-0. $78.

"A well-organized handbook. Recommended."
— *Choice, Association of College and Research Libraries, Apr '98*

"Recommended reference source."
— *Booklist, American Library Association, Mar '98*

"Recommended for public libraries."
—*American Reference Books Annual, 1998*

SEE ALSO *Congenital Disorders Sourcebook, Family Planning Sourcebook*

613

Prostate Cancer Sourcebook

Basic Consumer Health Information about Prostate Cancer, Including Information about the Associated Risk Factors, Detection, Diagnosis, and Treatment of Prostate Cancer

Along with Information on Non-Malignant Prostate Conditions, and Featuring a Section Listing Support and Treatment Centers and a Glossary of Related Terms

Edited by Dawn D. Matthews. 358 pages. 2001. 0-7808-0324-8. $78.

"Recommended reference source."
—*Booklist, American Library Association, Jan '02*

"A valuable resource for health care consumers seeking information on the subject....All text is written in a clear, easy-to-understand language that avoids technical jargon. Any library that collects consumer health resources would strengthen their collection with the addition of the *Prostate Cancer Sourcebook*."
— *American Reference Books Annual 2002*

∎

Public Health Sourcebook

Basic Information about Government Health Agencies, Including National Health Statistics and Trends, Healthy People 2000 Program Goals and Objectives, the Centers for Disease Control and Prevention, the Food and Drug Administration, and the National Institutes of Health

Along with Full Contact Information for Each Agency

Edited by Wendy Wilcox. 698 pages. 1998. 0-7808-0220-9. $78.

"Recommended reference source."
— *Booklist, American Library Association, Sep '98*

"This consumer guide provides welcome assistance in navigating the maze of federal health agencies and their data on public health concerns."
— *SciTech Book News, Sep '98*

∎

Reconstructive & Cosmetic Surgery Sourcebook

Basic Consumer Health Information on Cosmetic and Reconstructive Plastic Surgery, Including Statistical Information about Different Surgical Procedures, Things to Consider Prior to Surgery, Plastic Surgery Techniques and Tools, Emotional and Psychological Considerations, and Procedure-Specific Information

Along with a Glossary of Terms and a Listing of Resources for Additional Help and Information

Edited by M. Lisa Weatherford. 374 pages. 2001. 0-7808-0214-4. $78.

"An excellent reference that addresses cosmetic and medically necessary reconstructive surgeries. . . . The style of the prose is calm and reassuring, discussing the many positive outcomes now available due to advances in surgical techniques."
— *American Reference Books Annual 2002*

"Recommended for health science libraries that are open to the public, as well as hospital libraries that are open to the patients. This book is a good resource for the consumer interested in plastic surgery."
—*E-Streams, Dec '01*

"Recommended reference source."
—*Booklist, American Library Association, July '01*

∎

Rehabilitation Sourcebook

Basic Consumer Health Information about Rehabilitation for People Recovering from Heart Surgery, Spinal Cord Injury, Stroke, Orthopedic Impairments, Amputation, Pulmonary Impairments, Traumatic Injury, and More, Including Physical Therapy, Occupational Therapy, Speech/ Language Therapy, Massage Therapy, Dance Therapy, Art Therapy, and Recreational Therapy

Along with Information on Assistive and Adaptive Devices, a Glossary, and Resources for Additional Help and Information

Edited by Dawn D. Matthews. 531 pages. 1999. 0-7808-0236-5. $78.

"This is an excellent resource for public library reference and health collections."
—*American Reference Books Annual, 2001*

"Recommended reference source."
— *Booklist, American Library Association, May '00*

∎

Respiratory Diseases & Disorders Sourcebook

Basic Information about Respiratory Diseases and Disorders, Including Asthma, Cystic Fibrosis, Pneumonia, the Common Cold, Influenza, and Others, Featuring Facts about the Respiratory System, Statistical and Demographic Data, Treatments, Self-Help Management Suggestions, and Current Research Initiatives

Edited by Allan R. Cook and Peter D. Dresser. 771 pages. 1995. 0-7808-0037-0. $78.

"Designed for the layperson and for patients and their families coping with respiratory illness. . . . an extensive array of information on diagnosis, treatment, management, and prevention of respiratory illnesses for the general reader." — *Choice, Association of College and Research Libraries, Jun '96*

"A highly recommended text for all collections. It is a comforting reminder of the power of knowledge that good books carry between their covers."
— *Academic Library Book Review, Spring '96*

"A comprehensive collection of authoritative information presented in a nontechnical, humanitarian style for patients, families, and caregivers."
— *Association of Operating Room Nurses, Sep/Oct '95*

Sexually Transmitted Diseases Sourcebook, 1st Edition

Basic Information about Herpes, Chlamydia, Gonorrhea, Hepatitis, Nongonoccocal Urethritis, Pelvic Inflammatory Disease, Syphilis, AIDS, and More

Along with Current Data on Treatments and Preventions

Edited by Linda M. Ross. 550 pages. 1997. 0-7808-0217-9. $78.

■

Sexually Transmitted Diseases Sourcebook, 2nd Edition

Basic Consumer Health Information about Sexually Transmitted Diseases, Including Information on the Diagnosis and Treatment of Chlamydia, Gonorrhea, Hepatitis, Herpes, HIV, Mononucleosis, Syphilis, and Others

Along with Information on Prevention, Such as Condom Use, Vaccines, and STD Education; And Featuring a Section on Issues Related to Youth and Adolescents, a Glossary, and Resources for Additional Help and Information

Edited by Dawn D. Matthews. 538 pages. 2001. 0-7808-0249-7. $78.

"Recommended for consumer health collections in public libraries, and secondary school and community college libraries."
— American Reference Books Annual 2002

"Every school and public library should have a copy of this comprehensive and user-friendly reference book."
— Choice, Association of College & Research Libraries, Sep '01

"This is a highly recommended book. This is an especially important book for all school and public libraries." — AIDS Book Review Journal, Jul-Aug '01

"Recommended reference source."
— Booklist, American Library Association, Apr '01

"Recommended pick both for specialty health library collections and any general consumer health reference collection." — The Bookwatch, Apr '01

■

Skin Disorders Sourcebook

Basic Information about Common Skin and Scalp Conditions Caused by Aging, Allergies, Immune Reactions, Sun Exposure, Infectious Organisms, Parasites, Cosmetics, and Skin Traumas, Including Abrasions, Cuts, and Pressure Sores

Along with Information on Prevention and Treatment

Edited by Allan R. Cook. 647 pages. 1997. 0-7808-0080-X. $78.

". . . comprehensive, easily read reference book."
— Doody's Health Sciences Book Reviews, Oct '97

SEE ALSO Burns Sourcebook

Sleep Disorders Sourcebook

Basic Consumer Health Information about Sleep and Its Disorders, Including Insomnia, Sleepwalking, Sleep Apnea, Restless Leg Syndrome, and Narcolepsy

Along with Data about Shiftwork and Its Effects, Information on the Societal Costs of Sleep Deprivation, Descriptions of Treatment Options, a Glossary of Terms, and Resource Listings for Additional Help

Edited by Jenifer Swanson. 439 pages. 1998. 0-7808-0234-9. $78.

"This text will complement any home or medical library. It is user-friendly and ideal for the adult reader."
— American Reference Books Annual, 2000

"A useful resource that provides accurate, relevant, and accessible information on sleep to the general public. Health care providers who deal with sleep disorders patients may also find it helpful in being prepared to answer some of the questions patients ask."
— Respiratory Care, Jul '99

"Recommended reference source."
— Booklist, American Library Association, Feb '99

■

Sports Injuries Sourcebook

Basic Consumer Health Information about Common Sports Injuries, Prevention of Injury in Specific Sports, Tips for Training, and Rehabilitation from Injury

Along with Information about Special Concerns for Children, Young Girls in Athletic Training Programs, Senior Athletes, and Women Athletes, and a Directory of Resources for Further Help and Information

Edited by Heather E. Aldred. 624 pages. 1999. 0-7808-0218-7. $78.

"While this easy-to-read book is recommended for all libraries, it should prove to be especially useful for public, high school, and academic libraries; certainly it should be on the bookshelf of every school gymnasium." — E-Streams, Mar '00

"Public libraries and undergraduate academic libraries will find this book useful for its nontechnical language." — American Reference Books Annual, 2000

■

Stress-Related Disorders Sourcebook

Basic Consumer Health Information about Stress and Stress-Related Disorders, Including Stress Origins and Signals, Environmental Stress at Work and Home, Mental and Emotional Stress Associated with Depression, Post-Traumatic Stress Disorder, Panic Disorder, Suicide, and the Physical Effects of Stress on the Cardiovascular, Immune, and Nervous Systems

Along with Stress Management Techniques, a Glossary, and a Listing of Additional Resources

Edited by Joyce Brennfleck Shannon. 600 pages. 2002. 0-7808-0560-7. $78.

Substance Abuse Sourcebook

Basic Health-Related Information about the Abuse of Legal and Illegal Substances Such as Alcohol, Tobacco, Prescription Drugs, Marijuana, Cocaine, and Heroin; and Including Facts about Substance Abuse Prevention Strategies, Intervention Methods, Treatment and Recovery Programs, and a Section Addressing the Special Problems Related to Substance Abuse during Pregnancy

Edited by Karen Bellenir. 573 pages. 1996. 0-7808-0038-9. $78.

"A valuable addition to any health reference section. Highly recommended."
— *The Book Report, Mar/Apr '97*

". . . a comprehensive collection of substance abuse information that's both highly readable and compact. Families and caregivers of substance abusers will find the information enlightening and helpful, while teachers, social workers and journalists should benefit from the concise format. Recommended."
— *Drug Abuse Update, Winter '96/'97*

SEE ALSO Alcoholism Sourcebook, Drug Abuse Sourcebook

■

Transplantation Sourcebook

Basic Consumer Health Information about Organ and Tissue Transplantation, Including Physical and Financial Preparations, Procedures and Issues Relating to Specific Solid Organ and Tissue Transplants, Rehabilitation, Pediatric Transplant Information, the Future of Transplantation, and Organ and Tissue Donation

Along with a Glossary and Listings of Additional Resources

Edited by Joyce Brennfleck Shannon. 628 pages. 2002. 0-7808-0322-1. $78.

■

Traveler's Health Sourcebook

Basic Consumer Health Information for Travelers, Including Physical and Medical Preparations, Transportation Health and Safety, Essential Information about Food and Water, Sun Exposure, Insect and Snake Bites, Camping and Wilderness Medicine, and Travel with Physical or Medical Disabilities

Along with International Travel Tips, Vaccination Recommendations, Geographical Health Issues, Disease Risks, a Glossary, and a Listing of Additional Resources

Edited by Joyce Brennfleck Shannon. 613 pages. 2000. 0-7808-0384-1. $78.

"Recommended reference source."
— *Booklist, American Library Association, Feb '01*

"This book is recommended for any public library, any travel collection, and especially any collection for the physically disabled."
— *American Reference Books Annual, 2001*

Women's Health Concerns Sourcebook

Basic Information about Health Issues That Affect Women, Featuring Facts about Menstruation and Other Gynecological Concerns, Including Endometriosis, Fibroids, Menopause, and Vaginitis; Reproductive Concerns, Including Birth Control, Infertility, and Abortion; and Facts about Additional Physical, Emotional, and Mental Health Concerns Prevalent among Women Such as Osteoporosis, Urinary Tract Disorders, Eating Disorders, and Depression

Along with Tips for Maintaining a Healthy Lifestyle

Edited by Heather E. Aldred. 567 pages. 1997. 0-7808-0219-5. $78.

"Handy compilation. There is an impressive range of diseases, devices, disorders, procedures, and other physical and emotional issues covered . . . well organized, illustrated, and indexed." — *Choice, Association of College and Research Libraries, Jan '98*

SEE ALSO Breast Cancer Sourcebook, Cancer Sourcebook for Women, 1st and 2nd Editions, Healthy Heart Sourcebook for Women, Osteoporosis Sourcebook

■

Workplace Health & Safety Sourcebook

Basic Consumer Health Information about Workplace Health and Safety, Including the Effect of Workplace Hazards on the Lungs, Skin, Heart, Ears, Eyes, Brain, Reproductive Organs, Musculoskeletal System, and Other Organs and Body Parts

Along with Information about Occupational Cancer, Personal Protective Equipment, Toxic and Hazardous Chemicals, Child Labor, Stress, and Workplace Violence

Edited by Chad T. Kimball. 626 pages. 2000. 0-7808-0231-4. $78.

"As a reference for the general public, this would be useful in any library." — *E-Streams, Jun '01*

"Provides helpful information for primary care physicians and other caregivers interested in occupational medicine. . . . General readers; professionals."
— *Choice, Association of College & Research Libraries, May '01*

"Recommended reference source."
— *Booklist, American Library Association, Feb '01*

"Highly recommended." — *The Bookwatch, Jan '01*

Worldwide Health Sourcebook

Basic Information about Global Health Issues, Including Malnutrition, Reproductive Health, Disease Dispersion and Prevention, Emerging Diseases, Risky Health Behaviors, and the Leading Causes of Death

Along with Global Health Concerns for Children, Women, and the Elderly, Mental Health Issues, Research and Technology Advancements, and Economic, Environmental, and Political Health Implications, a Glossary, and a Resource Listing for Additional Help and Information

Edited by Joyce Brennfleck Shannon. 614 pages. 2001. 0-7808-0330-2. $78.

"Named an Outstanding Academic Title."

—*Choice, Association of College & Research Libraries, Jan '02*

"Yet another handy but also unique compilation in the extensive Health Reference Series, this is a useful work because many of the international publications reprinted or excerpted are not readily available. Highly recommended."

—*Choice, Association of College & Research Libraries, Nov '01*

"Recommended reference source."

—*Booklist, American Library Association, Oct '01*

Teen Health Series
Helping Young Adults Understand, Manage, and Avoid Serious Illness

Diet Information for Teens
Health Tips about Diet and Nutrition

Including Facts about Nutrients, Dietary Guidelines, Breakfasts, School Lunches, Snacks, Party Food, Weight Control, Eating Disorders, and More

Edited by Karen Bellenir. 399 pages. 2001. 0-7808-0441-4. $58.

"Full of helpful insights and facts throughout the book. ... An excellent resource to be placed in public libraries or even in personal collections."
—*American Reference Books Annual 2002*

"Recommended for middle and high school libraries and media centers as well as academic libraries that educate future teachers of teenagers. It is also a suitable addition to health science libraries that serve patrons who are interested in teen health promotion and education." —*E-Streams, Oct '01*

"This comprehensive book would be beneficial to collections that need information about nutrition, dietary guidelines, meal planning, and weight control. ... This reference is so easy to use that its purchase is recommended." —*The Book Report, Sep-Oct '01*

"This book is written in an easy to understand format describing issues that many teens face every day, and then provides thoughtful explanations so that teens can make informed decisions. This is an interesting book that provides important facts and information for today's teens." —*Doody's Health Sciences Book Review Journal, Jul-Aug '01*

"A comprehensive compendium of diet and nutrition. The information is presented in a straightforward, plain-spoken manner. This title will be useful to those working on reports on a variety of topics, as well as to general readers concerned about their dietary health." —*School Library Journal, Jun '01*

■

Drug Information for Teens
Health Tips about the Physical and Mental Effects of Substance Abuse

Including Facts about Alcohol, Anabolic Steroids, Club Drugs, Cocaine, Depressants, Hallucinogens, Herbal Products, Inhalants, Marijuana, Narcotics, Stimulants, Tobacco, and More

Edited by Karen Bellenir. 400 pages. 2002. 0-7808-0444-9. $58.

Mental Health Information for Teens
Health Tips about Mental Health and Mental Illness

Including Facts about Anxiety, Depression, Suicide, Eating Disorders, Obsessive-Compulsive Disorders, Panic Attacks, Phobias, Schizophrenia, and More

Edited by Karen Bellenir. 406 pages. 2001. 0-7808-0442-2. $58.

"In both language and approach, this user-friendly entry in the *Teen Health Series* is on target for teens needing information on mental health concerns." — *Booklist, American Library Association, Jan '02*

"Readers will find the material accessible and informative, with the shaded notes, facts, and embedded glossary insets adding appropriately to the already interesting and succinct presentation." —*School Library Journal, Jan '02*

"This title is highly recommended for any library that serves adolescents and parents/caregivers of adolescents." —*E-Streams, Jan '02*

"Recommended for high school libraries and young adult collections in public libraries. Both health professionals and teenagers will find this book useful." — *American Reference Books Annual 2002*

"This is a nice book written to enlighten the society, primarily teenagers, about common teen mental health issues. It is highly recommended to teachers and parents as well as adolescents." — *Doody's Review Service, Dec '01*

■

Sexual Health Information for Teens
Health Tips about Sexual Development, Human Reproduction, and Sexually Transmitted Diseases

Including Facts about Puberty, Reproductive Health, Chlamydia, Human Papillomavirus, Pelvic Inflammatory Disease, Herpes, AIDS, Contraception, Pregnancy, and More

Edited by Deborah A. Stanley. 400 pages. 2002. 0-7808-0445-7. $58.

Health Reference Series

Adolescent Health Sourcebook

AIDS Sourcebook, 1st Edition

AIDS Sourcebook, 2nd Edition

Alcoholism Sourcebook

Allergies Sourcebook, 1st Edition

Allergies Sourcebook, 2nd Edition

Alternative Medicine Sourcebook,
1st Edition

Alternative Medicine Sourcebook,
2nd Edition

Alzheimer's, Stroke & 29 Other
Neurological Disorders Sourcebook,
1st Edition

Alzheimer's Disease Sourcebook,
2nd Edition

Arthritis Sourcebook

Asthma Sourcebook

Attention Deficit Disorder Sourcebook

Back & Neck Disorders Sourcebook

Blood & Circulatory Disorders
Sourcebook

Brain Disorders Sourcebook

Breast Cancer Sourcebook

Breastfeeding Sourcebook

Burns Sourcebook

Cancer Sourcebook, 1st Edition

Cancer Sourcebook (New), 2nd Edition

Cancer Sourcebook, 3rd Edition

Cancer Sourcebook for Women,
1st Edition

Cancer Sourcebook for Women,
2nd Edition

Cardiovascular Diseases & Disorders
Sourcebook, 1st Edition

Caregiving Sourcebook

Childhood Diseases & Disorders
Sourcebook

Colds, Flu & Other Common Ailments
Sourcebook

Communication Disorders
Sourcebook

Congenital Disorders Sourcebook

Consumer Issues in Health Care
Sourcebook

Contagious & Non-Contagious
Infectious Diseases Sourcebook

Death & Dying Sourcebook

Depression Sourcebook

Diabetes Sourcebook, 1st Edition

Diabetes Sourcebook, 2nd Edition

Diet & Nutrition Sourcebook,
1st Edition

Diet & Nutrition Sourcebook,
2nd Edition

Digestive Diseases & Disorder
Sourcebook

Disabilities Sourcebook

Domestic Violence & Child Abuse
Sourcebook

Drug Abuse Sourcebook

Ear, Nose & Throat Disorders
Sourcebook

Eating Disorders Sourcebook

Emergency Medical Services
Sourcebook

Endocrine & Metabolic Disorders
Sourcebook

Environmentally Induced Disorders
Sourcebook

Ethnic Diseases Sourcebook

Family Planning Sourcebook

Fitness & Exercise Sourcebook,
1st Edition

Fitness & Exercise Sourcebook,
2nd Edition

Food & Animal Borne Diseases
Sourcebook

Food Safety Sourcebook

Forensic Medicine Sourcebook

Gastrointestinal Diseases & Disorders
Sourcebook